CLINICAL SONOGRAPHY

CLINICAL

SONOGRAPHY

A PRACTICAL GUIDE

Roger C. Sanders
M.A., B.M., B.Ch.(Oxon), M.R.C.P., F.R.C.R.
Associate Professor of Radiology and Urology,
The Johns Hopkins University School of Medicine;
Director, Section of Abdominal Ultrasound,
The Johns Hopkins Hospital, Baltimore

with
Joan Campbell, R.T.(R), R.D.M.S.,
Susan M. Guidi, R.T.(N), R.D.M.S.,
Patricia May Kaplan, R.T.(R), R.D.M.S.,
Mimi Maggio, R.T.(R), R.D.M.S.,
Mary B. Silberstein, R.T.(R), R.D.M.S.,
Nancy A. Smith, R.T.(R), R.D.M.S., and
Irma L. Wheelock, R.T.(R), R.D.M.S.,
all of the Section of Abdominal
Ultrasound of The Johns Hopkins
Hospital, Baltimore

Little, Brown and Company
Boston/Toronto

Library of Congress Catalog Card No.
83-80548

ISBN 0-316-77010-8

Printed in the United States of America

SEM

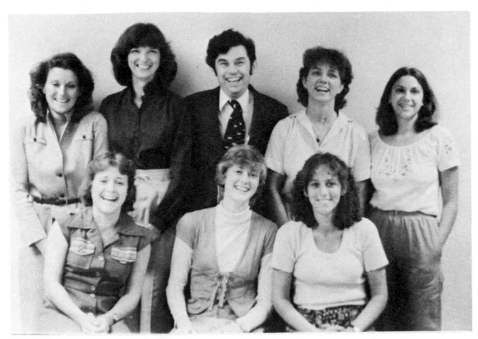

Standing (L–R): Susan Guidi, Irma Wheelock, Roger Sanders, Joan Campbell, Nancy Smith

Sitting (L–R): Patricia Kaplan, Mary Silberstein, Mimi Maggio

PREFACE

Our motive for writing this book was the feeling that existing sonographic texts use an organ (e.g., liver) or disease (e.g., pancreatitis) approach rather than focusing on the clinical problem (e.g., right upper quadrant pain) as it presents to the sonographer. Most books are geared to physicians rather than sonographers and do not tackle the nuts and bolts of how to run a sonography department on a day-to-day basis.

The group of sonographers and sonologists at Johns Hopkins has been together for some years, and we felt that pooling the technical approaches that we have evolved might help others who are just beginning to become sonographers. Other sonography textbooks often describe pathologic, physiologic, or anatomic processes that cannot be seen visually or that have no ultrasonic impact. We decided to put our book squarely into a clinical context by describing only those phenomena that have an ultrasonic aspect. The reader, therefore, will not find details of pancreatic enzyme physiology or how the exchange mechanism in the kidney functions, but you will find out why there are little white marks all over the picture one morning or how to obtain decent views of that pancreas that seems so inaccessible.

We would like to think that our book is the sort of book that will be used in the lab as the patient is being examined rather than studied at night for theoretical knowledge before the registry exam (although we hope it will have value in that area as well).

Numerous individuals have helped with the production of this book. We feel particularly grateful to Ed Krajci, M.D., who went through much of the book with a fine tooth comb making editorial changes; to Joan Batt, who devoted hours of her time to the typing of innumerable versions; to Ed Lipsit, M.D., Mike Hill, M.D., Frank Leo, B.S.E.E., Natalie Benningfield, R.D.M.S., and George Keffer, R.T.(R), who helped eliminate some of the errors, both in text and ideas; and to our artists, Tom Xenakis, assisted by Ranice Crosby, who have been very patient and inventive with numerous diagram versions.

R. C. S.

CONTENTS

APPENDIXES

CLINICAL SONOGRAPHY

1. INTRODUCTION

ROGER C. SANDERS

In no other field of imaging is the role of the technologist (more properly known as the sonographer) in assisting the physician (the sonologist) as critical as it is in ultrasound. Because the images are fraught with technical artifacts and only a selection of the images obtained are captured permanently, it is hard to tell from the final pictures how comprehensive and conscientious a study was performed. Sonographers act as physician's assistants. This book is a cooperative venture between a sonologist and a group of sonographers in an effort to describe the approach that we believe sonographers should adopt and the knowledge that they should possess.

The chapters are organized with a statement of the diagnostic problem to be considered and a brief overview of the place of ultrasound in the context of the clinical problem. Anatomy and technique are then described, followed by a description of the pathological appearances of the area in question. Pitfalls are specified, and further areas for examination are suggested if pathology is found.

Each patient should be approached with the intention of finding answers to diagnostic problems rather than merely looking at the organ that is specified on the requisition. The reality of a patient examination is that the patient does not stroll into the emergency room and announce that he has a pseudocyst in his pancreas; instead, he complains of epigastric pain. Perhaps the doctor, alerted by the smell of gin on the patient's breath, refers him to ultrasound for a pancreatic sonogram. A pseudocyst is found in the head of the pancreas, but an informed sonographer would not stop there. Continued investigation might reveal a common bile duct compressed by the pseudocyst, which is causing biliary dilatation proximal to the level of the pancreas. A sonogram is completed when it has answered the posed question and followed through on the implications the answer may have created.

It is not our intention to set standard routines for scanning average patients. Anyone who has performed several ultrasonic examinations will understand that there are no "average" patients where sonographic internal anatomy is concerned. A good understanding of standard scanning techniques is essential, but it is even more important to know how to adjust your technique to suit each patient's needs. If conventional views are not adequate, it is often necessary to use or even invent special views to demonstrate anatomy. However, different techniques, especially poor techniques, may create artifacts or deceptive appearances that may simulate pathology. Only the person wielding the transducer can prove whether or not an echo is "real."

The sonographer can see what doctors can only feel and laboratory tests can only suggest. It is therefore important that the sonographer identify the mass that is being questioned by the clinician and place markers on the ultrasonic image to indicate where the mass is located. The sonographer should attempt to define which organ is responsible for pain; for example, ultrasonic identification of the gallbladder as the focal site of pain can be the key to clinical management. The solution is often more evident to the sonographer, who has to modify scanning techniques to show an unusually placed "interface," than it is to a physician reading the films. However, we believe that in the most effective laboratory, the physician sonologist should be as good or better a technologist than the sonographers, because separating artifacts from pathology is such an important part of the interpretation of a sonogram.

2. BASICS

Physics

MIMI MAGGIO
ROGER C. SANDERS

SONOGRAM ABBREVIATIONS

Bl Bladder

D Diaphragm

Gbl Gallbladder

K Kidney

L Liver

Th Thyroid

Ut Uterus

KEY WORDS

Acoustic Impedance. Density of tissue times the speed of sound in tissue. The speed of sound waves in body tissue is relatively constant, approximately 1540 meters per second.

Amplitude. Strength or height of the wave measured in decibels (db).

Attenuation. Progressive weakening of the sound beam as it travels through body tissue caused by scatter, absorption, and reflection.

Beam. Directed acoustic field produced by a transducer.

Cycle. Per second frequency at which the crystal vibrates. The number of cycles per second determines frequency.

Crystal. Substance within the transducer that converts electrical impulses into sound waves and vice versa.

Decibel (db). A unit used to express the intensity of amplitude of sound waves; does not specify voltage.

Focusing. Helps to increase the intensity and narrow the width of the beam at a chosen depth.

Focal Zone. That depth in the sound beam where resolution is highest.

Fraunhofer Zone (far field). Area where transmitted beam begins to diverge.

Frequency. Number of times the wave is repeated per second as measured in Hertz. Usable frequencies lie between 1.6 and 10 million per second in the abdomen.

Fresnel Zone (near field). Area close to the transducer where the beam form is uneven.

Hertz (Hz). Standard unit of frequency; equal to 1 cycle per second.

Interface. Occurs whenever two tissues of different acoustic impedance are in contact.

Megahertz (MHz). 1,000,000 Hz.

Piezoelectric Effect. Effect caused by crystals, such as lead zirconate, changing shape when in an electrical field or when mechanically stressed, so that an electrical impulse can generate a sound wave or vice versa.

Power (acoustic). Quantity of energy generated by the transducer expressed in watts.

Pulse Repetition Rate. The number of times per second that transmit-receive cycles occur.

Resolution. Ability to distinguish between two adjacent structures (interfaces).

Specular Reflector. Reflection from a smooth surface at right angles to the sound beam.

Transducer (probe). A device capable of converting energy from one form to another (see Piezoelectric Effect). In ultrasound the term is used to refer to the crystal and the surrounding housing.

Velocity. Speed of the wave, depending on tissue density. The speed of sound in soft tissues is between 1500 and 1600 meters per second. Velocity is standardized at 1540 meters per second on instruments in the United States.

Wavelength. Distance the wave travels in a single cycle. As frequency becomes higher, wavelengths become smaller.

3

PHYSICS FOR SUCCESSFUL SCANNING

In order to obtain the best image possible, some basic fundamentals about ultrasound waves must be understood and used.

Audible Sound Waves

Audible sound waves lie within a 20- to 20,000-Hz range. Ultrasound uses sound waves with a far greater frequency (i.e., between 1 and 30 MHz).

Sound Wave Propagation

Sound waves do not exist in a vacuum, and propagation in gases is poor because the molecules are widely separated. The closer the molecules, the faster the sound wave moves through a medium, so bone and metals conduct sound exceedingly well (Fig. 2-1).

EFFECT ON IMAGE

Lung and bowel containing air conduct sound so poorly that they cannot be imaged with ultrasound instruments. Structures behind them cannot be seen. A neighboring soft-tissue or fluid-filled organ must be used as a window from which to image a structure that is obscured by air (Fig. 2-2 A,B).

Gel or mineral oil must be placed between the transducer and the patient; otherwise sound will not be transmitted across the air-filled gap.

Bone conducts sound at a much faster speed than soft tissue. Because ultrasound instruments cannot accommodate the difference in speed between soft tissue and bone, current systems do not image bone or structures covered by bone.

The Pulse Echo Principle

Because the crystal in the transducer is electrically pulsed, it changes shape and vibrates, thus producing the sound beam that propagates through tissues. The crystal emits sound for a brief moment and then waits for the returning echo that is reflected from the structures in the plane of the sound beam (Fig. 2-3). When the echo is received, the crystal again vibrates, generating an electrical voltage comparable to the strength of the returning echo.

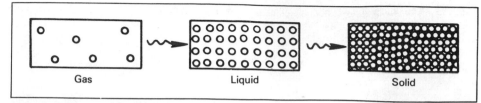

FIGURE 2-1. Sound propagation is worse in gas because molecules are widely separated. It is better in liquids and best in solids.

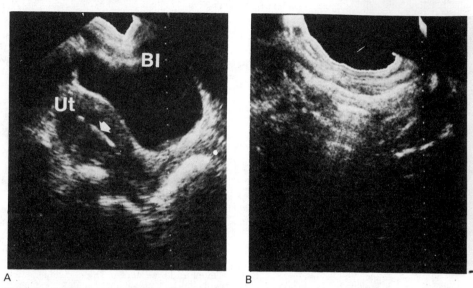

FIGURE 2-2. Effects on image. A. Distending the urinary bladder (Bl) serves as a window for imaging the uterus. Note IUD (arrow) in uterus (Ut) (see Chapter 25). B. With an empty urinary bladder, nothing can be visualized.

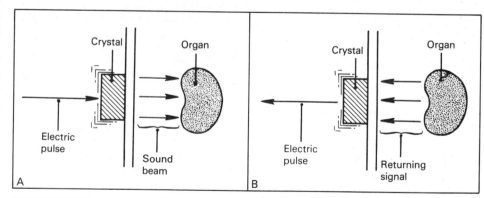

FIGURE 2-3. The pulse-echo principle. A. The electrical pulse strikes the crystal and produces a sound beam, which propagates through the tissues. B. Echoes arising from structures are reflected back to the crystal, which in turn vibrates, generating an electrical impulse comparable to the strength of the returning echo.

Beam Angle to Interface

The strength of the returning echo is related to the angle at which the beam strikes the acoustic interface. The more nearly perpendicular the beam is, the stronger the returning echo; smooth interfaces at right angles are known as specular reflectors (Fig. 2-4A). Echoes reflecting at other angles are known as scatter (Fig. 2-4B).

EFFECT ON IMAGE

Demonstrating the borders of a body structure requires placement of the transducer so that the beam will strike the borders more or less at a right angle. It is worthwhile attempting to image a structure from different angles to bring out interfaces (Fig. 2-5). Some smaller echoes return from structures that are not at right angles to the beam and can partially obscure the borders of a structure (Fig. 2-5).

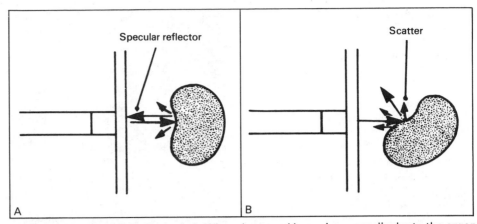

FIGURE 2-4. Angle of sound beams. A. When the sound beam is perpendicular to the organ interface, specular echoes will be produced. B. When the sound beam is not perpendicular to the organ interface, scatter is seen.

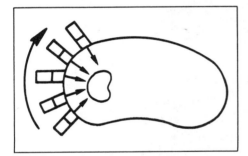

FIGURE 2-5. It is possible to image a structure at several different angles with a B-scanner when compound scanning.

Tissue Acoustic Impedance

The strength of the returning echo depends on the differences in acoustic impedance between the various tissues in the body. Acoustic impedance relates to tissue density; the greater the difference in density between two structures, the stronger the returning echo.

EFFECT ON THE IMAGE

Structures of differing acoustic impedance (such as the gallbladder and the liver) are much easier to distinguish from one another than structures of similar acoustic texture (e.g., kidney and liver) (Fig. 2-6).

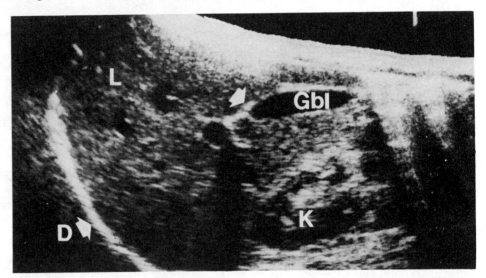

FIGURE 2-6. Tissue acoustic impedance. The bright interfaces at the gallbladder (Gbl) and the diaphragm (D) (arrows) are due to large differences in acoustic impedance (density) from the liver (L). The kidney (K), which is similar in texture to the liver, is not as easy to see.

Absorption and Scatter

Because much of the sound beam is absorbed or scattered as it travels through the body, it undergoes progressive weakening (attenuation).

EFFECT ON IMAGE

Transducers are chosen according to the structure being examined and the size of the patient. The highest possible frequency should be used because this will result in superior resolution. Low frequencies permit greater penetration. Pediatric patients can be examined at 5 MHz; lower frequencies (e.g., 2.5 MHz) may be needed for larger patients (Fig. 2-7A,B).

Transducer Focal Zone

The shape of the transducer crystal can be altered to focus the beam. With a static scanner three different focal areas are usually used—long focus (8 to 12 cm), medium focus (4 to 8 cm), and short focus (2 to 5 cm). The three standard frequencies (2.5, 3.5, and 5 MHz) come in different focal zones, but generally 5 MHz is used with a short focus, 3.5 MHz with a medium focus, and 2.25 MHz with a long focus. Quarter-wave transducers match the thickness of the lens to the wavelength to produce greater output and higher resolution.

EFFECT ON IMAGE

High resolution demands selection of the right frequency as well as a transducer with the proper focal zone; for example, it is useless to examine the thyroid at a depth of 3 cm with a long-focus transducer (Fig. 2-8A–C).

Transducer Face Diameter

The wider the diameter of the transducer face for a given frequency, the more it can be focused. However, the transducer itself becomes more cumbersome.

EFFECT ON IMAGE

A 19-mm-wide transducer has a longer focal zone and therefore finer resolution than a 13-mm transducer. However, the smaller transducer face is more convenient for use between the ribs and in other limited access areas.

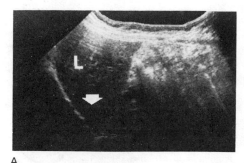
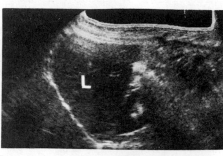

A   B

FIGURE 2-7. Transducers. A. A longitudinal scan using a 3.5 MHz transducer did not penetrate to the posterior aspect of the liver (L). B. A 2.25-MHz transducer penetrates adequately in the obese patient.

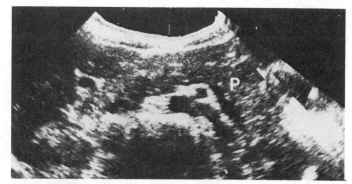

A

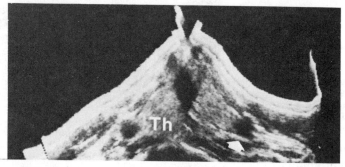

B

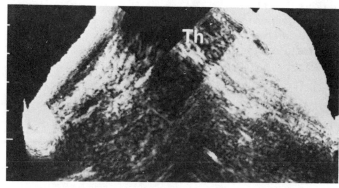

C

FIGURE 2-8. Transducer focal zones. A. A superficial pancreas (P) is seen very well with a 5-MHz short-focus transducer. B. A thyroid (Th) scan using a 7.5-MHz water-path transducer. Note carotid artery (arrow). C. Poor quality thyroid (Th) scan with a 2.25-MHz long-focus transducer.

Beam Profile

The sound beam varies in shape and resolution. Close to the skin it suffers from the effect of turbulence, and resolution here is poor. Beyond the focal zone the beam widens.

EFFECT ON IMAGE

Outside the focal zone, information that appears to be present in the near field may really be an artifact. Structures beyond the focal zone are distorted and seen poorly. A structure as small as a pinhead may appear to be half a centimeter wide (Fig. 2-8C).

SELECTED READING

Kremkau, F. W. (Ed.). *Diagnostic Ultrasound: Physical Principles and Exercises.* New York: Grune & Stratton, 1980.

McDicken, W. N. *Diagnostic Ultrasonics: Principles and Use of Instruments* (2nd ed.). Toronto: Wiley, 1981.

3. INSTRUMENTATION

MIMI MAGGIO
ROGER C. SANDERS

KEY WORDS

A-Mode (Amplitude Modulation). A one-dimensional image displaying the amplitude (strength) of the returning echo signals along the vertical axis and the time (the distance from the transducer) along the horizontal axis (Fig. 3-1).

Annular Array. A type of real-time system.

Arm. The transducer on B-scan systems is attached to a gantry, which is known as the transducer arm. It has three joints within it.

B-Mode (Brightness Modulation). A method of displaying the intensity (amplitude) of an echo by varying the brightness of a dot to correspond to echo strength (Fig. 3-2).

B-Scanner (Contact Scanner, Articulated Arm Scanner, Static Scanner). The transducer is attached to a fixed gantry and moved around the patient manually. Image creation takes 15 to 45 seconds.

CRT (Cathode Ray Tube). Term used to describe the television image.

Doppler. (1) *Continuous* Within the Doppler probe head are two transducers. One emits a continuous beam of ultrasound, and one receives the signal when it returns. Alterations in frequency of the returning signal allow the detection of motion. (2) *Pulsed* When used on an intermittent basis to coincide with the phases of the cardiac cycle the Doppler phenomenon allows creation of a two-dimensional image.

Electronically Steered System. Electrical excitation of many transducers in sequence causes a flicker-free real-time image and allows manipulation of the beam direction.

Frame Rate (Image Rate). Rate at which the image is refreshed in a real-time system display. Most real-time systems have a frame rate of more than 30 per second. At lower frame rates the image flickers.

Freeze Frame. Control that preserves the image for photography or prolonged evaluation.

Gantry. A mechanical structure to which the transducer is attached. Standard on B-scanners.

Mechanically Steered System. The physical movement of a transducer or mirror causes the sound beam to sweep through the tissue, providing a real-time image.

Monitor. Term used for the TV display.

Oscilloscope. Term used for the TV display.

Phased Array. Many small transducers are electronically coordinated to produce a focus wave front. A wide field of view is obtained by electronically delaying the return of some signals.

Radial Scanning. Method of scanning used in prostatic scanners in which the transducer rotates in a circle.

Real-Time (Dynamic Imaging). Type of imaging in which the image is created so many times per second that a cinematic view of the tissues is obtained.

Scan Converter. Portion of the imaging system in which the echoes are converted to a television image: (1) analog scan converters provide a transient image only; (2) digital scan converters store the image so that postprocessing of the image can be performed. These are much more stable than analog scan converters.

A-MODE

A-mode (amplitude mode; Fig. 3-1) is the most basic form of diagnostic ultrasound; a single beam of ultrasound is analyzed. The distance between the transducer and a structure determines where an echo is seen along the time axis. Time and distance are interchangeable; because an echo (sound wave) is assumed to travel at a constant speed in body tissue (1540 m/sec), the time it takes for the echo to return to the transducer can be converted to a distance. Isolated use of the A-mode is almost obsolete but is still useful under the following circumstances:

1. To determine whether an echo-free structure is fluid-filled or contains solid homogeneous material (Fig. 3-3A–C)
2. To determine whether a structure is pulsatile (Fig. 3-4)
3. To aid in cyst puncture
4. For use in echoencephalography

B-MODE

A-mode signals can be converted to dots that vary in size depending on the strength of the signal (see Fig. 3-2). Multiple B-mode images form a B-scan image (see Fig. 3-6).

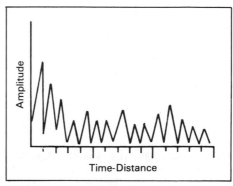
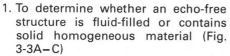

FIGURE 3-1. A-mode display. The strength of the acoustic interface is shown by the size of the echo.

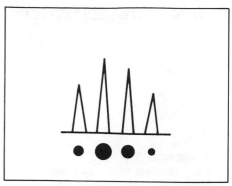

FIGURE 3-2. B-mode. The amplitude of an echo is displayed as the brightness of a dot comparable to the echo strength on the A-mode display.

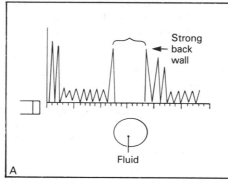
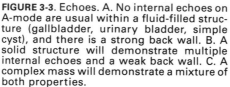

FIGURE 3-3. Echoes. A. No internal echoes on A-mode are usual within a fluid-filled structure (gallbladder, urinary bladder, simple cyst), and there is a strong back wall. B. A solid structure will demonstrate multiple internal echoes and a weak back wall. C. A complex mass will demonstrate a mixture of both properties.

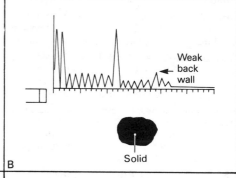
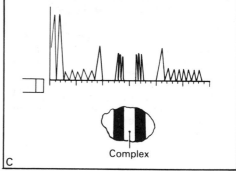

FIGURE 3-4. When the sound beam passes through a pulsatile structure, the A-mode echoes due to the arterial walls will move in, A, and out, B (arrows).

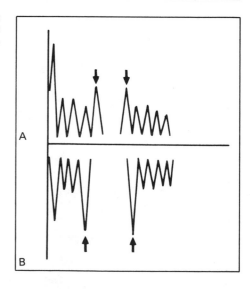

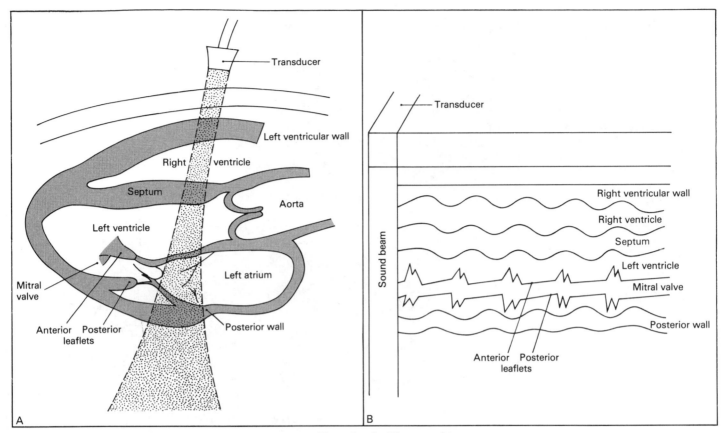

FIGURE 3-5. M-mode. A. Diagram demonstrating the sound beam angled through specific heart structures. B. The M-mode read-out of those structures within the sound beam.

M-MODE

If a series of B-mode dots are displayed on a moving time base, the motion of mobile structures can be observed. This process forms the basis of echocardiography (Fig. 3-5A,B).

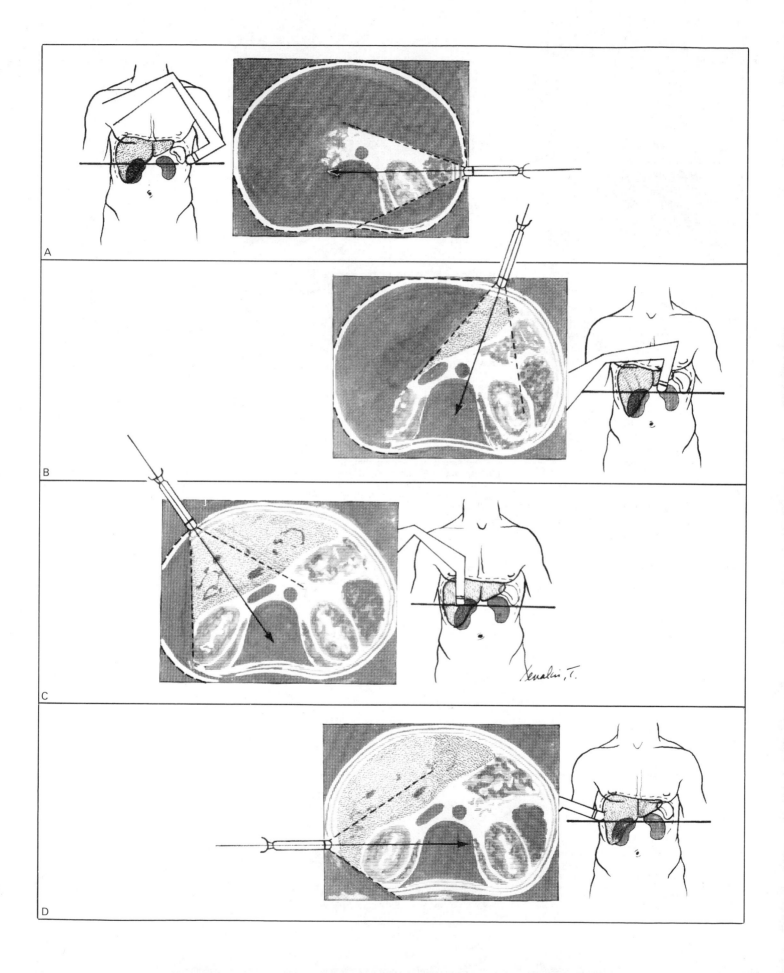

A

B

C

D

B-SCAN (ARTICULATED ARM SCANNING, STATIC SCANNING, CONTACT SCANNING)

This technique creates a two-dimensional cross-section of the body that is obtained by summing many A-mode beams and converting the echoes to dots of a brightness that varies with the strength of the echo. As the transducer is moved across the body, dots are created and are retained on the oscilloscope by the use of a scan converter (memory) (Fig. 3-6A–D).

The basic design of all B-scanners is similar. The transducer is attached to an arm, which has three joints within it. The transducer arm can be moved so that the transducer moves along an oblique, a transverse, or a longitudinal axis. If desirable, motion in a series of steps at set intervals in any given plane can be achieved along the arm. Positional information is recorded, and images can be easily reproduced. This differs from real-time systems, in which the exact plane cannot be systematically reduplicated. The B-scan image, which takes some 15 to 20 seconds to create by manually moving the transducer around the body, is displayed on the TV monitor on the main console of the system (Fig. 3-6). In the TV image there are numerous shades of gray, which can be varied by the use of pre- and postprocessing controls that allow certain levels of gray to be accentuated.

Although B-scanners are difficult to use and do not give a cinematic image, they have the following advantages:

1. A large field of view can be examined, so the complete outline of a mass and the neighboring structures can be seen.

2. The transducer face is relatively small and can be placed in small areas (e.g., between ribs); inaccessible regions that are not approachable with real-time can be seen.
3. Because the transducer arm can reproduce a precise section that was seen previously, tracing the outlines of a mass on serial ultrasonic images when the study is reviewed is simpler.
4. A complete contour image of the body, used by some clinicians for planning radiotherapy, can be obtained.

REAL-TIME

Real-time systems provide an immediate image of the body and allow the examiner to see movement. In our view the ideal system is a static scanner with real-time of two different types (linear array and mechanical sector scanner).

Some advantages of real-time are the following:

1. The scanning plane that best demonstrates the area of interest can be rapidly located.
2. The entire examination can be done very quickly because there is constant visual feedback on the display screen.
3. The course of extended structures such as vessels can be followed, allowing them to be traced to their origin.
4. Movement observation may allow organ identification (i.e., mass versus bowel).
5. Infants, children, and uncooperative patients can be examined more easily than with the conventional B-mode scanner, because they need not suspend their respiration or remain immobile during the study. Acute conditions and critically ill patients can be studied by means of portable scanners.
6. A real-time examination is less dependent upon the skill of the operator because the scan is repetitive and to some extent automated.

Mechanically Steered Systems

ROTARY TYPE (WHEEL)

One or more transducer elements are arranged in a wheel-like housing that moves the beam through an arc-shaped sector field (Fig. 3-7). The small size of the transducer face design allows use between intercostal spaces, so organs such as the liver and heart can be imaged. A variant of this system is a housing that contains three wheels.

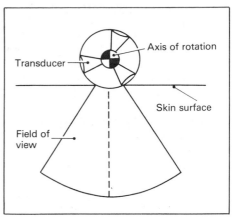

FIGURE 3-7. Mechanical rotary sector scanner.

OSCILLATING TRANSDUCER (WOBBLER)

The drive motor and transducer are housed in a small container. The motor drives the transducer back and forth, producing a pie-shaped beam (Fig. 3-8).

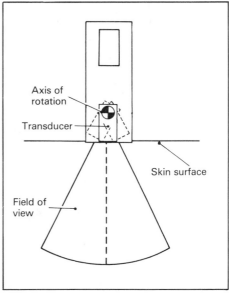

FIGURE 3-8. Oscillating transducer (wobbler).

FIGURE 3-6. Sequence of diagrams showing development of transverse view of upper abdomen by B-scanning. A. A sound beam angled through the left side of the abdomen. B. Sound beam angled toward the center of the abdomen. C. Sound beam angling through the right side of the abdomen. D. Sound beam completing the scan.

TRANSDUCER WITH OSCILLATING MIRROR

In this system the transducer is stationary, but the beam is moved by oscillating a mirror that reflects the sound. The mirror is capable of focusing the sound beam at a specific area. The image is pie-shaped (Fig. 3-9).

Electronically Steered Systems

LINEAR SEQUENCED ARRAYS

This system consists of a set of 64 to 128 transducer elements mounted in line. The elements are pulsed sequentially in groups of four or five to produce a rectangular field (Fig. 3-10). (Several small transducers act in the same way as one large one, whereas one small transducer would be subject to considerable beam spread.)

It is possible to improve the resolution of the sound beam in a linear array by electronic focusing.

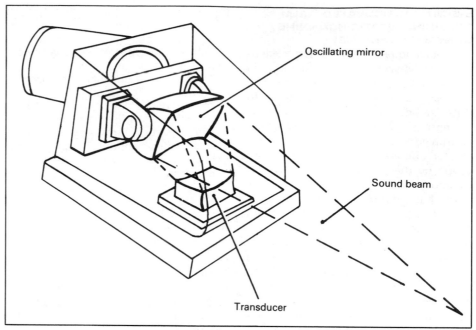

FIGURE 3-9. Stationary transducer with oscillating mirror.

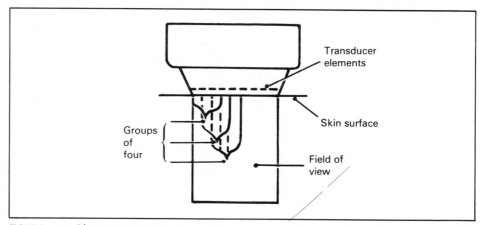

FIGURE 3-10. Linear sequenced array. There are multiple transducer elements pulsed in groups of four or five.

PHASED (STEERED) ARRAY

This system produces a wedge-shaped field that is particularly useful in cardiac imaging (Fig. 3-11A,B) because simultaneous M-mode tracings can be obtained. It uses electronic delay techniques similar to those used for electronic focusing of linear arrays. Some phased array systems offer beam steering.

ANNULAR ARRAY TRANSDUCER

This system employs crystals of varying thicknesses, thereby producing different frequencies in the sound beam. The transducer is electronically focused at several depths. The beam is reflected off an oscillating acoustic mirror into a water bath (Fig. 3-12).

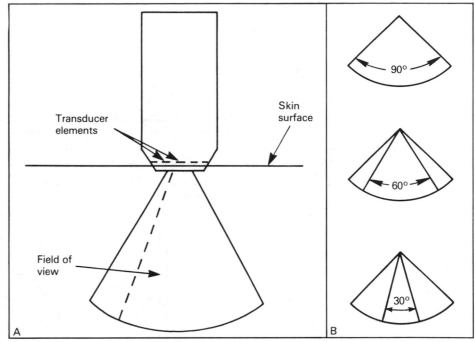

FIGURE 3-11. Wedged-shaped field. A. Phased (steered) array. B. Different size fields of view. Smaller fields give better resolution.

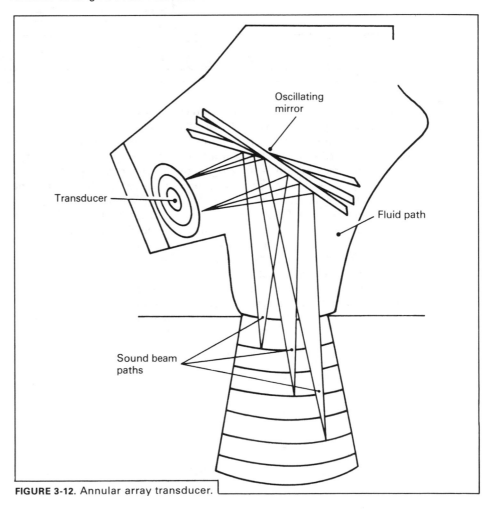

FIGURE 3-12. Annular array transducer.

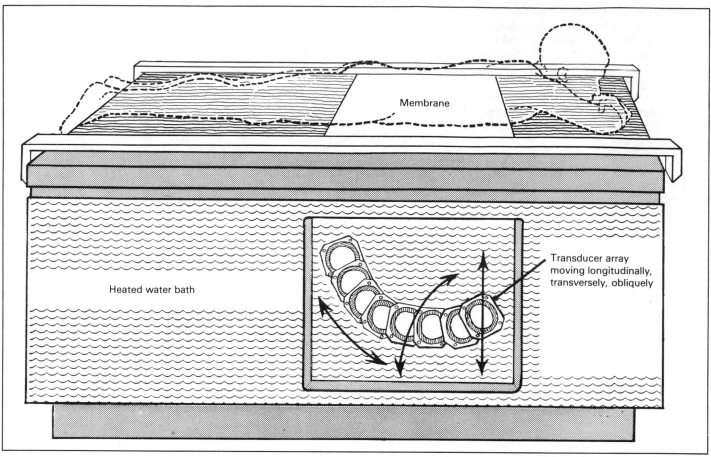

Membrane

Heated water bath

Transducer array moving longitudinally, transversely, obliquely

Small Parts Scanners

These systems are usually lightweight, hand-held, real-time probes capable of high resolution using a 7.5- or 10-MHz transducer in a water or oil bath. All types of real-time systems have been used as small parts scanners. They are designed for visualizing the fine detail of superficial structures, usually at a depth of less than 4 cm from the skin surface (i.e., thyroid, carotid arteries, or testes, or pediatric conditions). They can be obtained either as stand-alone systems or as add-on transducers to a standard system.

Automated Systems

A series of transducers is located in a water bath at some distance from the patient. The patient immerses an organ such as the breast or testicle in the water bath or lies on a plastic membrane above the transducers. The transducers rotate in an arc automatically. The operator has to control only the instrument settings and the number of transducers to be used at any given time. Because the transducers are located at a considerable distance from the patient, a relatively low frequency such as 2.25 MHz can be finely focused (Fig. 3-13).

FIGURE 3-13. Octoson. The patient lies on a warm membrane over a water bath; an array of transducers in the water bath can be moved by the sonographer in a longitudinal, transverse, or oblique axis. Each transducer covers a 15° angle.

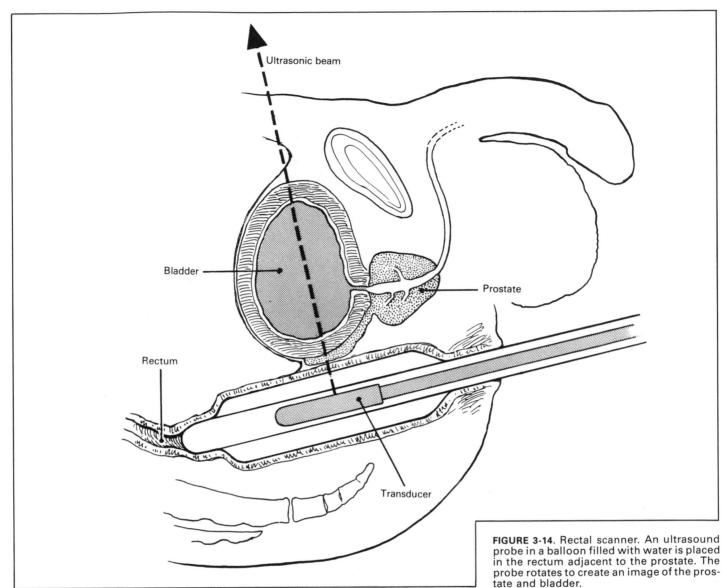

Ultrasonic beam

Bladder

Prostate

Rectum

Transducer

FIGURE 3-14. Rectal scanner. An ultrasound probe in a balloon filled with water is placed in the rectum adjacent to the prostate. The probe rotates to create an image of the prostate and bladder.

Rectal Systems (Radial Systems)

The transducer is placed on the end of a rod, which rotates through a 360-degree angle. This rod is inserted into the rectum and is surrounded by a balloon containing water. Views of the prostate and bladder can be obtained with this system (Fig. 3-14).

Doppler

Doppler has been added to a variety of systems. By analyzing the difference in frequency between emitted and received signals with continuous wave ultrasound, motion can be detected and blood vessels recognized (Fig. 3-15). An idea of flow can be obtained with some modern systems using pulsed Doppler.

FIGURE 3-15. Doppler transducer. The probe is placed on the skin and angled in the direction opposite to that of the blood flow. Continuous wave ultrasound is used. The constant monitoring of the returning sound waves allows detection of flow by an alteration in the pitch of the ultrasound waves.

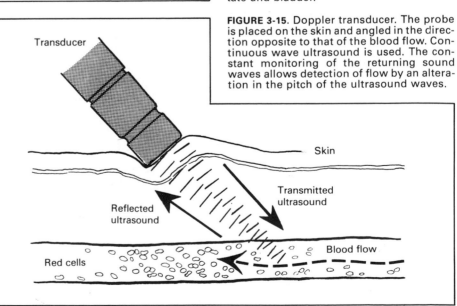

Transducer

Skin

Transmitted ultrasound

Reflected ultrasound

Red cells

Blood flow

Doppler is particularly valuable in the carotid artery. Recognition of a typical pattern of flow in the external and internal carotid arteries is possible, and with a pulsed Doppler system the examiner can get an idea of the percentage of flow compared with normal. The Doppler signal can be converted into an audible signal, which has a typical sound for veins and for patent and obstructed arteries.

SELECTED READING

Lateral resolution. *Aero-Tech Reports,* Vol. 1, No. 3, Krautkramer-Branson, 1978,

McDicken, W.N. *Diagnostic Ultrasonics: Principles and Use of Instruments* (2nd ed). Toronto: Wiley, 1981.

Sensitivity 1 (Transducer Sensitivity). *Aero-Tech Reports,* Vol. 1, No. 4, Krautkramer-Branson, 1979.

Ultrasonic transducer performance parameters effects on diagnostic imaging: Axial resolution. *Aero-Tech Reports,* Vol. 1, No. 1, Krautkramer-Branson, 1978.

4. KNOBOLOGY

MIMI MAGGIO
ROGER C. SANDERS

SONOGRAM ABBREVIATIONS

Bl Bladder

K Kidney

L Liver

Ut Uterus

KEY WORDS

Attenuator. Opposite of gain; when the attenuator is turned up, fewer echoes will be displayed.

B-Scan (Static Scan). A two-dimensional cross-sectional image displayed on a TV screen in which the brightness of the echoes and their position on the screen is determined by the movement of a transducer and the time it takes the echoes to return to the transducer.

Delay. Sets the depth at which the TGC (time gain compensation—see below) slope commences; used to depress artifactual echoes in the near field.

Field of View. Allows four or five choices to the sonographer to make maximal use of the screen's potential resolution and yet display all of the relevant area (i.e., 1:1, 2:1, 3:1, 4:1, 5:1 imaging display).

Gain, Power. Measure of the strength of the ultrasound signal throughout the image.

Horizontal, Vertical. Controls that place the image in the desired position on the screen.

Knee. Region of the curve where the slope changes markedly.

Main Bang. Strong echoes derived from the transducer/skin interface shown in the first 1 or 2 cm of the image.

Oscilloscope (CRT). Screen used to display the A-mode, the B-scan image, and TGC characteristics.

Range. Varies the depth at which the echoes are optimally displayed.

Time Gain Compensation Curve (TGC), Time Compensation Gain (TCG), Swept Gain Compensation (SGC). Controls that compensate for the loss (attenuation) of the sound beam as it passes through tissue.

USE OF KNOBS

The basic knowledge of knobology is interchangeable between different types of systems, although additional knobs are required for static scanning, real-time, or M-mode. The critical knobs are those concerned with gain (power, output), time gain compensation, erase, centering, left and right movement, freeze frame, and write. Learning to use these knobs effortlessly is an important part of the art of ultrasonic scanning.

A-Mode

Most modern systems incorporate A-mode. Should one wish to use A-mode alone (e.g., for cyst puncture), the controls needed are (1) an on-off switch (power), (2) a switch that directs the system to the A-mode transducers rather than to B-scan, real-time, or M-mode, and (3) gain and TGC controls.

B-Scan

B-scanning requires detailed use of the TGC controls.

POWER OUTPUT (GAIN OR ATTENUATION)

This control affects the echoes throughout the ultrasonic field by regulating the amount of sound sent through the transducer (gain) or varying the strength of the signal after it has come back to the transducer (attenuation). An alteration in the size of all echoes occurs when the gain is changed (Fig. 4-1 A–D). The gain control is usually calibrated in decibels (db)—an arbitrary measure of sound amplitude. Some versions have a smaller central control for fine adjustment.

Too much overall gain is dangerous. One can fill in fluid-filled structures such as vessels and the gallbladder and lose the outline and texture of the organs (Fig. 4-1A,B).

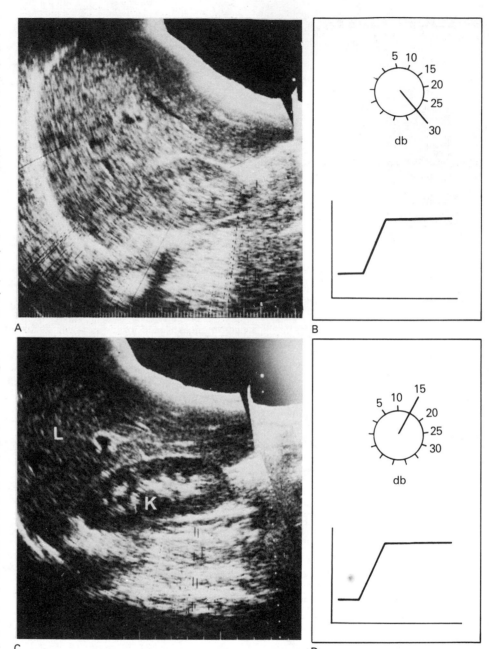

FIGURE 4-1. Power output (gain or attenuation). A. Too much overall gain causes too many echoes in the liver and right kidney. B. Power-gain (db) levels are high. C. With reduced gain, the liver (L) and right kidney (K) are now outlined well. D. The overall power-gain (db) has been decreased but the TGC is unchanged.

TIME GAIN COMPENSATION (GAIN CURVE, SWEPT GAIN, TGC/SGC)

There are four controls to most time gain compensation curves (Fig. 4-2). These knobs attempt to compensate for the acoustic loss that occurs by absorption, scatter, and reflection and to show structures of the same acoustic strength as echoes of the same size whatever their depth.

SLOPE RATE (SLOPE). Echoes from distant tissues are smaller than those from near structures due to reflection, absorption, and scatter. The echoes from the structures near the transducer are therefore artificially reduced by the use of "slope." Ideally, echoes from distant structures of the same acoustic strength as those from near structures should be represented in the same fashion. Experienced sonographers can set the slope so that this is more or less achieved (Fig. 4-3). The severity of the slope varies between different individuals because the amount of sound attenuation differs greatly depending on, for example, the amount of fat within the liver. The site of the knee (far end of the slope) is critical in displaying an even texture throughout an organ such as the liver. Subtle metastatic lesions in the liver will be missed if the liver texture is not evenly displayed. Without the use of the TGC a structure may have too few or too many echoes. For example, a mass behind the uterus could be missed or mistaken for bowel (Fig. 4-3A,B).

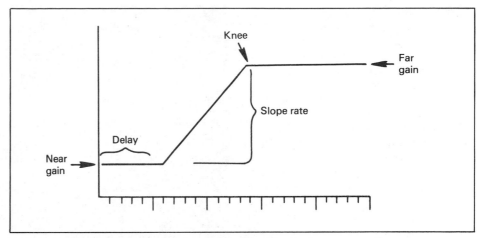

FIGURE 4-2. Diagram showing components of the time gain compensation curve.

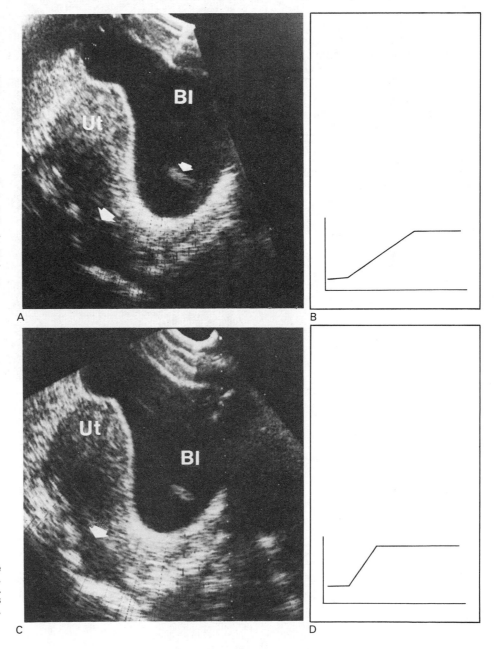

FIGURE 4-3. Slope rate. A. Echoes behind the uterus (Ut) are not being visualized (arrows). B. The slope rate is suppressed too much. C. With better slope adjustment, the ovary is imaged posterior to the uterus (Ut) (arrow). D. Correct adjustment of the slope rate.

SLOPE START (DELAY). Because the echoes from the skin and subcutaneous tissues are rather strong and of little relevance to the image, the point at which the slope starts is often delayed by 2 to 3 cm. This distance is prescribed by the slope-start control. This control is of more value with B-scanners than with other systems. In real-time the first few centimeters are often filled with useless artifacts because of reverberation.

The slope-start (delay) control is especially helpful in large patients who have a lot of subcutaneous fat. The near echoes can be suppressed to a sufficient depth to cut down on the artifacts that fat often causes in the near field (Fig. 4-4).

NEAR GAIN (INITIAL GAIN). Near gain controls the strength of the echoes in the near field. In most systems the entire slope will be moved up or down as this knob is altered (see Fig. 4-2).

If all the near field echoes were displayed, the image would be swamped with echoes in the near field (Fig. 4-5) because there would be too many echoes from small structures. Too little near gain yields an image with too little near field information (Fig. 4-5E,F).

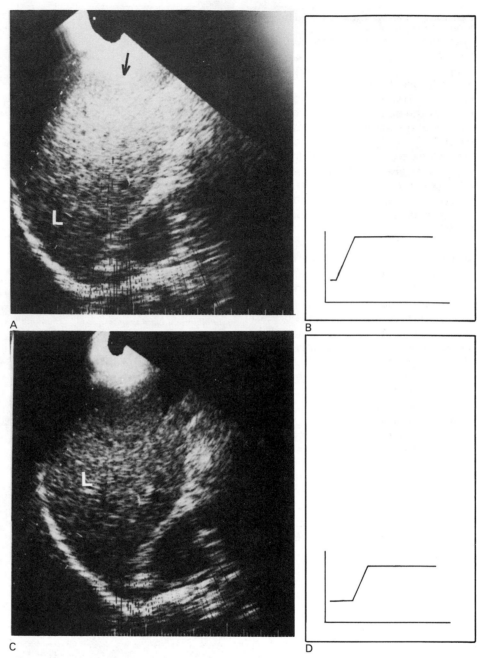

FIGURE 4-4. Slope-start (delay) control. A,B. Excess echoes in the near field due to incorrect setting of the delay control. C,D. Correct adjustment of the delay control yields a high quality image.

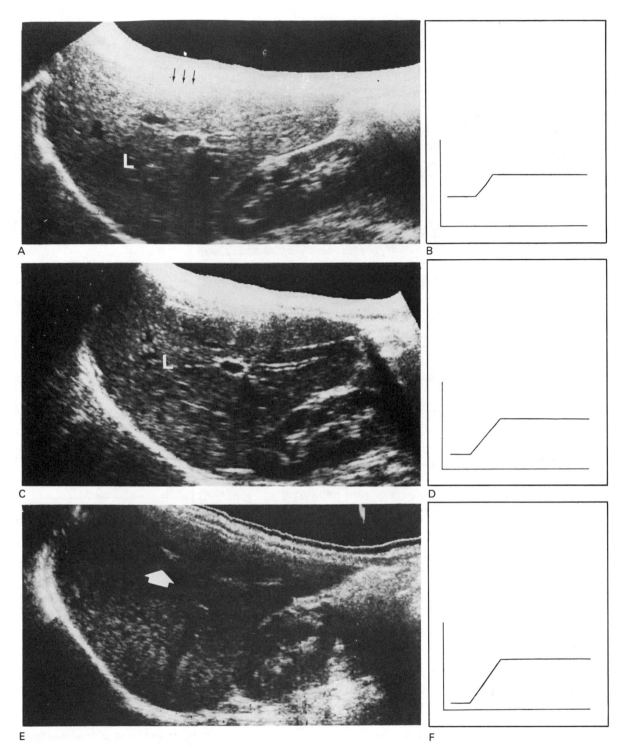

FIGURE 4-5. Near gain (initial gain). A,B. Too much near gain (arrows). C,D. Correct adjustment of the near gain control without slope adjustment. E,F. Too little near gain (arrow).

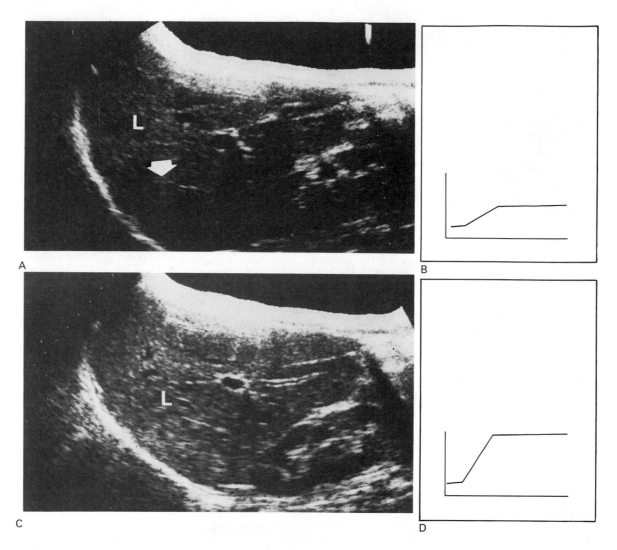

FAR GAIN. This control affects only the echoes beyond the slope endpoint and is responsible for the strength of the distant echoes in the image (Fig. 4-6).

TGC DISPLAY ON SEPARATE SCREEN

Alongside an A-mode display it is routine to show the time gain compensation curve. Having the time gain compensation and A-mode display visible when performing a static scan or a real-time examination is a great aid in maintaining good scanning technique.

PRE- AND POSTPROCESSING CONTROLS

These controls, which usually have about four settings, are used to alter the image by accentuating different echo levels (e.g., low-level echoes, or high-level echoes) or by producing a linear gray scale display as opposed to the logarithmic scale that is used routinely on most instruments. These controls are occasionally used clinically when a more detailed look at texture is required; for example, accentuating the low-level echoes can help bring out subtle tumors in the liver (see Chapter 8, Fig. 8-9).

PREPROCESSING. The preprocessing control assigns gray scale values to the different strengths of the returning echoes before the image is displayed.

POSTPROCESSING. The postprocessing control allows emphasis of different echo levels in the image after it has been displayed on the screen (e.g., low-level echoes can be emphasized).

FIGURE 4-6. Far gain. A,B. Too few echoes in the distal part of the liver (L [arrow]) caused by too much far field suppression. C,D. After correct adjustment of the far field setting without changing slope, the liver (L) is well displayed.

REJECT

Reject is useful in M-mode to clean up the image and to get rid of apparently artifactual echoes. Reject is rarely or never used in B-scanning because it tends to eliminate true gray scale information by cutting out a few low-level shades of gray.

TEST PATTERN

A test pattern introduces a range of gray scale bars on the screen. It is used mainly for establishing photographic settings.

CALIPERS

Usually two calipers are used as variable markers, which allow measurements of structures in centimeters.

ZOOM

The zoom places a box on the screen. The material seen within the box can be expanded to fill the entire screen. It should be used with caution; the number of television lines used in the boxed area is unaltered and magnified, so the blown-up image looks coarse and has poor resolution.

MEASUREMENT FEATURES

Centimeter markers provide a scale of dots 1 cm apart at any position when superimposed on the B-scan image.

VIDEO INVERT

The video invert feature allows one to select a "positive" or "negative" image (i.e., a white or black background). We usually use the negative polarity (black background) because it allows better detection of subtle abnormalities in texture, for example, metastatic lesions in the liver.

TRANSDUCER SELECTION

Selection must be used on some machines to match the gain controls and sound filtering to a given transducer, that is, a 3.5-MHz setting has to be used with a 3.5-MHz transducer.

Real-Time

Controls used only with real-time are the following:

FRAME RATE

With some systems a slow frame rate is used for high quality photography. In most systems the image is more or less flicker-free at the standard frame rate (more than 30 per second), and this option is not available.

IMAGE WIDTH

With some systems one has the option of using a 45°, 60°, or 90° angle. With smaller widths the frame rate is higher and the real-time resolution is finer. With wider angles the image is more convenient, but there is a slower scanning speed or inferior resolution.

FREEZE FRAME

When this button is depressed, the real-time image is maintained on the screen. There is usually some degradation in image quality between the real-time and the frozen image.

IMAGE PLACEMENT CONTROL

Because the real-time image is relatively small, many systems now allow two linear array real-time images to be placed side by side on the screen, thus creating a larger field of view or allowing comparison between, for example, the left and right kidneys.

TAPE

The tape control has to be activated to set in action videotaping or playback of the image.

RECORD

The record button is used to videotape the image.

SELECTED READING

Bartrum, R., and Crow, H. C. (Eds.). *Real-Time*. Philadelphia: Saunders, 1983.

McDicken, W. N. *Diagnostic Ultrasonics: Principles and Use of Instruments* (2nd ed.). Toronto: Wiley, 1981.

5. BASIC PRINCIPLES

NANCY A. SMITH

SONOGRAM ABBREVIATIONS

Ao	Aorta
Du	Duodenum
F	Fibroid
GBl	Gallbladder
IVC	Inferior vena cava
K	Kidney
L	Liver
P	Pancreas
S	Spine
SMa	Superior mesenteric artery
Sp	Spleen
Spa	Splenic artery
Spv	Splenic vein
St	Stomach
Trans	Transducer
Ut	Uterus

KEY WORDS

Anechoic. Without internal echoes. Not necessarily cystic unless there is good thorough transmission.

B-Scanning. Term used to describe the use of an articulated arm scanner for examining a patient.

Complex. A mass that has both fluid-filled and echogenic areas.

Cyst. Spherical fluid-filled structure with a well-defined wall.

Cystic. In ultrasound, the word *cystic* does not necesssarily refer to a cyst. The term is used by some (inaccurately) to describe any fluid-filled structure (e.g., urine-filled bladder or bile-filled gallbladder; Fig. 5-1).

Echogenic. Describes a structure that produces echoes. Usually a relative term. For example, Figure 5-1 shows the normal texture of the liver and kidney; the liver is slightly more echogenic. A change in the normal echogenicity signifies a pathologic condition (Fig. 5-1).

Echogram. Term used by some to describe an ultrasonic examination.

Echo-Free. See *Anechoic* (above).

Echolucent. Without internal echoes; not necessarily cystic.

Echopenic. A few echoes within a structure; less echogenic. The normal kidney is echopenic relative to the liver (Fig. 5-1).

Echo-Poor. See *Echopenic* (above).

Echo-Rich. See *Echogenic* (above).

Enhancement (acoustic). Because sound traveling through a fluid-filled structure is barely attenuated, the structures distal to a cystic lesion appear to have more echoes than neighboring areas. Also referred to as *through transmission* (see below and Fig. 5-2).

Fluid-Fluid Level. Interface between two fluids with different acoustic characteristics. This interface forms a level that varies with position (see Chapter 22).

Gain. The strength of the echoes throughout the image can be varied by changing the power output from the system.

Homogeneous. Of uniform composition. The normal texture of several parenchymal organs is homogeneous (e.g., liver, thyroid, and pancreas).

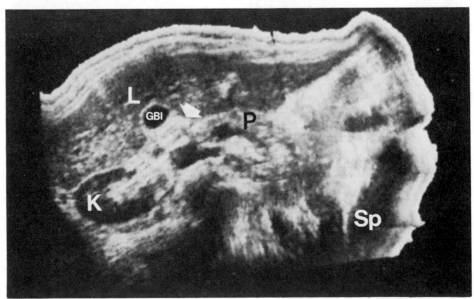

FIGURE 5-1. Transverse section of the upper abdomen showing the usual echogenicity of the organs in a young adult. Note that the pancreas (P) contains more echoes than the liver (L) and that the liver is slightly more echogenic than the kidneys (K) and the spleen (Sp). The gallbladder (GBl), a "cystic" (fluid-filled) structure, shows acoustic enhancement behind it, in the region of the duodenum (arrow).

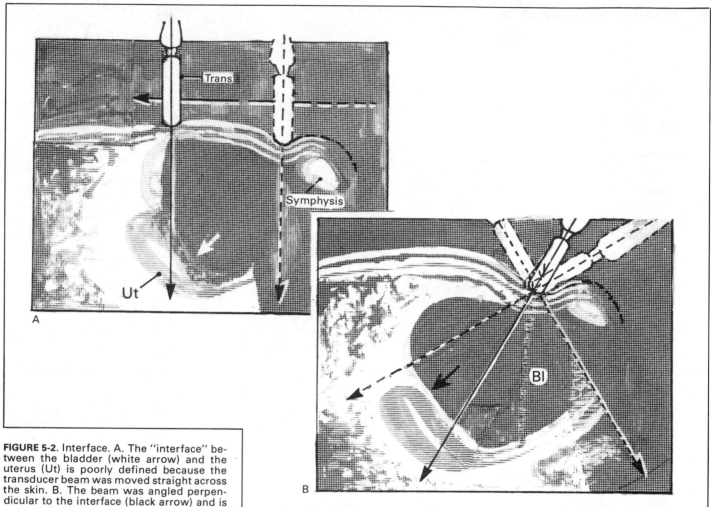

FIGURE 5-2. Interface. A. The "interface" between the bladder (white arrow) and the uterus (Ut) is poorly defined because the transducer beam was moved straight across the skin. B. The beam was angled perpendicular to the interface (black arrow) and is now well seen.

Interface. Strong echoes that delineate the boundary of organs, caused by the difference between the acoustic impedance of the two adjacent structures; an interface is usually more pronounced when the transducer is perpendicular to it (Fig. 5-2A,B).

Noise. Artifact, usually due to using too much gain, that occurs when echoes are seen in organs that do not really contain any interfaces (e.g., bladder).

Overwriting. Occurs when too many echoes are produced by repeated scanning over an area. The overabundance of echoes does not result from too much gain but from "writing" or scanning, over a given area more than is necessary (Fig. 5-3).

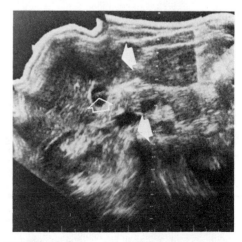

FIGURE 5-3. Overwriting artifact due to scanning over the same area twice (arrows).

Real-Time. Systems that create images so rapidly (i.e., more than 30 per second) that a cinematic view of an organ appears to be obtained.

Reverberation. An artifact that results from a strong echo returning from a large acoustic interface to the transducer. This echo returns to the tissues again, causing additional echoes parallel to the first.

Ring Down. Extreme form of reverberation artifact that occurs when a long series of echoes caused by a very strong acoustic interface and consequent reverberations are seen.

Scan. Verb—to perform an ultrasound scan. Noun—a sonographic examination.

Shadowing. Failure of the sound beam to pass through an object. This blockage is caused by reflection or absorption of the sound and may be partial or complete. For example, air bubbles in the duodenum allow poor transmission of the sound beam because most of the sound is reflected. A hard calcified gallstone does not allow any sound to pass through, and shadowing is pronounced (Fig. 5-4). These degrees of acoustic shadowing may help in diagnosis.

Solid (homogeneous). A mass that has uniform low-level echoes within it because the cellular tissues are acoustically very similar. A far wall echo can be made out, but it is not as well defined as the back wall of a cyst (Fig. 5-5).

Sonodense. A structure that transmits sound poorly.

Sonogenic. Handsome ultrasound image (like *photogenic*), for example, a good example of vascular anatomy.

Sonologist. A physician who specializes in ultrasound.

Sonogram. An ultrasound examination.

Sonographer. A technologist who specializes in ultrasound.

Sonolucent (anechoic). Without echoes. Not necessarily cystic unless there is good through transmission.

Specular Reflector. Structure that creates a strong echo because it interfaces at right angles to the sound beam and has a significantly different acoustic impedance from a neighboring structure.

Texture. The echo pattern within an organ such as the liver or kidney.

Through Transmission. The amount of sound passing through a structure (Fig. 5-1). Same as *Enhancement* (see above).

Transonicity. Term used to indicate the amount of sound passing through a mass or cyst, usually qualified as good or bad. Same as *Enhancement.*

Trendelenburg. A recumbent patient is tilted so that the feet are higher than the head.

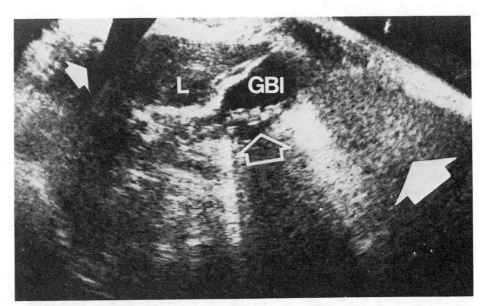

FIGURE 5-4. The acoustic shadowing from the stones in the gallbladder (GBI) is "sharp" (open arrow), whereas the shadowing from the bowel gas is "soft" (large arrow). Note the compounding technique (small arrow). L = liver.

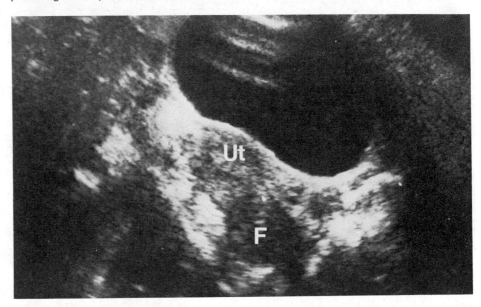

FIGURE 5-5. The fibroid (F) in the uterus (Ut) is a solid homogeneous mass. Because sound is attenuated, the far wall interface is weak, and there are internal echoes.

TERMS RELATING TO ORIENTATION

Anatomic Terms

See Figures 5-6, 5-7, 5-8.

Superior, Cranial, Cephalad, Rostral. Interchangeable terms denoting a structure closer to the patient's head.

Inferior or Caudal. Terms denoting a structure closer to the patient's feet.

Anterior or Ventral. Structure lying toward the front of the patient.

Posterior or Dorsal. Structure lying toward the back of the patient.

Medial or Mesial. Structure lying toward the midline.

Lateral. Structure lying away from the midline.

Prone. The patient lies on the front.

Supine. The patient lies on the back.

Proximal. Near.

Distal. Away from.

Quadrant. The abdomen is divided into four quarters, each known as a quadrant.

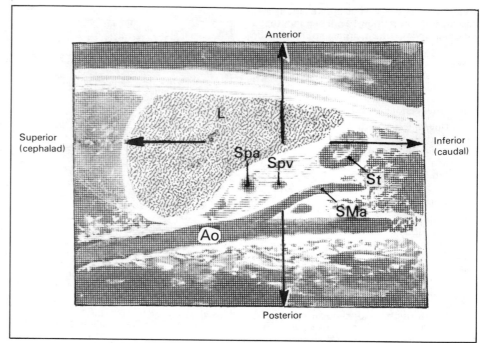

FIGURE 5-7. A longitudinal scan to the left of the midline showing normal structures and orientation.

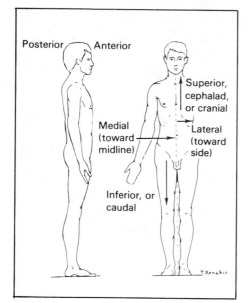

FIGURE 5-6. Standard labeling nomenclature used to show where structures lie in relation to each other.

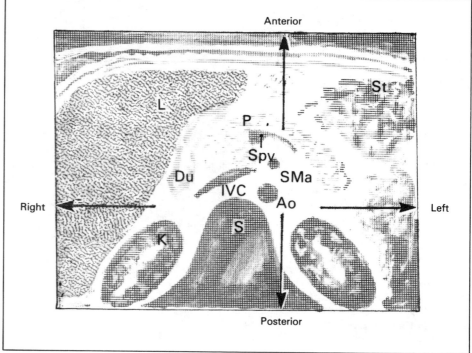

FIGURE 5-8. Transverse scan. The sonographic right and left are the opposite of the viewer's right and left.

TERMS RELATING TO LABELING

The American Institute of Ultrasound in Medicine (AIUM) has established standards for labeling studies so that a sonogram done in Columbus, Ohio, can be interpreted with no misunderstanding in Baltimore, Maryland.

Longitudinal Scans (Sagittal)

See Figure 5-9. The planes to the right or the left of the midline may be designated as right (R) or left (L) plus the distance in centimeters. Another accepted method is to use the midline as a reference (ML) with + indicating the right and − indicating the left.

LONGITUDINAL REFERENCE POINTS

See Figure 5-6.

ML Midline
Decub Decubitus

This term is least muddling if marked as "right side up" or "left side up" (Fig. 5-10).

Coronal

A long axis scan is performed from the patient's side (i.e., in the decubitus position; Fig. 5-10) or transversely in the neonatal head (see Chapter 40).

Transverse

The reference is first established and the distance in centimeters is marked with + for the superior direction and − for the inferior planes.

TRANSVERSE REFERENCE POINTS

See Figure 5-11.

N Notch (the sternal notch in thyroid scanning)
X Xiphoid—inferior tip of the sternum
IC or *C* Iliac crest, or crest
Umb or *U* Umbilicus
Sym, S, P, or *SP* Symphysis pubis

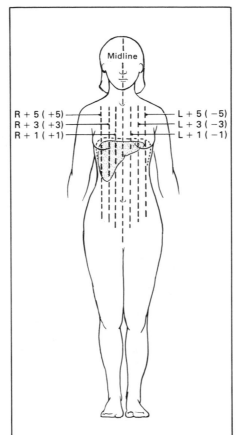

FIGURE 5-9. Longitudinal planes are labeled with the midline as the reference point.

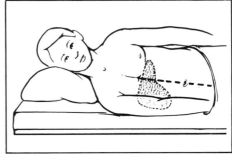

FIGURE 5-10. Left coronal, right decubitus, or left-side-up view.

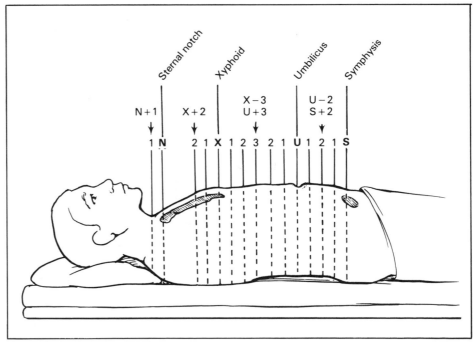

FIGURE 5-11. Transverse planes with reference points.

SCANNING TECHNIQUES

B-scanner (Static Scanning)

B-scanning is not obsolete. Although not easy to perform, it provides a much more complete picture of how a structure relates to other organs, and the picture is of high quality.

LINEAR SCAN

A linear scan is made when the transducer is perpendicular to the table top; the transducer face is in full contact with the body without angling the transducer. The transducer is held in the same position for the full sweep (Fig. 5-12).

SECTOR SCAN (ARC SCAN)

A sector scan is made when the transducer is not moved across the skin surface but left in place and angled to achieve a scan. The result is a wedge-shaped image (Fig. 5-13). This type of maneuver is used to achieve an image between ribs and under gas. This term is also used for the pie-shaped image produced by some real-time systems.

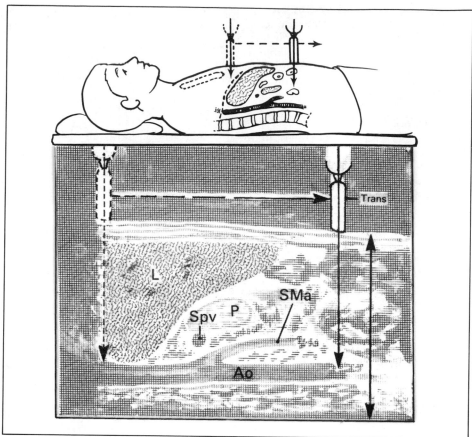

FIGURE 5-12. A linear scan.

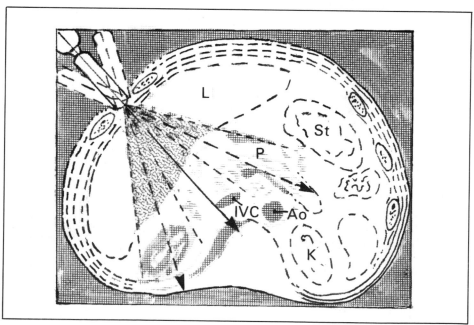

FIGURE 5-13. A sector scan.

COMPOUND SECTOR

Compound sector scans are multiple sector scans that overlap to create a compound image. This maneuver is an effective way to demonstrate an area partially obscured by ribs and gas, but artifacts are usually produced by the crossing of echoes from different directions (Fig. 5-14).

SINGLE PASS

For textured organs such as the liver, a single pass technique is used. With this technique the transducer is moved over a structure only once. Subtle lesions such as liver metastases that may be concealed by compound scanning may be revealed by a single pass; however, interfaces may be missed (Fig. 5-15).

Linear Arrays

Linear array real-time systems are most useful in obstetric work, where there are no ribs to be avoided, and the large superficial increased field of view is especially valuable. Real-time is indispensable for speed and accuracy in obstetric scanning. Fetuses are notoriously uncooperative when being photographed and must be chased. Specific fetal anatomic structures such as the long axis of the spine or the biparietal diameter are demonstrated best with real-time.

Sector Scanners

Sector scanners are more versatile than linear arrays. Because the relatively small scanning head can be placed intercostally, the long axis of the common bile duct, pancreas, or kidney can be readily found. A sector scan can demonstrate an aortic aneurysm well; however, it may not show the location of the aneurysm in relation to the rest of the aorta. A comparison between the texture of the kidney and the liver can be shown beautifully with a sector scan, but a diagnosis of hepatomegaly may be missed. A static B-scan gives the "whole picture"; a combined approach is the ideal.

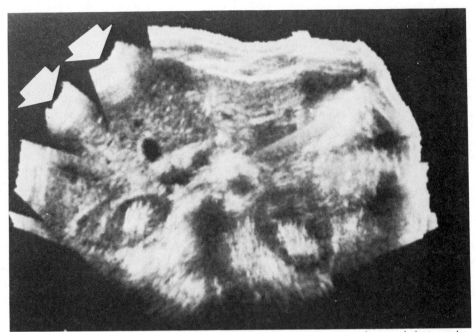

FIGURE 5-14. Compound scan made up of several short sector scans (arrows) that produce one complete image.

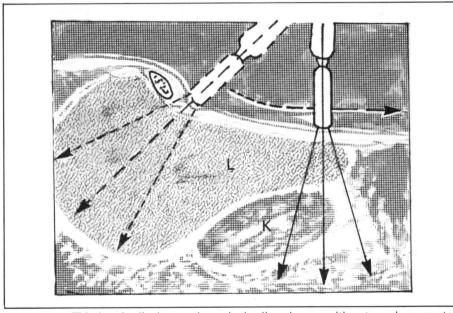

FIGURE 5-15. This longitudinal scan through the liver began with a transducer sectored against the 12th rib, then straightened into a linear scan. In this fashion the liver is seen with a single pass.

PATIENT PREPARATION

Most organs do not require specific patient preparation.

GALLBLADDER, LIVER AND PANCREAS

Only water should be given by mouth for the preceding 8 hours so that the gallbladder is distended. Even if only the liver and pancreas are being examined, it is still useful to have the gallbladder as a landmark.

PELVIS

The patient should drink several glasses of water and not void so that the bladder is present as an acoustic window through which to see the pelvic structures.

PATIENT-SONOGRAPHER INTERACTION

Because sonography requires so much time and patient contact, a sonographer is in an excellent position to elicit pertinent information from the patient. Talk to your patient! Not only will this relieve anxiety, it will reassure the patient that you are interested in figuring out just what is wrong, as indeed you are.

The request information that is provided with outpatients is limited, so it is very important to draw them out. Leading questions such as "What kind of trouble are you having?" or "Is this the first time you have been in the hospital?", can trigger a flood of information that can be relayed to the physician. With inpatients it should be standard procedure to read the synopsis of a patient's history in the chart. However, investigation of a decreased hematocrit can become more focused if a patient suddenly remembers that he fell down the stairs last week and hit the left side.

A sonographer cannot answer direct questions from patients about their condition. For legal reasons such questions must be evaded and passed on to the referring physician or, with the agreement of the referring physician, to the sonologist.

SONOGRAPHER-PHYSICIAN INTERACTION

The physician should be informed about any problems encountered during scanning that may pertain to pathology. For instance, if a 2.25-MHz transducer was required to scan the liver of a small patient, or if a surprisingly high gain setting was needed, perhaps the patient has a fatty liver.

Perhaps one of the most significant contributions a sonographer can make to the diagnosis is to determine the source of a localized area of pain. The sonographer is in a unique position to see what lies directly beneath the patient's most tender spot. A good example is the patient with right upper quadrant pain in whom no gallstones are found. The presence of acute pain at the site of the gallbladder makes acute cholecystitis likely. Also, the borders of a mass that can be felt should be placed on the image by putting dot markers on either side.

6. ANATOMY WITH EMPHASIS ON VESSELS

IRMA L. WHEELOCK

SONOGRAM ABBREVIATIONS

Ao	Aorta
Azv	Azygos vein (ascending lumbar vein)
Ca	Celiac artery
CBD	Common bile duct
CHa	Common hepatic artery
CHD	Common hepatic duct
CIa	Common iliac artery
Cr	Crus
Du	Duodenum
Gda	Gastroduodenal artery
GBl	Gallbladder
Hea	Hepatic artery
Hev	Hepatic vein
IMa	Inferior mesenteric artery
IMv	Inferior mesenteric vein
IVC	Inferior vena cava
K	Kidney
L	Liver
LGa	Left gastric artery
LGv	Left gastric vein
LHev	Left hepatic vein
LPv	Left portal vein
LRa	Left renal artery
LRv	Left renal vein
MHev	Middle hepatic vein
P	Pancreas
PHa	Proper hepatic artery
Pv	Portal vein
RGv	Right gastric vein
RHev	Right hepatic vein
RPv	Right portal vein
RRa	Right renal artery
RRv	Right renal vein
S	Spine
SGv	Splenogastric vein
SMa	Superior mesenteric artery
SMv	Superior mesenteric vein
Spa	Splenic artery
Spv	Splenic vein
St	Stomach

A clear understanding and an ability to demonstrate vascular anatomy are essential to an ultrasonic examination of the upper abdomen. Alterations of normal vessel size and location may be the key to detecting or localizing pathology.

ARTERIES

Aorta (abdominal). Main trunk of the arterial system (Figs. 6-1 and 6-5). It is anterior to the spine and bifurcates into the right and left common iliac arteries at the level of the umbilicus.

Celiac Artery (Axis, Trunk). This artery arises just below the liver from the anterior aorta and is only 2 to 3 cm in length (Figs. 6-1, 6-2, and 6-5). It almost immediately divides into the splenic, left gastric, and common hepatic arteries.

Gastroduodenal Artery. Originates from the common hepatic trunk and supplies the stomach and duodenum (Figs. 6-1, 6-2, and 6-4 A,B). It is a landmark delineating the antero-lateral aspect of the head of the pancreas.

Left Gastric Artery. Arises from the superior margin of the celiac axis and can be seen for only 1 or 2 cm (Figs. 6-1 and 6-2); supplies the stomach.

Hepatic Artery (Common). Originates from the celiac trunk (Figs. 6-1 and 6-2). Supplies the stomach, pancreas, duodenum, liver, gallbladder, and greater omentum. Divides into the proper hepatic and gastroduodenal arteries.

Hepatic Artery (Proper). Originates from the common hepatic artery and supplies the liver and gallbladder (Figs. 6-1 and 6-2); runs medial to the common bile duct and anterior to the portal vein into the liver within the porta hepatis.

Inferior Mesenteric Artery (IMa). Originates from the abdominal aorta close to the umbilicus (Fig. 6-1). Supplies the left portion of the transverse colon, the descending and sigmoid colon, and part of the rectum. It is not usually seen on the sonogram except at its origin.

Renal Arteries (Right and Left). Originate from the abdominal aorta at about the level of the superior mesenteric artery (Fig. 6-1); the right renal artery runs posterior to the inferior vena cava. They supply the kidney, adrenals, and ureters and are often best seen when the patient is in the appropriate decubitus position.

Replaced Right Hepatic Artery. A variant hepatic arterial supply originating from the superior mesenteric artery (Fig. 6-3).

Superior Mesenteric Artery (SMa). Originates from the anterior abdominal aorta just below the celiac axis and runs parallel to the aorta (Figs. 6-1 to 6-5). Supplies the small bowel, cecum, ascending colon, and part of the transverse colon and is a major landmark for localization of the pancreas.

Splenic Artery. Originates from the celiac trunk (Figs. 6-1, 6-2, and 6-5). Supplies the pancreas, spleen, stomach, and greater omentum and runs superior to the body and tail of the pancreas throughout most of its course. It is quite a tortuous vessel and may be difficult to visualize completely on one section.

FIGURE 6-1. Commonly visualized vessels arising from the aorta are the celiac artery (Ca), splenic artery (Spa), left gastric artery (LGa), common hepatic artery (CHa), proper hepatic artery (PHa), gastroduodenal artery (Gda), right and left renal arteries (RRa, LRa), superior mesenteric artery (SMa), inferior mesenteric artery (IMa), and below the bifurcation at the level of the fourth lumbar vertebra, the right and left iliac arteries (CIa). Only the portion of the aorta below the diaphragm is visualized on an abdominal study.

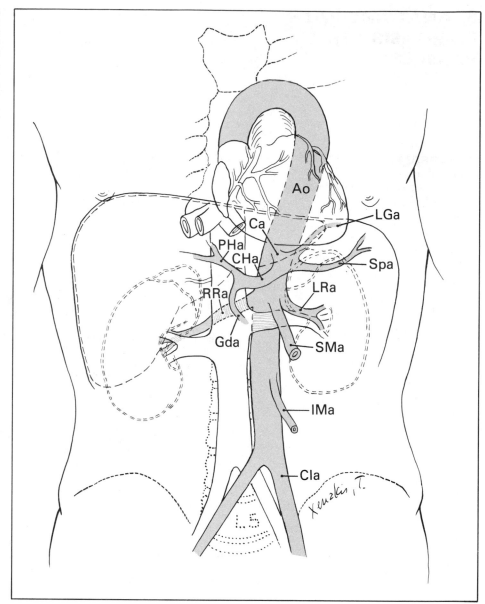

FIGURE 6-2. The vessel leaving the aorta closest to the diaphragm is the celiac artery (Ca). This vessel is a 1- to 2-cm trunk, which bifurcates into the splenic (Spa) and hepatic arteries (CHa). The hepatic artery (CHa) again bifurcates into the proper hepatic artery (PHa) and gastroduodenal artery (Gda). The superior mesenteric artery arises from the anterior surface of the aorta at a level just inferior to the celiac artery (Ca). The less frequently visualized left gastric artery (LGa) originates from the celiac artery (Ca).

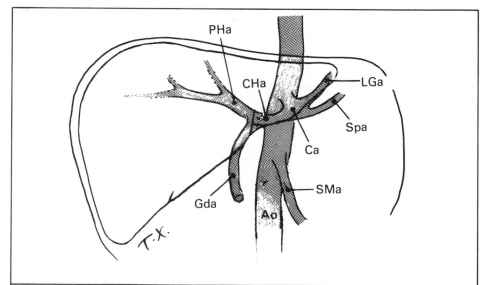

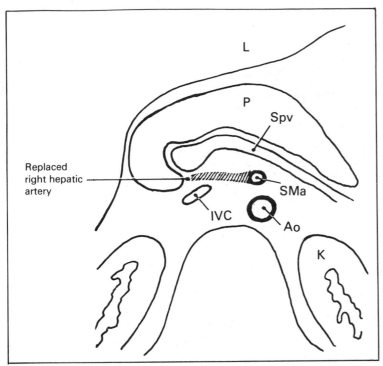

FIGURE 6-3. At the level of the splenic vein (Spv) and pancreas (P), a normal variant can sometimes be visualized. The replaced right hepatic artery originates from the superior mesenteric artery (SMa) to supply the liver.

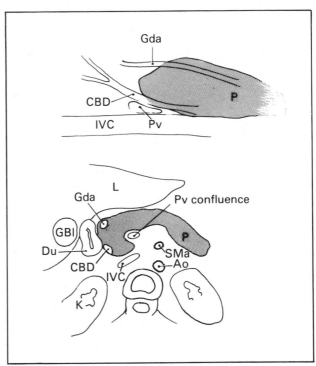

FIGURE 6-4. The gastroduodenal artery (Gda) outlines the antero-lateral margin of the head of the pancreas (P), whereas the common bile duct (CBD) marks the postero-lateral margin. A. Longitudinal. B. Transverse.

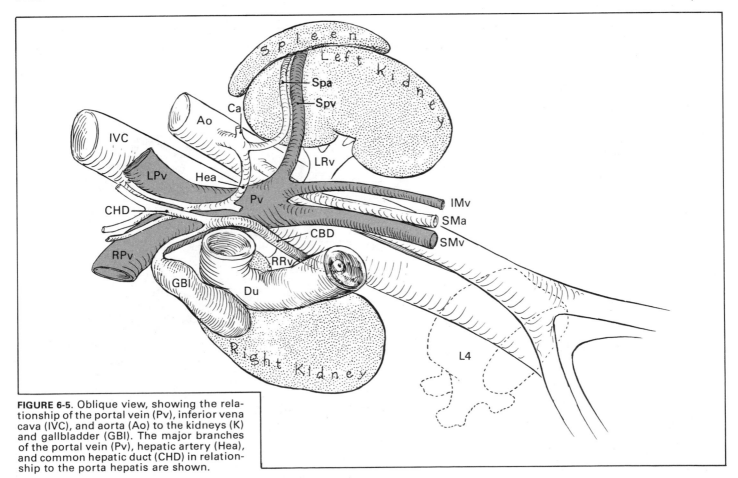

FIGURE 6-5. Oblique view, showing the relationship of the portal vein (Pv), inferior vena cava (IVC), and aorta (Ao) to the kidneys (K) and gallbladder (GBl). The major branches of the portal vein (Pv), hepatic artery (Hea), and common hepatic duct (CHD) in relationship to the porta hepatis are shown.

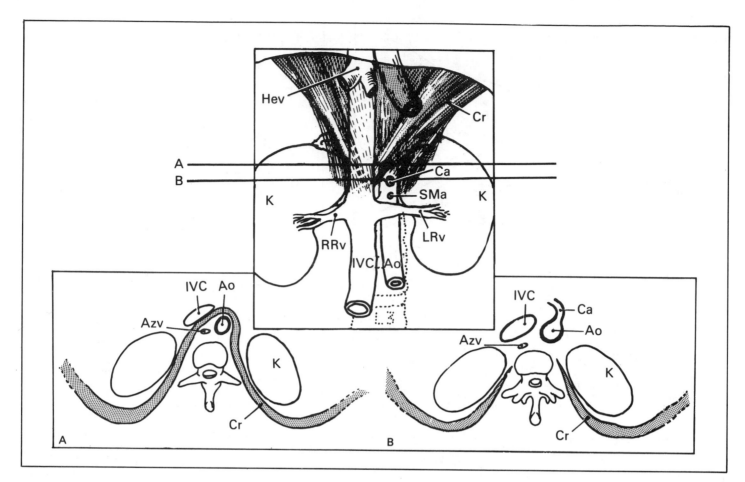

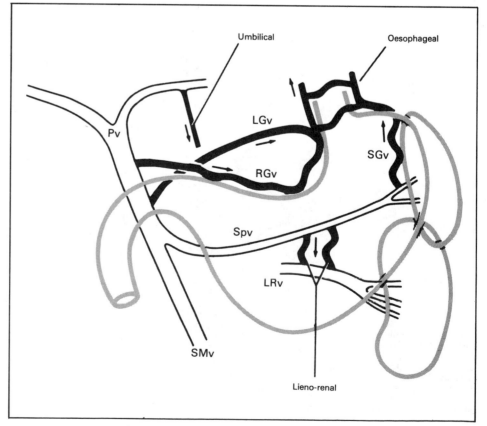

FIGURE 6-6. The crus of the diaphragm (Cr) can be visualized anterior to the aorta above the level of the celiac artery (Ca). Below that level it extends along the lateral aspects of the vertebral columns only. A. A transverse section at a higher level shows the crus posterior to the IVC and anterior to the aorta. The infrequently visualized ascending lumbar vein (Azv) is seen posterior to the crus. B. At a lower level, transversely, the crus is seen only at the lateral vertebral margins extending posteriorly.

FIGURE 6-7. Diagram showing the collateral routes established when portal hypertension exists. (Reprinted with permission from *Ultrasound Imaging: Liver, Spleen, and Pancreas.* Cosgrove, D., and McCready, R. John Wiley: 1982.)

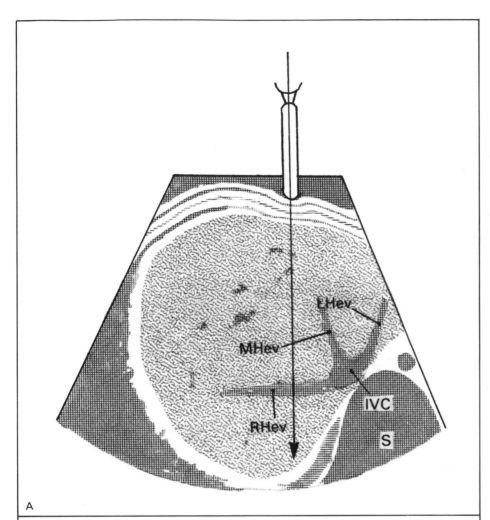

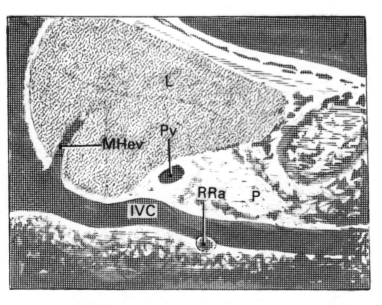

VEINS

Ascending Lumbar Vein. Lies posterior to the inferior vena cava and is not usually seen unless the patient has congestive failure (Fig. 6-6).

Collaterals. Vessels that develop when portal vein pressure is increased (e.g., by thrombosis). Collaterals are seen in the region of the pancreas, around the esophagogastric junction (anterior to the upper portion of the aorta), and in the porta hepatis (Fig. 6-7).

Coronary Vein. Connects the splenic vein to the region of the esophagus. Can be seen in only 10 to 20% of normal people and measures less than 4 mm. Dilates in portal hypertension.

Hepatic Veins. Drain the liver and empty into the inferior vena cava just below the diaphragm (Figs. 6-8 A,B and 6-13). They have poorly defined borders and branch away from the diaphragm. There are three main veins, of which two, the left and the middle, have a common trunk into the inferior vena cava.

Inferior Vena Cava. Returns blood from the lower half of the body and enters the right atrium of the heart (Figs. 6-5, 6-6 and 6-8B). There is a marked change in caliber with respiration (Fig. 6-12).

Inferior Mesenteric Vein (IMv). Vein of highly variable size (Fig. 6-5). It is usually small and runs to the left of the superior mesenteric vein to join the splenic vein.

Portal System. Composed of the superior and inferior mesenteric veins, splenic vein, and portal vein.

FIGURE 6-8. Hepatic veins. A. Transverse view, using a slightly cephalad angulation. The left (LHev), middle (MHev), and right (RHev) hepatic veins can be imaged as they empty into the inferior vena cava (IVC) just beneath the right diaphragm. B. Longitudinal view. The middle hepatic vein (MHev) is shown as it empties into the IVC at the level of the right diaphragm. The main branch of the portal vein (Pv) is seen in its extrahepatic location just superior to the head of the pancreas (P). The right renal artery (RRa) is visualized posterior to the IVC.

Portal Vein. Collects blood from the digestive tract and empties into the liver (Fig. 6-9). Formed by the junction of the splenic vein and the superior mesenteric vein. A large left branch supplies the left lobe of the liver (Fig. 6-9), the right portal vein has a major branch coming off just superior to the gallbladder (Fig. 6-10). Portal veins have echogenic borders and branch away from the porta hepatis.

Renal Veins. Drain the kidneys and empty into the inferior vena cava (IVC) (Figs. 6-1, 6-5, 6-6 and 6-11). The left is much longer than the right and may be dilated before it passes between the superior mesenteric artery and the aorta, a condition that should not be confused with adenopathy.

Splenic Vein. Collects blood from the spleen and part of the stomach (Fig. 6-3, 6-5, and 6-9). It runs posterior to the middle of the pancreas to join the superior mesenteric vein to form the portal vein and is a pancreatic landmark.

Superior Mesenteric Vein (SMv). Drains the cecum, transverse and sigmoid colon, and small bowel (Figs. 6-5, 6-9, and 6-11). Ascends in the mesenteric sheath just anterior to the aorta to join the splenic vein at the "confluence" behind the head of the pancreas. It too is a pancreatic landmark.

Umbilical Vein. Not normally visible but can be seen in portal hypertension as a sonolucent center in the ligamentum teres (Fig. 6-7).

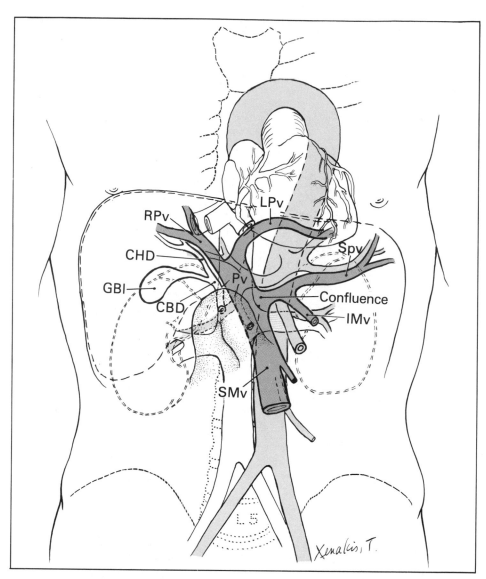

FIGURE 6-9. The splenic vein (Spv) and superior mesenteric vein (SMv) join (at the confluence) to form the main portal vein (Pv). The portal vein then branches into the liver, forming the left portal vein (LPv) and the right portal vein (RPv).

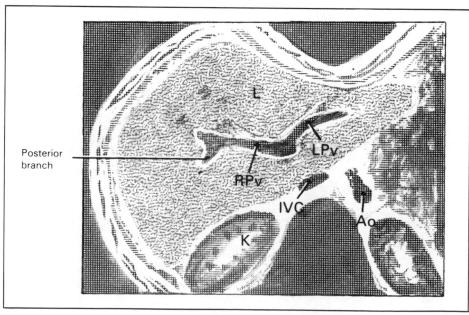

FIGURE 6-10. Transverse view within the liver (L). The portal vein branches into the left (LPv) and right portal veins (RPv). The right vein again bifurcates the posterior branch supplying the posterior right lobe of the liver.

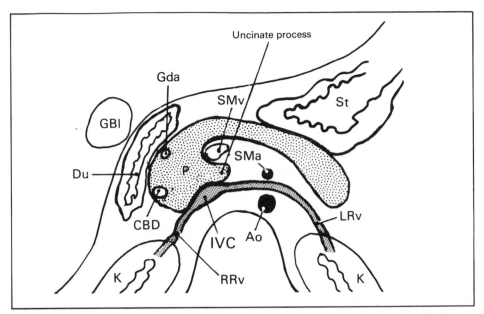

FIGURE 6-11. Many vascular structures can be visualized on a transverse section in the midabdomen. The inferior vena cava (IVC) gives rise to the right (RRv) and left renal veins (LRv); the latter passes between the aorta (Ao) and the superior mesenteric artery (SMa). Anterior to the inferior vena cava lies the superior mesenteric vein (SMv). The pancreas (P) can be imaged anterior to these vessels. The gastroduodenal artery (Gda) and the common bile duct (CBD) assist in outlining the lateral margin of the head of the pancreas. When empty, the walls of the antrum of the stomach (St) and the duodenum (Du) are seen as echo-free linear structures. The gallbladder (GBl) is lateral to the duodenum.

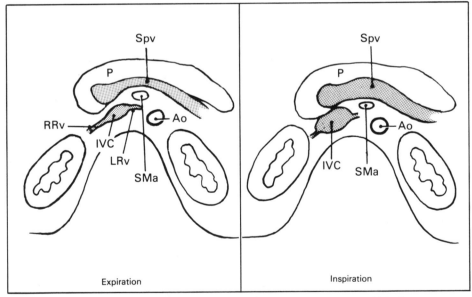

FIGURE 6-12. Venous structures should dilate with deep inspiration or the Valsalva maneuver. This can be helpful to confirm the venous nature of the vessels or perhaps to enlarge the vein to make it easier to image.

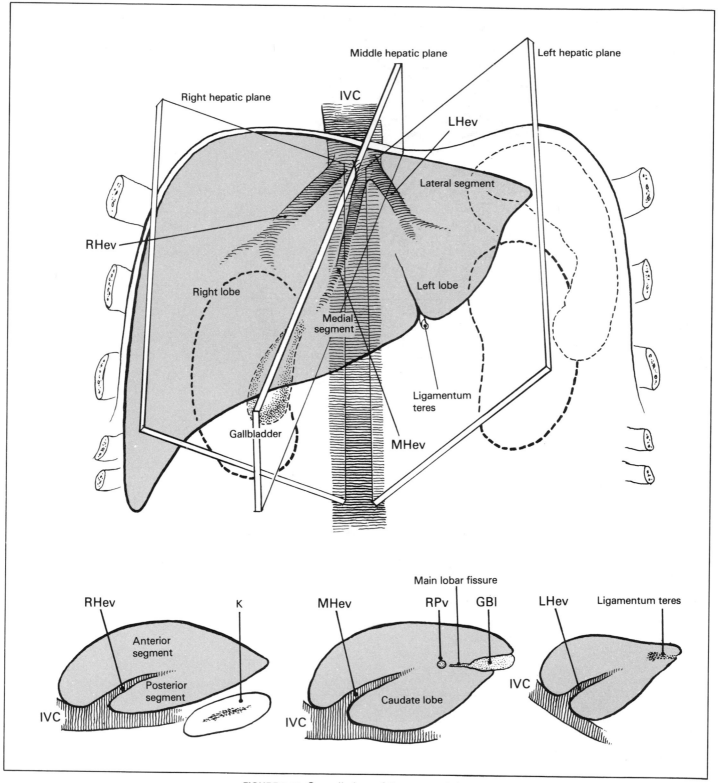

FIGURE 6-13. Overall view of the upper abdomen showing the liver, spleen, gallbladder, and kidneys. The hepatic veins represent the divisions between the lobes and segments of the liver. The middle hepatic vein divides the right and left lobes of the liver. The left hepatic vein separates the medial and lateral segments of the left lobe; the right hepatic vein separates the anterior and posterior segments of the right lobe of the liver. The gallbladder represents the inferior end of the separation between right and left lobes of the liver; the ligamentum teres represents the inferior end of the separation between the medial and lateral segments of the left lobe.

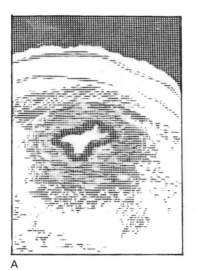 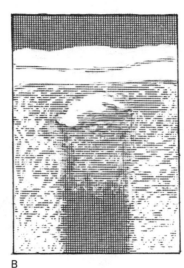 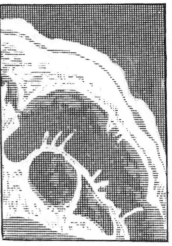

A   B   C

FIGURE 6-14. Gut can have a number of different manifestations. A. When empty, there is an echo-free wall around an echogenic center. B. When gas-filled, there is acoustic shadowing. C. When fluid-filled, one may be able to make out the haustral markings or valvulae conniventes in the wall of the fluid-filled bowel.

OTHER LINEAR STRUCTURES

Crus of the Diaphragm. A tubular muscular structure seen anterior to the aorta and posterior to the inferior vena cava above the level of the celiac axis and SMa (Fig. 6-6).

Ligamentum Teres. Echogenic structure in the left lobe of the liver (a remnant of the ductus venosum) in which the umbilical vein runs (Fig. 6-13).

Ligamentum Venosum. Echogenic line anterior to the caudate lobe of the liver.

Fissure Between the Right and Left Lobes of the Liver (main lobar fissure). Seen only between the gallbladder and the right portal vein (Fig. 6-13).

Hilum of the Spleen. Echogenic structure in the center of the medial border of the spleen; it represents the site of vessel entrance.

Porta Hepatis. Echogenic areas surrounding the portal veins, hepatic artery, and common bile duct.

GUT

The gut has three principal manifestations (Fig. 6-14).

EMPTY

An echogenic center is surrounded by a thin sonolucent ring (e.g., the antrum of the stomach usually has this appearance).

GAS-FILLED

Acoustic shadowing is present. The shadow has an irregular border, a poorly defined source, and some internal echoes, or, alternatively, it forms a banding pattern (see Chapter 45).

FLUID-FILLED

Sausage-shaped, fluid-filled structures are seen. Sometimes one can make out the valvulae conniventes or the haustral markings if there is a large amount of fluid in distended loops of bowel.

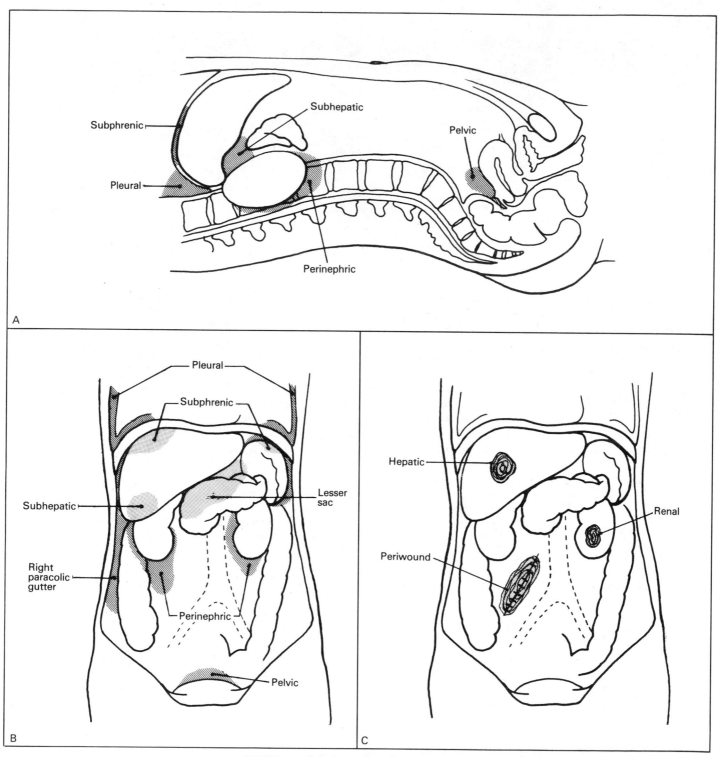

FIGURE 6-15. A,B. A number of spaces exist in the abdomen where fluid may collect. Common sites for fluid collection are the pelvic, subphrenic, subhepatic, paracolic gutter, and lesser sac areas. Fluid may collect around the kidneys or in the pleural space. C. Sites where abscesses may form are the spaces already mentioned, as well as within the liver or kidney and around incisions.

SPACES

There are a number of potential spaces in the abdomen where fluid can collect and where abscesses commonly form (Fig. 6-15).

1. *Right subphrenic.* Between the diaphragm and the dome of the liver.
2. *Subhepatic (Rutherford Morrison's pouch).* Between the inferior posterior aspect of the liver and the right kidney.
3. *Left subphrenic.* Between the spleen and the left hemidiaphragm.
4. *Lesser sac.* A large potential space mainly anterior to the pancreas and posterior to the stomach.
5. *Pelvic cul-de-sac.* Posterior to the uterus and anterior to the rectum.
6. *Paracolic gutters.* Along the flanks lateral to the colon.
7. *Perinephric.* There are various spaces around the kidneys that are described in detail in chapter 21.

MUSCLES

Some large muscles form a sort of framework on which the intra-abdominal structures lie.

PSOAS MUSCLES

These muscles lie alongside the spine and join the iliacus muscles in the pelvis.

QUADRATUS LUMBORUM

These muscles form the posterior wall of the abdomen behind the kidneys.

INTERNAL AND EXTERNAL OBLIQUE MUSCLES

These form the anterior and lateral walls of the abdomen.

RECTUS SHEATH

This muscle lies along the anterior aspect of the abdomen and is an important site of hematoma and abscess development (see Figs. 15-1 and 15-2).

PITFALLS

1. Excessive pressure with the transducer can collapse the walls of vessels so that they become invisible.
2. Expiration views may not allow visualization of vessels such as the inferior vena cava that can be seen on inspiration.

SELECTED READING

Carlsen, E. N., and Filly, R. A. Newer ultrasonic anatomy in the upper abdomen. *J. Clin. Ultrasound* 4:85, 1976.

Chafetz, N., and Filly, R. A. Portal and hepatic veins: Accuracy of margin echoes for distinguishing intrahepatic vessels. *Radiology* 130:725–728, 1979.

Filly, R. A., and Laing, F. C. Anatomic variation of portal venous anatomy in the porta hepatis: Ultrasonographic evaluation. *J. Clin. Ultrasound* 6:73–142, 1978.

Heap, S. W. The cross-sectional anatomy of the vessels and ducts of the upper abdomen. *Australas. Radiol.* 24:32, 1980.

Netter, F. H. *Digestive System: Upper Digestive Tract*, Part I, Vol. 3, CIBA (The Collection of Medical Illustrations). New York: CIBA Pharmaceuticals. Pp. 56–61.

Ralls, P. W., Quinn, M. F., and Rogers, W. Sonographic anatomy of the hepatic artery. *A.J.R.* 136:1059–1063, 1981.

Sample, W. F. Techniques for improved delineation of normal anatomy of the upper abdomen and high retroperitoneum with gray-scale ultrasound. *Radiology* 124:197–202, 1977.

7. EPIGASTRIC PAIN (UPPER ABDOMINAL PAIN)

Pancreatitis?

SUSAN M. GUIDI
ROGER C. SANDERS

SONOGRAM ABBREVIATIONS

Ao	Aorta
Ca	Celiac artery, axis
CD	Common duct
Du	Duodenum
GBl	Gallbladder
Gda	Gastroduodenal artery
Hea	Hepatic artery
IVC	Inferior vena cava
K	Kidney
L	Liver
LRv	Left renal vein
P	Pancreas
PD	Pancreatic duct
Pv	Portal vein
RRv	Right renal vein
S	Spine
SMa	Superior mesenteric artery
SMv	Superior mesenteric vein
Sp	Spleen
Spa	Splenic artery
Spv	Splenic vein
St	Stomach

KEY WORDS

Epigastrium. Upper abdominal region overlying the area of the stomach; adj., *epigastric.*

Hyperlipidemia. Congenital condition in which there are elevated fat levels that cause pancreatitis.

Ileus. Dilated loops of bowel that do not show any evidence of peristalsis. Ileus is associated with many abdominal problems (e.g., pancreatitis, sickle cell crisis, prolonged bowel obstruction).

Pancreatic Ascites. If a pancreatic pseudocyst bursts, the fluid pools in the same sites as ascites but contains dangerous enzymes. This is a very rare event.

Pancreatic Pseudocyst. Accumulation of pancreatic juice within or outside the pancreas.

Pancreatitis. Inflammation of the pancreas. (1) *Acute*—edematous swelling of the pancreas with severe upper abdominal pain, (2) *chronic*—chronic changes due to repeated attacks with resultant fibrosis, stone formation, and permanent damage, (3) *hemorrhagic*—greatly swollen pancreas with inflammation and bleeding, (4) *phlegmonous*—much enlarged pancreas with spread of the inflammatory process into the neighboring structures.

Peptic Ulcer Disease (PUD). An ulcer of the stomach or duodenum.

Serum Amylase. An enzyme that is elevated at some point during the clinical course of acute pancreatitis. It may also be elevated in other conditions such as penetrating peptic ulcer.

Uncinate Process. Portion of the head of the pancreas that lies posterior to the superior mesenteric vein.

Urinary Amylase. Enzyme that remains elevated longer than serum amylase in patients with acute pancreatitis.

THE CLINICAL PROBLEM

Epigastric pain, whether acute or chronic, is frequently caused by peptic ulcer or pancreatitis. Acute cholecystitis and hepatic disorders such as abscesses may also be characterized by epigastric pain (see Chapter 10). A rarer cause of epigastric pain is an aortic aneurysm (see Chapter 15). Uncomplicated peptic ulcer has no useful sonographic features, but fortunately all the other diseases do.

Acute Pancreatitis

Alcoholics and patients with blunt mid-abdominal trauma, gallbladder stones, and congenital conditions such as hyperlipidemia are predisposed to the development of acute pancreatitis. Pain can be so intense that exploratory surgery is often considered, although the best treatment is nonsurgical. A sonographic diagnosis of pancreatitis may prevent dangerous surgery.

The serum amylase level is commonly elevated in acute pancreatitis, although this finding is not specific for this condition. Because pancreatitis may be associated with ileus, gas may be present in large quantities. Acute pancreatitis may lead to the following complications: (1) pancreatic pseudocyst, (2) pancreatic abscess, (3) pancreatic ascites, or (4) common bile duct obstruction.

Chronic Pancreatitis

Patients present with pain similar to that which occurs in acute pancreatitis, but the pain is more persistent and not as severe. The condition occurs most frequently in alcoholics after multiple episodes of acute pancreatitis. These patients may be difficult to examine because of other sequelae of alcoholism such as delirium tremens (DTs). In addition, the liver may be a poor acoustic window because of fatty changes in it.

Pseudocysts

Fluid collections (commonly termed pseudocysts) occur frequently with pancreatitis. These collections are the result of the pancreatic edema that develops in pancreatitis. Such collections may breech their thin covering owing to autodigestion of the pancreas and neighboring organs by enzymes. Collections are commonly found within (1) the lesser sac, (2) the anterior pararenal space, (3) liver, (4) spleen, (5) mediastinum, and (6) mesentery. Ultrasound can be useful for (1) detection of pseudocysts, (2) serial follow-up of the evolution of a collection, and (3) diagnostic aspiration or therapeutic percutaneous drainage of a collection.

Pancreatic Carcinoma

A history of weight loss, chronic severe abdominal pain, and possible epigastric mass suggests carcinoma of the pancreas. Except for lesions involving the ampulla and common duct (see Chapter 11), symptoms are of such late onset that curative surgical treatment is impossible owing to local invasion or metastatic spread.

Because this grim disease is notorious for lymphatic and hematogenous spread, which has usually occurred by the time of diagnosis, the sonographer should not only evaluate the biliary tree but also search for enlarged lymph nodes and metastases to the liver. Ultrasound (1) detects the presence of a mass, particularly if the distal pancreatic duct is dilated, (2) delineates the size of the tumor, (3) establishes the degree of local and metastatic spread, (4) assists radiation therapy by mapping out tumor port sites, and (5) guides percutaneous biopsy of a mass.

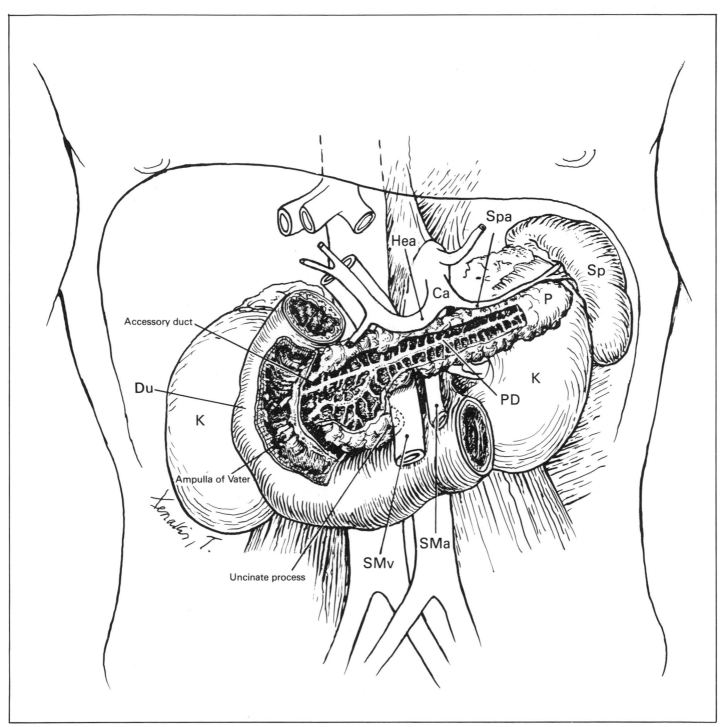

FIGURE 7-1. Diagram showing the relationship of the pancreas (P) to the celiac artery (Ca), duodenum (Du), kidneys (K), and spleen. Note that the pancreatic duct (PD) runs through the center of the pancreas to the ampulla of Vater. The splenic artery (Spa) lies superior to the pancreas.

ANATOMY

The pancreas is a long, thin gland that lies posterior to the stomach and the left lobe of the liver. It is divided into the head, neck, body, and a tail that usually abuts on the spleen.

An understanding of pancreatic anatomy is based upon the relationship of the pancreas to the vessels that surround the pancreas (Figs. 7-1 and 7-2).

SPLENIC VEIN

Located posterior to the center of the body and the tail of the pancreas, the splenic vein joins the superior mesenteric vein (SMv) to form the portal vein (Figs. 7-2 and 7-3B).

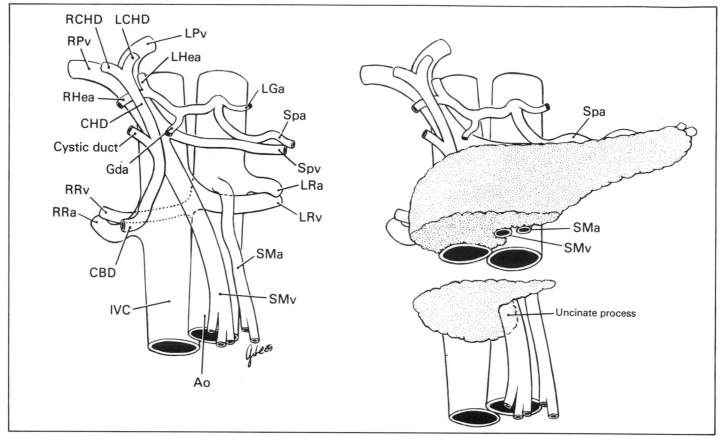

FIGURE 7-2. Diagram showing the relationship of the vessels to the pancreas. The "exploded" view through the uncinate process shows the relationship of the superior mesenteric artery and the vein to the uncinate process.

SPLENIC ARTERY

The splenic artery traverses the superior margin of most of the pancreas (the body and tail) to enter the splenic hilum (Figs. 7-1, 7-2, and 7-3B).

SUPERIOR MESENTERIC ARTERY (SMA)

The SMa is visible on transverse views as a sonolucent dot surrounded by an echogenic area posterior to the body of the pancreas (Figs. 7-2 and 7-3A).

It runs anterior to the aorta and is not in contact with the uncinate lobe of the pancreas. The SMa originates approximately at the level of the pancreas (Figs. 7-2 and 7-3A,B).

LEFT RENAL VEIN

This vein runs approximately 1 cm posterior to the body of the pancreas between the superior mesenteric artery and the aorta (Figs. 7-2 and 7-3).

SUPERIOR MESENTERIC VEIN (SMV)

The SMv is located posterior to the neck of the pancreas and anterior to the uncinate process (Figs. 7-1, 7-2, and 7-3).

INFERIOR VENA CAVA

The inferior vena cava lies posterior to the head of the pancreas in most people (Figs. 7-2 and 7-3).

COMMON BILE DUCT

This duct runs in the superior posterior portion of the pancreatic head (Figs. 7-2, 7-3A, 7-4, and 7-5).

GASTRODUODENAL ARTERY

The gastroduodenal artery lies in the anterior portion of the head of the pancreas (Figs. 7-2, 7-3, and 7-4).

PANCREATIC DUCT

This duct, which has a maximum normal size of 2 mm, extends through the pancreas. An accessory duct may also be seen (Fig. 7-1).

AMPULLA OF VATER

The entrance of the pancreatic duct and the common bile duct into the duodenum is called the ampulla of Vater (Fig. 7-1).

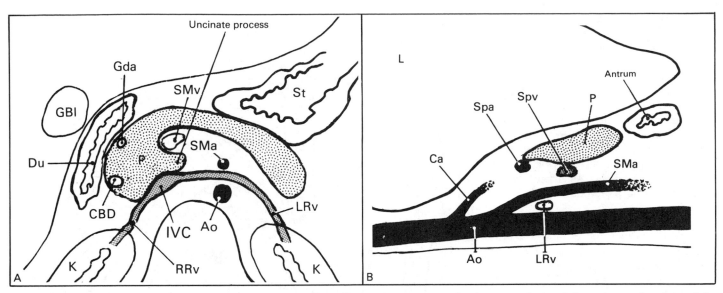

FIGURE 7-3. Transverse view of pancreas. A. Transverse section. The uncinate process lies between the superior mesenteric vein and the inferior vena cava (IVC). The gallbladder (GBl), duodenum (Du), and pancreas (P) form a constant threesome. The superior mesenteric vein (SMv) lies medial to the head of the pancreas. The gastroduodenal artery (Gda) and common bile duct (CBD) lie in the lateral aspect of the head of the pancreas. B. Diagram showing the relationship of the pancreas (P) to the splenic vein (Spv), splenic artery (Spa), and superior mesenteric artery (SMa).

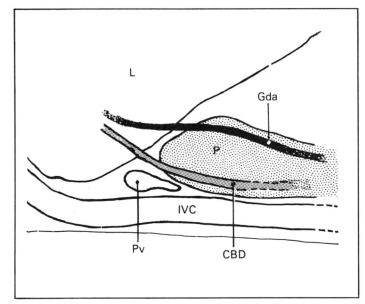

FIGURE 7-4. Longitudinal section through head of the pancreas (P) showing the normal location of the gastroduodenal artery (Gda) and common bile duct (CBD).

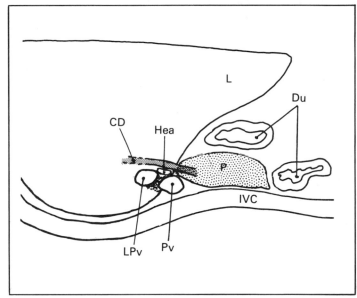

FIGURE 7-5. Diagram of the structures in the porta hepatis showing the common duct passing anterior to the hepatic artery and the main and left portal veins passing into the head of the pancreas.

Relationship to Other Organs

The relationship of the gallbladder, duodenum, and head of the pancreas to other organs remains constant, although the pancreatic head may lie further to the left than the inferior vena cava. The tail of the pancreas is of variable length and may not reach the splenic hilum. The antrum of the stomach lies anterior and somewhat inferior to the pancreas. As a rule, the left lobe of the liver acts as an ultrasonic window for the pancreas (Fig. 7-6).

Texture

The pancreas in most adults is a little more echogenic than the liver. In older people the pancreas may be especially echogenic owing to fatty changes. In fact, the pancreas in older people may be normal yet so echogenic that it is difficult to distinguish from the surrounding retroperitoneal fat. In children, on the other hand, the normal pancreas may be less echogenic than the liver.

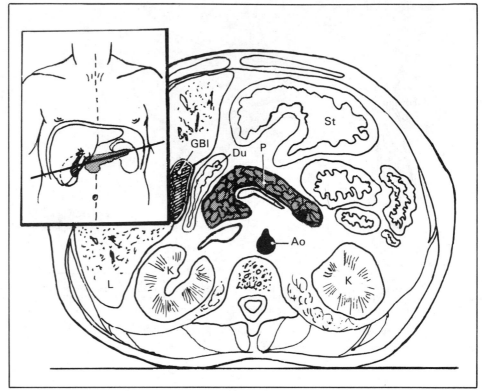

FIGURE 7-6. Transverse section showing the usual axis of the pancreas in relation to the kidneys (K), duodenum (Du), and gallbladder (GBl).

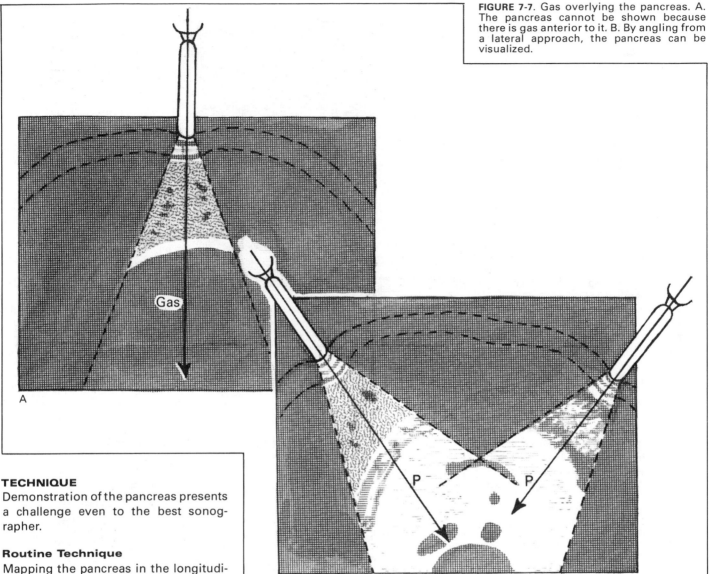

FIGURE 7-7. Gas overlying the pancreas. A. The pancreas cannot be shown because there is gas anterior to it. B. By angling from a lateral approach, the pancreas can be visualized.

TECHNIQUE
Demonstration of the pancreas presents a challenge even to the best sonographer.

Routine Technique
Mapping the pancreas in the longitudinal plane will reveal the oblique direction of the pancreas. Find the pancreas anterior to the aorta and to the inferior vena cava to get an idea of its axis, and then direct the transducer obliquely along this axis to show the vascular landmarks (Fig. 7-6). Angling in a caudal fashion through the liver may be helpful. High-frequency transducers (5.0 MHz) may be necessary to scan a superficially situated pancreas.

Gas Problems
If there is gas overlying the pancreas, water in the stomach can provide an acoustic window for the pancreas. Fat administration as given for a gallbladder examination (e.g., Neocholex) may be used to prevent peristalsis and stomach emptying. About 1 quart of water is given immediately after fat administration. Glucagon can be used instead of fat (Fig. 7-7).

Performing the scan with the patient in an erect position may increase the chances of demonstrating the pancreas because the liver descends from beneath the ribs and can be used as an acoustic window. Placing the patient in the right posterior oblique or left posterior oblique position may also shift bowel gas away from the pancreas (See Figs. 7-7A,B below). Angulation of the transducer in a transverse plane either cephalad or caudad may circumvent pockets of gas.

Pancreas Versus Duodenum
Real-time is useful in distinguishing the bowel from a mass, particularly in the region of the head of the pancreas where the duodenum and the pancreas can look very similar.

Possible Pseudocyst Versus Stomach
Filling the stomach with tap water will allow the sonographer to distinguish the stomach from a cystic mass such as a pseudocyst in the left upper quadrant. Tap water will be echogenic at first owing to microbubbles but will later become echo-free. When pancreatitis is suspected, the patient often has a nasogastric tube in position and cannot be given fluids. However, water may be injected through the nasogastric tube and later withdrawn after optimal views of the pancreas have been obtained.

Displaying the Pancreatic Tail

The left-side-up position looking through the kidney should be routine when the sonographer is searching for a pancreatic pseudocyst (see Chapter 16). The tail of the pancreas may also be demonstrated in the prone position using the spleen and left kidney as a window.

PATHOLOGY

Acute Pancreatitis

During an initial attack, the findings include the following:

1. *Textural changes.* The pancreas is less echogenic than normal.
2. *Enlargement.* May be focal or diffuse. A width of more than 3 cm for the head and tail is considered indicative of enlargement owing to edema or inflammation. Smaller increases can indicate pancreatitis if the pancreas was originally small; therefore, symmetry of the gland is important (Fig. 7-8).

   A pancreatic head or tail that is wider than the width of the vertebral body is also said to be abnormally large. The pancreas may be massively enlarged if phlegmonous or hemorrhagic pancreatitis is present.
3. *Focal enlargement.* Focal enlargement is possible with local widening and sonolucency in focal acute pancreatitis.

When acute pancreatitis is superimposed on chronic pancreatitis, ultrasonic changes may not be seen.

Chronic Pancreatitis

See Figure 7-9. There are four ultrasonic features.

1. *Irregular pancreatic outline.*
2. *Dilatation of the pancreatic duct* (over 2 mm).
3. *Calculi* can be identified as small groups of dense echoes, often with acoustic shadowing.
4. *Focal enlargement* with patchy groups of echoes.

In the more advanced stages, there is a generalized decrease in the size of the pancreas with increased echogenicity because of fibrosis. Acute on chronic pancreatitis may show features of both conditions.

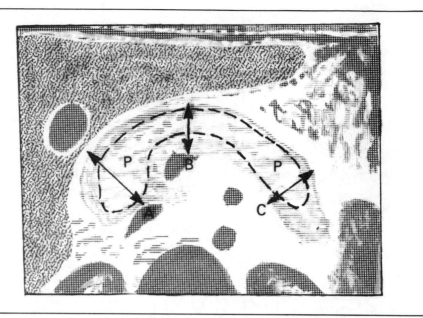

FIGURE 7-8. In pancreatitis the pancreas swells and becomes more sonolucent than usual. The dotted lines show the normal size of the pancreas; the arrows (A,B,C) show the increase that occurs with pancreatitis. The pancreas is normally considered to have an upper size limit of 1.5 cm at the level of the body and of 3 cm at the head and tail.

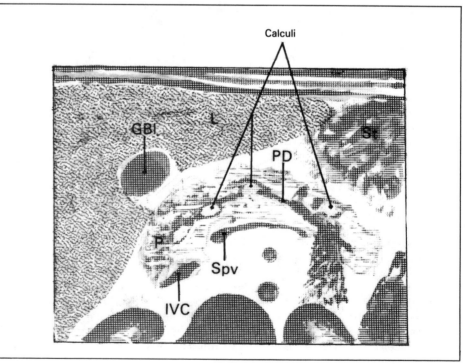

FIGURE 7-9. In chronic pancreatitis, calculi develop within the pancreas (some with acoustic shadowing), and the pancreatic duct enlarges. The outline of the pancreas is more irregular, and its overall echogenicity is increased.

Pseudocyst

A pseudocyst usually appears as a circular echo-free mass with good through transmission. The most common location is in the lesser sac anterior to the tail of the pancreas (Fig. 7-10). The head of the pancreas is the next most common location.

Less commonly, pseudocysts may have internal echoes, fluid-fluid levels, or irregular borders, particularly when hemorrhage or superinfection is present.

Pseudocysts may be multiple and may dissect into neighboring structures, notably the liver, spleen, or mediastinum. Septation within a pseudocyst may be seen. Infection can occur but may not alter the sonographic pattern.

Pancreatic Cancer

Typically, there is a hypoechoic sonolucent mass that is less echogenic than the surrounding pancreas. The mass may be too small to cause changes in the pancreatic outline, but can be recognized by the irregular borders and a difference in acoustic texture (Fig. 7-11).

Cystadenomas

These rare neoplasms may be benign or malignant and may be recognizable because they contain cysts. They may be confused with pancreatic pseudocysts.

Islet Cell Tumors

These tumors produce a hormone that causes hypoglycemic episodes. They can grow to a large size if they do not produce hormones and are generally echo-free.

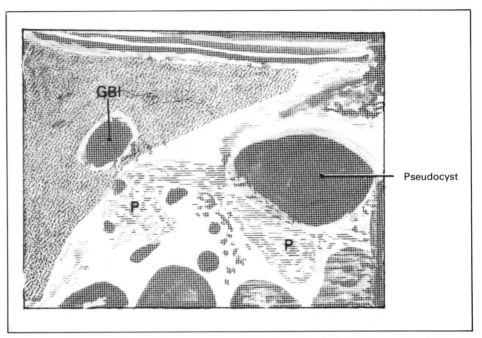

FIGURE 7-10. Pancreatic pseudocysts are usually large, echo-free structures that lie in the region of the lesser sac. They show good through transmission. They can lie in many other locations.

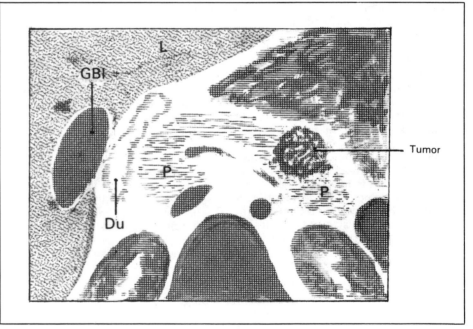

FIGURE 7-11. Pancreatic carcinomas are generally less echogenic than the normal pancreas, with irregular borders. They can develop anywhere in the pancreas, but when located in the pancreatic head, their presence soon becomes evident by causing biliary duct obstruction.

PITFALLS

1. *The posterior wall of the stomach* can be mistaken for the pancreatic duct. However, the stomach wall can be traced around the entire outline of the stomach (Fig. 7-12).

2. *The pancreas becomes more echogenic with age* due to fatty changes. Do not confuse aging changes with chronic pancreatitis. The outline of the pancreas remains smooth in normal old age. Fatty changes, unlike chronic pancreatitis, cause an even pancreatic echogenicity.

3. *Left lobe of the liver versus pancreas.* The echogenic line around the left portal vein may be mistaken for the posterior aspect of the liver. Thus, the posterior portion of the left lobe of the liver may be wrongly identified as the pancreas.

4. *Cyst versus pseudocyst.* Cystic structures near the pancreas are not always pseudocysts. Make sure that the cystic structure is not a fluid-filled stomach, colon, or renal cyst.

5. *Splenic artery versus pancreatic duct.* The splenic artery may be confused with the pancreatic duct and occasionally runs through the center of the pancreas. Examine it with real-time to see if the apparent duct connects with the celiac axis and pulsates.

6. *Gallbladder versus pseudocyst.* Confusion between a gallbladder and a pseudocyst may occur; a gallbladder will contract with fat administration, but a pseudocyst will not.

7. *Duodenum versus head of pancreas.* The duodenum may be mistaken for a mass in the head of the pancreas when the gut is filled with echogenic contents. Using real-time, identify the location of the common duct and the gastroduodenal artery. Give the patient fluid by mouth to identify the duodenum.

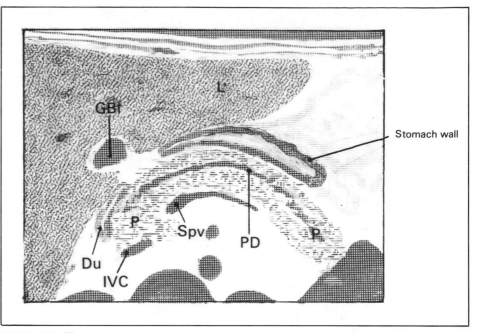

FIGURE 7-12. The posterior wall of the stomach can be mistaken for a dilated pancreatic duct if the site of the pancreas is not carefully identified. The posterior wall of the stomach does not reach as far to the right as the pancreatic duct (PD).

WHERE ELSE TO LOOK

1. If a *mass* in the head of the pancreas is noted, make sure that the common bile duct, gallbladder, and pancreatic duct are not obstructed and dilated.

2. A *mass* in the pancreas may be a carcinoma. Look for liver metastases and para-aortic or porta hepatis nodes.

3. If *pancreatitis* is found, look for the other stigmata of alcoholism, such as (1) altered liver texture due to cirrhosis, hepatitis, or fatty liver, (2) splenomegaly, (3) portal hypertension, shown by a dilated splenic vein, portal vein, superior mesenteric and coronary veins, and evidence of collaterals (extra vessels around the pancreas), and (4) ascites that may be caused by liver disease or pancreatic ascites (i.e., a ruptured pseudocyst).

SELECTED READING

Bowie, J. D., and MacMahon, H. Improved techniques in pancreatic sonography. *Semin. Ultrasound* 1:170–178, 1980.

Cosgrove, D. O., and McCready, V. R. (Eds.). *Ultrasound Imaging: Liver, Spleen, Pancreas.* Toronto: Wiley, 1982.

Johnson, M. L., and Mack, L. A. Ultrasonic evaluation of the pancreas. *Gastrointest. Radiol.* 3:257–266, 1978.

Marks, W. M., Filly, R. A., and Callen, P. W. Ultrasonic evaluation of normal pancreatic echogenicity and its relationship to fat deposition. *Radiology* 137:475–479, 1980.

Weinstein, B. J., and Weinstein, D. P. Ultrasonographic evaluation of the pancreas. *CRC Crit. Rev. Diagn. Imaging* 18:81–120, 1982.

8. COLD DEFECTS ON LIVER SCAN

Possible Metastases to Liver

NANCY A. SMITH
ROGER C. SANDERS

SONOGRAM ABBREVIATIONS

Ao	Aorta
Ca	Celiac artery
CD	Common duct
D	Diaphragm
GBl	Gallbladder
Hev	Hepatic vein
IVC	Inferior vena cava
K	Kidney
L	Liver
LHev	Left hepatic vein
MHev	Middle hepatic vein
Pv	Portal vein
RHev	Right hepatic vein
RPv	Right portal vein
S	Spine
Sp	Spleen
St	Stomach

KEY WORDS

Ameboma. Abscess caused by amebic infection. Common in Mexico and southern United States.

Alpha-Fetoprotein (AFP). Biochemical marker that, when elevated, may indicate liver metastases.

Carcinoembryonic Antigen (CEA). Biochemical tumor marker that, when elevated, may indicate liver metastases.

Caudate Lobe. Lobe of the liver that lies posterior to the left lobe, anterior to the inferior vena cava.

Cold Defect. Area of decreased radionuclide uptake on nuclear liver-spleen scan.

Echinococcal Cyst. Infected cyst caused by hydatid disease. Frequently calcified. Seen in individuals who are in contact with sheep and dogs.

Hemangioma. Benign tumor of the liver, which is highly vascular, making biopsy dangerous.

Hepatoblastoma. Liver tumor that is common in childhood.

Hepatoma. Tumor of the liver that is associated with cirrhosis. Common in the Far East and Africa.

Hydatid. See *Echinococcal cyst* (above).

Ligamentum Teres. Echogenic focus in the left lobe of the liver; remnant of the fetal ductus venosus (see Fig. 8-17).

Quadrate Lobe. Obsolete term for the medial segment of the left lobe of the liver.

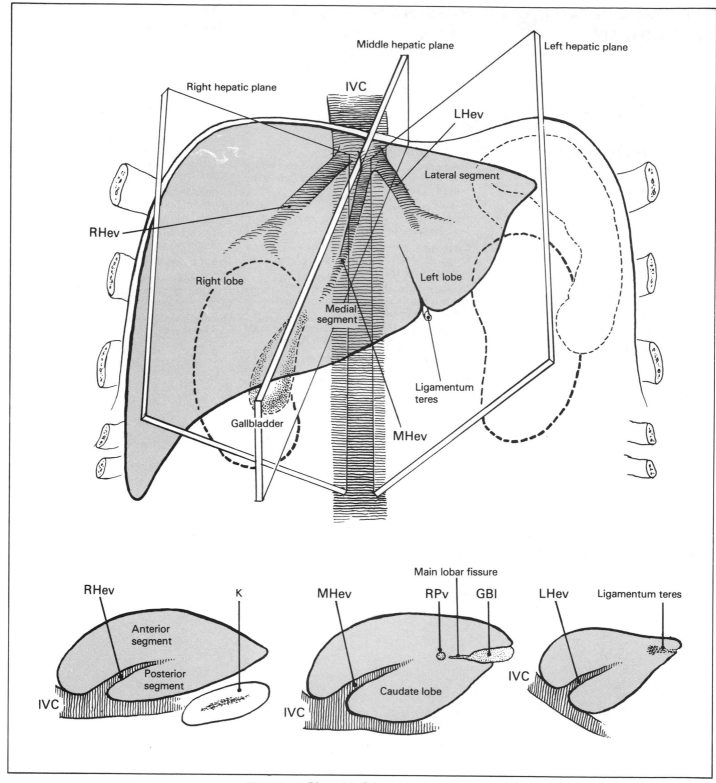

FIGURE 8-1. Diagram of the lobes and segments of the liver. The middle hepatic vein separates the left and right lobes. The left hepatic vein separates the lateral and medial segments of the left lobe. The right hepatic vein separates the anterior and posterior segments of the right lobe. The caudate lobe can be seen only on sagittal sections. The right hepatic vein and the gallbladder form the junction between the right and left lobes of the liver. The left hepatic vein and ligamentum teres separate the medial and lateral segments.

THE CLINICAL PROBLEM

A common ultrasonic question is whether or not there are metastatic lesions within the liver. Clinical findings that suggest a hepatic mass are a palpable nodule in the liver, hepatomegaly, and sudden onset of ascites. Liver metastases may be suspected because biochemical tumor markers (CEA and AFP) are elevated. Alternatively, a patient may be referred because a previous nuclear medicine liver-spleen scan showed a cold defect. Possible causes of focal defects on a liver-spleen scan are cysts, primary or secondary liver tumors, abscesses, hematomas, and a number of normal variants. Normal variants that may cause confusion on the liver scan include

1. Thinning of the left lobe of the liver
2. Rib impressions
3. A kidney lying more anteriorly than usual
4. A prominent gallbladder in the gallbladder fossa
5. Hepatic veins

Primary liver tumors may be suspected in cirrhotic patients who have a rapid downhill course if liver function tests become rapidly worse. Delineation of the precise site of a primary liver tumor is important because it influences resectability. If both right and left lobes are involved, a tumor cannot be resected. The margins between the individual segments of each lobe can be defined with ultrasound.

ANATOMY

Liver Architecture

The liver is divided into three lobes—right, left, and caudate lobes (Fig. 8-1). A fissure known as the ligamentum teres, in which lies a remnant of the fetal umbilical vein, separates the left lobe into two segments. The medial segment of the left lobe of the liver was formerly known as the quadrate lobe. This is now an obsolete term. The division between the right and left lobes is not visible except at a point superior to the gallbladder, where an echogenic line seems to connect the right portal vein to the gallbladder fossa (the main lobar fissure). More superiorly, the demarcation

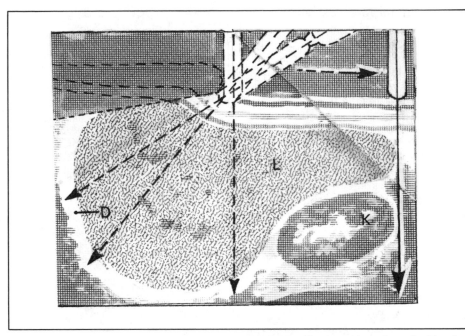

is along the line of the middle hepatic vein. The left hepatic vein separates the two segments of the left lobe of the liver, and the right hepatic vein separates the two segments of the right lobe. There is a marked separation between the caudate lobe, which lies posterior to the left lobe, and the rest of the liver because of a fissure where the ligamentum venosum lies.

The liver is surrounded by peritoneum except for a segment known as the bare area posterior to the dome of the liver where fluid cannot collect. Elsewhere, particularly in the right subhepatic space anterior to the kidney and inferior to the diaphragm, there are potential sites for abscess or ascitic collections (see Fig. 6-15).

TECHNIQUE

B-scan static views are best for documenting a liver study because they show the complete liver.

FIGURE 8-2. The transducer is rocked in place against the costal margin before straightening into a linear scan. In this way more of the liver is demonstrated.

Longitudinal-Sagittal View

Longitudinally, the liver can usually be seen best on deep inspiration. By angling the transducer up under the costal margin, first sectoring and then straightening out to a linear scan, the diaphragm can usually be seen as well (Fig. 8-2). Because of the great difference in size, a high-frequency (5-MHz) transducer may be used for the left lobe of the liver, and a 3.5-MHz transducer may be appropriate for the right lobe.

Longitudinal-Intercostal View

The sagittal technique will not be adequate if the liver is small or is too high up under the ribs. An alternative is an intercostal scan. Often multiple-sector scans are necessary to show the entire liver adequately (Fig. 8-3).

Oblique-Longitudinal (Right Oblique) View

An additional technique that is of value on longitudinal section in high small livers is to angle the scanning arm toward the patient and scan from the patient's side (Fig. 8-4). This projection can be helpful if the liver is inaccessible and is surrounded by lung and bowel. Comparison between the right kidney and the liver for texture is easy with this view.

Transverse View

Use a single sweep when scanning the liver in any direction. Transversely this is done by making a large sector under the ribs and a linear scan across the left lobe, usually on inspiration (Fig. 8-5). A long focus transducer should be chosen unless the area of interest is fairly superficial. The entire liver is usually visualized by a single sweep. The transducer must be angled sharply to show the lateral edge.

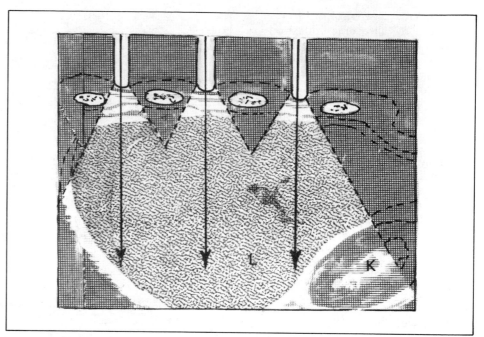

FIGURE 8-3. Multiple intercostal scans may be necessary and are often the best way to see the upper pole of the right kidney.

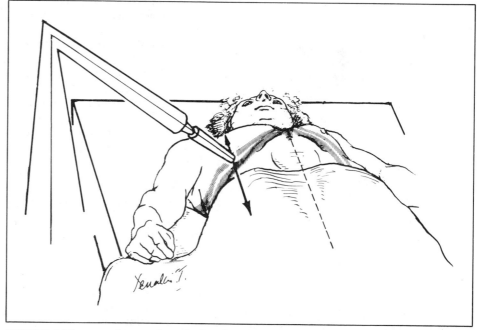

FIGURE 8-4. The scanning arm is angled until it is perpendicular to the sloping ribs. The angle varies with the patient's build; it is important to get good contact against the skin.

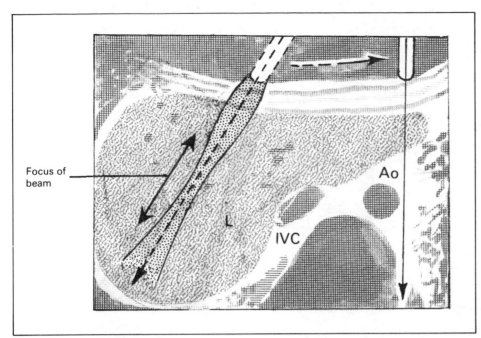

FIGURE 8-5. Transverse view of the liver. Primarily a linear scan, transverse views done in this fashion should use a focal zone that is long enough to include the patient's right lobe. Texture is best seen without overwriting.

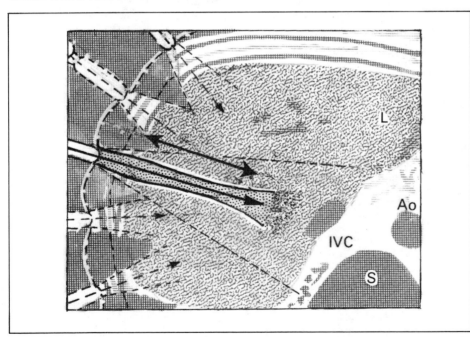

FIGURE 8-6. Multiple intercostal scans, usually done with a 13-mm face transducer, require less depth of focal zone, but care should be taken not to overwrite.

Transverse-Intercostal View

If the entire liver is hidden under the ribs, angling the arm cephalad on a transverse view will help, but only a few centimeters of the liver can be seen this way. Multiple-sector scans through the intercostal spaces are usually required (Fig. 8-6). A 13-mm transducer face is desirable to reach between the ribs. Because the depth to be penetrated from a lateral approach is less than that from an anterior approach, a medium focal zone is usually best (Fig. 8-6).

Right Costal Margin View (RCM)

A useful view for visualizing a large amount of liver and for assessing texture is the right costal margin view (Fig. 8-7). The dome of the liver can be reached by angling cephalad along a plane parallel to the costal margin on deep inspiration. The amount of cephalad angulation required on the scanning arm varies with liver size. The hepatic veins are well demonstrated with this projection, for which a single sweep should be used. Overwriting of the echoes is seldom diagnostic.

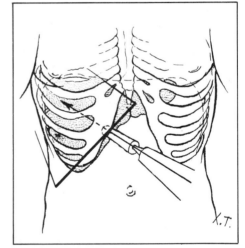

FIGURE 8-7. Right costal margin view. By angling up under the costal margin and scanning along that plane, large sweeps of the liver can be seen with a single pass. Far gain enhancement is usually required.

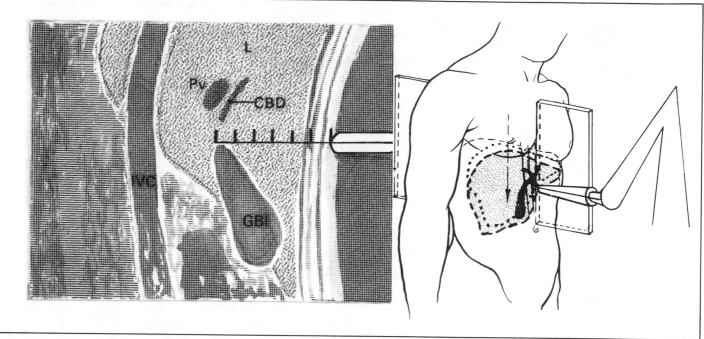

FIGURE 8-8. Gravity and redistribution of abdominal organs allow better access to the liver when the patient is upright.

Upright View

With a very small, high liver that provides limited access, the upright position may be helpful. This position allows the liver to fall somewhat and, coupled with inspiration, can bring it within reach of the beam (Fig. 8-8). Ideally, the patient stands, but this is practical only if the patient is relatively healthy. An alternative that is usually satisfactory is to have the patient sit or stand with support. The gallbladder can be visualized at the same time to check for layering of gallstones.

Decubitus View

If the patient is unable to sit up, the decubitus position may induce the liver to fall away from the ribs, which will make it accessible (see Chapter 9).

Pre- and Postprocessing

Pre- and postprocessing are worth using in liver sonograms to bring out subtle differences in texture related to metastases (Fig. 8-9).

Real-Time

Real-time is worth using when looking for liver metastases because sometimes such lesions can be seen better with real-time than with static scanning and vice versa. It is easy to scan the liver comprehensively with real-time but hard to effectively document the findings.

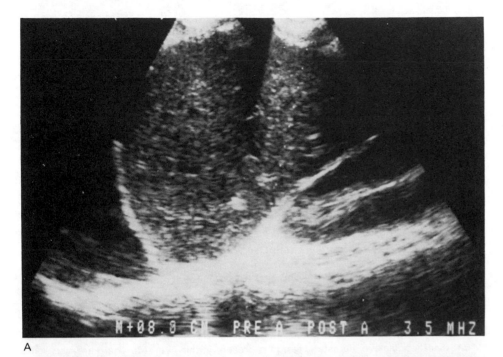

A

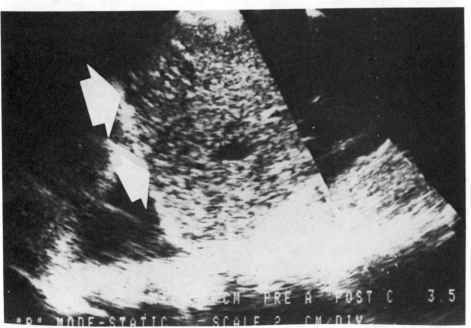

B

FIGURE 8-9. Pre- and post-processing of the echoes will enhance visualization of subtle lesions. This feature is particularly valuable in the liver. A. Two subtle echopenic metastases are poorly seen. B. After post-processing, the lesions are better seen (arrows).

PATHOLOGY

Metastases

Metastases are almost always multiple. Common patterns include the following:

1. *Bulls eye.* An echogenic center with a surrounding echopenic area (Fig. 8-10)
2. *Echopenic.* Less echogenic than the neighboring liver (Fig. 8-10)
3. *Echogenic.* More echogenic than the surrounding liver (this pattern tends to be associated with gastrointestinal carcinoma and may be calcified) (Fig. 8-11)
4. *Cystic.* Rare and impossible to distinguish from a benign cyst
5. *Diffuse.* Numerous echopenic lesions throughout the liver (Fig. 8-12)
6. *Necrotic.* Fluid-filled center with thick irregular walls (Fig. 8-13)

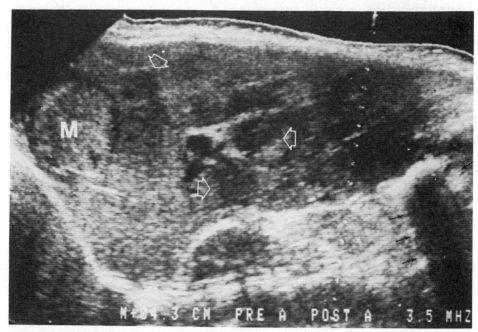

FIGURE 8-10. A bull's eye metastatic lesion is present in this liver (M). There are also some sonolucent metastatic lesions (arrows).

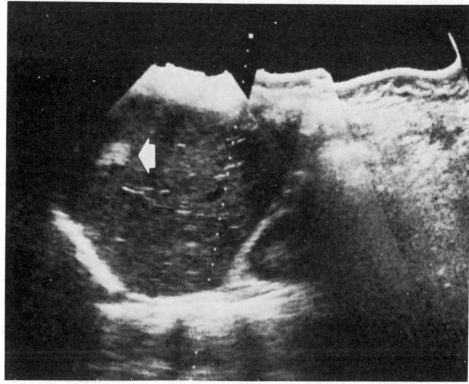

FIGURE 8-11. The echogenic focus is a metastatic lesion (arrow).

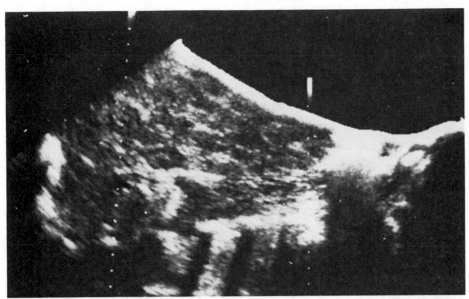

FIGURE 8-12. The entire liver parenchyma is involved with diffuse metastatic lesions.

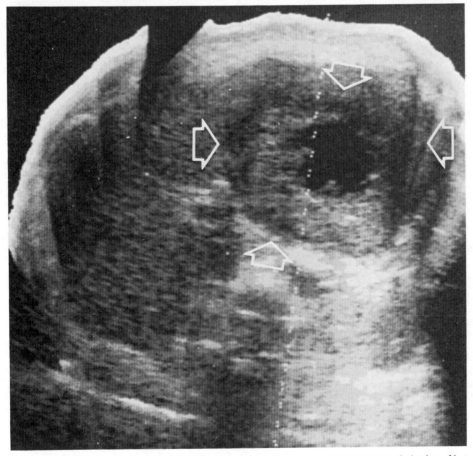

FIGURE 8-13. The large mass in the left lobe of the liver represents a metastatic lesion. Note the large central sonolucent area within the mass (arrows)—an area of necrosis.

Primary Liver Tumors

These are generally single lesions and may be echogenic or echopenic. Hemangiomas tend to be echogenic. A single small echogenic lesion in an asymptomatic patient is probably a hemangioma.

Cysts

Liver cysts are rather common and may be multiple. They usually have no internal echoes and show good through transmission. They usually have smooth borders but not always. Septa may be seen within. They usually have a thin echogenic wall.

Abscesses

Abscesses usually have an echopenic center with good through transmission and a slightly thickened wall; there may be internal echoes within. Amebic abscesses may be densely echogenic. Abscesses around the liver in subhepatic or subphrenic spaces are common, particularly in postoperative patients (see Chapter 12). Necrotic liver tumors also have fluid-filled centers and may be confused with abscesses, but they generally have thicker walls (Fig. 8-13).

Echinococcal (Hydatid) Cysts

These cysts, caused by a parasite, are generally fluid-filled; they consist of smaller cysts within a larger cyst. The walls of the daughter cyst appear as septa (Fig. 8-14). Echogenic areas may be present within hydatid cysts. Calcification within a "burnt-out" hydatid cyst is common.

Hematomas

Usually post-traumatic, hematomas appear as lesions that either contain low-level echoes or are echo-free. They usually have rather poor through transmission.

Polycystic Disease

Appearances are similar to those seen with polycystic kidney disease. The liver is enlarged, and there are multiple cysts of varying size and shape throughout the liver (Fig. 8-15).

Schistosomiasis

The echogenic zone around the portal veins is more pronounced owing to fibrosis.

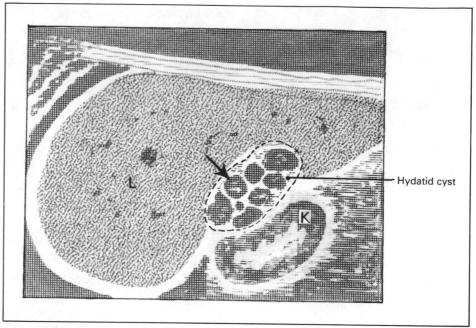

FIGURE 8-14. Longitudinal scan. A hydatid cyst, containing several daughter cysts, lies at the inferior aspect of the liver and displaces the kidney and its surrounding fat line posteriorly.

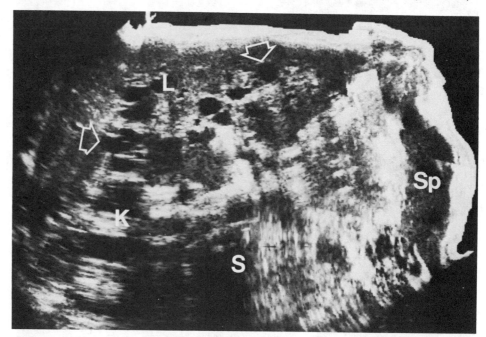

FIGURE 8-15. Transverse scan. Polycystic liver and kidneys are present. Note the numerous cysts within the liver and kidneys (arrows). The distinction between the two organs is difficult because of distortion of the anatomy caused by multiple cysts.

PITFALLS

Normal structures can mimic metastases.

1. *Perinephric fat.* A transverse section or right costal margin view may show perinephric fat without showing the kidney. This fat is usually echogenic but may be echopenic and may appear to be intrahepatic. A longitudinal section through the lesion will show it to be perirenal fat (Fig. 8-16).
2. *Ligamentum teres.* This remnant of the fetal umbilical vein is a fibrous structure surrounded by fat. It appears as an echogenic lesion in the left lobe of the liver (Fig. 8-17).

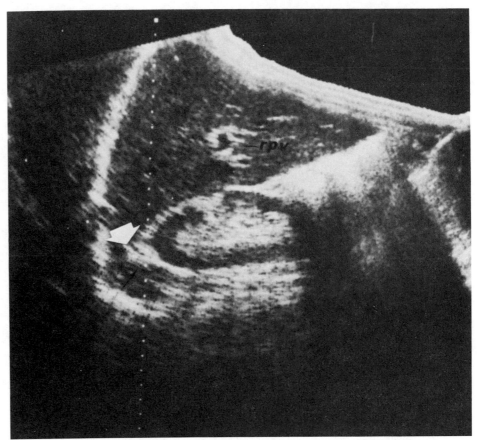

FIGURE 8-16. Worrisome echogenic focus (arrow), apparently in the liver. It actually represents perinephric fat.

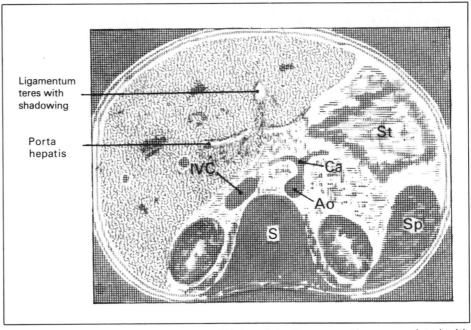

FIGURE 8-17. An echogenic focus in the left lobe of the liver, sometimes associated with acoustic shadowing, represents the ligamentum teres—a normal variant and remnant of the fetal umbilical vein.

3. *Dilated hepatic veins versus cysts.* On longitudinal scans cystic structures with poorly defined walls in the right lobe of the liver may represent hepatic veins. Real-time will show variations in size with inspiration. A transverse view will show that the apparent cyst is a tubular structure draining into the inferior vena cava. Enlarged hepatic veins are often associated with congestive failure, in which the size of the inferior vena cava will not vary much between inspiration and expiration (Fig. 8-18A,B).

4. *Fat-free area.* In fatty infiltration of the liver, the overall liver parenchyma is more echogenic than it should be by comparison with the kidney (See Chapter 11). There may be patchy areas free of fat that are less echogenic and can be mistaken for metastases. The only definite way to tell the difference between a metastatic lesion and a fat-free area is by means of a CT scan.

5. *Diaphragmatic leaflet.* The diaphragm may appear to be double in certain segments owing to its insertion into the ribs.

6. *Hypoechoic caudate and left lobes.* Owing to absorption and attenuation by fissures or the left portal vein, the caudate lobe and the posterior aspect of the left lobe of the liver may be less echogenic than the rest of the liver; this appearance is a normal variant.

7. *Gut versus metastasis.* Portions of the gut may lie between the liver and the diaphragm, causing acoustic shadowing. These bowel loops may be confused with metastatic lesions if careless scanning techniques are used.

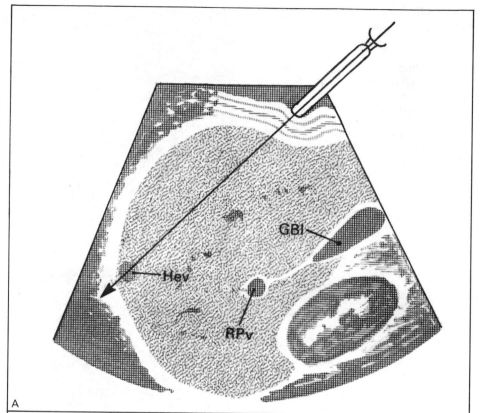

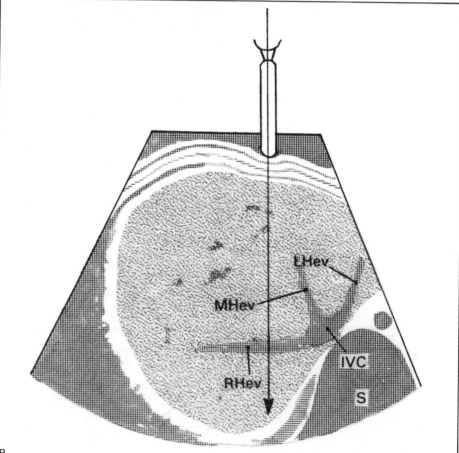

FIGURE 8-18. Dilated hepatic veins. A sonolucent structure in A, close to the diaphragm within the liver, may not represent a cyst. A transverse view, B, shows that this structure actually represents a dilated right hepatic vein.

WHERE ELSE TO LOOK

1. If echogenic metastatic lesions are seen, look throughout the bowel for a target lesion that suggests carcinoma of the colon or stomach (see Chapter 15).
2. If polycystic liver disease is seen, examine the kidneys, which are certain to show signs of the disease. Also examine the pancreas and spleen, which occasionally have cysts with polycystic liver disease.
3. If a malignancy or a metastatic lesion is found, the rest of the patient's abdomen should be surveyed for evidence of adenopathy or ascites.

SELECTED READING

Cosgrove, D. O., and McCready, V. R. (Eds.). *Ultrasound Imaging: Liver, Spleen, Pancreas.* Toronto: Wiley, 1982.

Kane, R. A. Sonographic anatomy of the liver. *Semin. Ultrasound* 2:190, 1981.

Marks, W. M., Filly, R. A., and Callen, P. W. Ultrasonic anatomy of the liver: A review with new applications. *J. Clin. Ultrasound* 7:137, 1979.

Mayes, G. B., and Bernardino, M. E. The role of ultrasound in the evaluation of hepatic neoplasms. *Semin. Ultrasound* 2:212–218, 1981.

Parulekar, S. G. Ligaments and fissures of the liver: Sonographic anatomy. *Radiology* 130:409–411, 1979.

Sarti, D. A., and Sample, W. F. (Eds.). *Diagnostic Ultrasound Text and Cases.* Boston: Hall, 1980.

Viscomi, G. N., Gonzalez, R., and Taylor, K. J. W. Histopathological correlation of ultrasound appearances of liver metastases. *J. Clin. Gastroenterol.* 3:395–400, 1981.

9. RIGHT UPPER QUADRANT MASS

NANCY A. SMITH
ROGER C. SANDERS

SONOGRAM ABBREVIATIONS

Ao   Aorta

Bl   Bladder

Ca   Celiac artery
CD   Common duct

GBl   Gallbladder

Hea   Hepatic artery

IMv   Inferior mesenteric vein
Ip   Iliopsoas muscle
IVC   Inferior vena cava

K   Kidney

L   Liver
LPuv   Left pulmonary vein

Pv   Portal vein

RPuv   Right pulmonary vein

S   Spine
SMa   Superior mesenteric artery
SMv   Superior mesenteric vein
Spa   Splenic artery
Spv   Splenic vein

KEY WORDS

Adenopathy. Multiple enlarged lymph nodes.

Budd-Chiari Syndrome. Thrombosis of the hepatic veins. Associated with ascites and liver failure.

Courvoisier's Law. See Chapter 11, Key Words.

Riedel's Lobe. Change in shape that occurs when the right lobe of the liver is longer than usual but the left is smaller—a normal variant.

THE CLINICAL PROBLEM

When a mass is felt in the right upper quadrant (RUQ), it is most often caused by an enlarged liver. Depending on the cause of hepatomegaly, the liver may take on various shapes or become hard and therefore easily palpable.

Lesions arising in the following organs may be responsible for a right upper quadrant mass—liver, mesenteric nodes, gallbladder, right kidney, adrenal, pancreas, gastrointestinal tract, abdominal wall, and retroperitoneal tissues. Even if a primary neoplasm cannot be seen, metastatic deposits in the liver or adrenals may grow to such an extent that they can be felt. Malignancies may be accompanied by ascites or enlarged nodes.

ANATOMY

The major structure in the right upper quadrant is the liver. This more or less triangular organ hugs the right diaphragm. The gallbladder hangs on its inferior aspect, and the right kidney lies to the right posteriorly (see Fig. 8-1). The porta hepatis (a fibrous structure containing the hepatic artery, portal vein, and common bile duct) enters the liver from its inferior aspect close to the midline. Adjacent to the porta hepatis are the duodenum, gallbladder, and head of the pancreas. The inferior vena cava runs through the posterior aspect of the center of the liver. The aorta lies just to the left of the midline behind the left lobe of the liver.

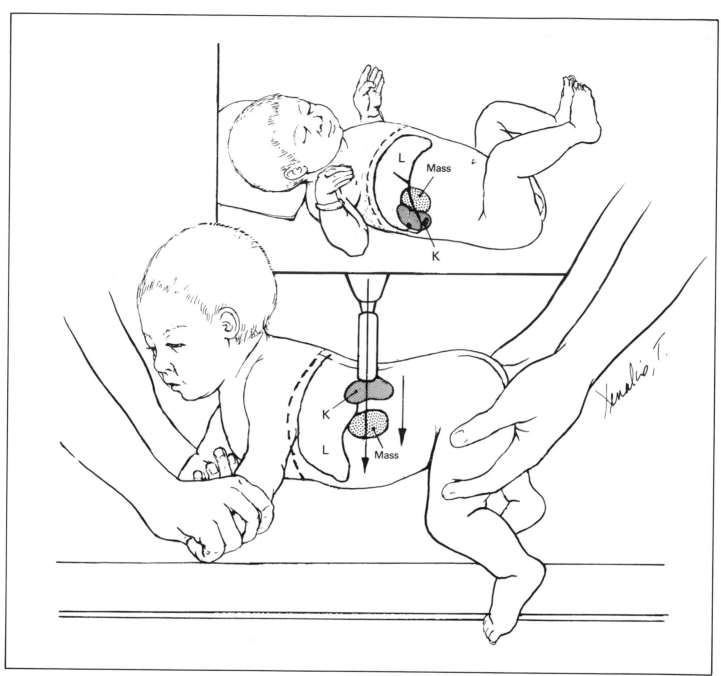

FIGURE 9-1. Diagram showing the sling position that can be used with infants and small children for assessment of a mass. The infant is held in the air by two assistants while scanning is performed. This position will cause a mass to drop away from an adjacent organ.

TECHNIQUE

1. Palpate the apparent mass and perform a scan in the fashion already described in Chapter 8 to determine the organ of origin. Use real-time plus palpation to decide on the anatomic relationship between the mass and the neighboring organs. Document your findings with static scans, because the mass will probably be too large for the field of view of a real-time system.

2. It may not be apparent whether a mass involves the liver. Placing the patient in an upright position and attempting to see between the mass and the liver with real-time may be helpful in deciding whether the mass is of hepatic origin. A decubitus view may help in patients who cannot stand. In such a position the mass may fall away from the liver and show a good interface, thus establishing an extrahepatic location.

3. In infants a sling position will create space that will allow a mass to fall away from the adjacent organs (Fig. 9-1).

PATHOLOGY

Liver

An abnormal liver is the usual cause of a RUQ mass.

POSITIONAL VARIANTS

The liver may lie in an unduly low position for no apparent reason, or it may be depressed owing to chest pathology.

ENLARGEMENT

The liver is considered enlarged if it measures more than 15 cm in length at a point midway between the spine and the right side of the body (Fig. 9-2). The left lobe does not extend very far across the midline and is usually smaller in patients with a large antero-posterior diameter.

If the organs are in a normal relationship, a simple assessment of liver enlargement can be made by noting whether the inferior aspect of the liver extends below the right kidney. There are many causes of focal masses in the liver, and these are described in detail in Chapter 8.

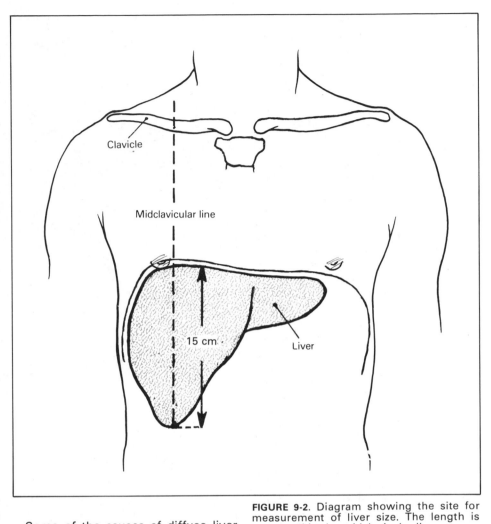

FIGURE 9-2. Diagram showing the site for measurement of liver size. The length is measured in the midclavicular line.

Some of the causes of diffuse liver disease, notably fatty liver and acute hepatitis, can cause hepatomegaly. In such a case there will be a generalized alteration in sonographic appearance (described in Chapter 11). The Budd-Chiari syndrome, which is caused by clot in the hepatic veins or inferior vena cava, is a rare cause of an enlarged and tender liver.

Porta Hepatis Nodes

Nodes can cause a RUQ mass, particularly when they are clustered in the porta hepatis. Typically, they are not limited to the porta hepatis but surround and straighten the celiac axis and the superior mesenteric artery. If nodes are caused by lymphoma, they are generally echo-free.

Gallbladder

If the cystic duct or common duct is obstructed, the gallbladder may become so enlarged that it is palpable. A right upper quadrant mass coupled with jaundice and absence of pain is known as Courvoisier's sign; it indicates obstruction of the common duct, usually caused by carcinoma of the pancreas.

Gastrointestinal Tumors

Mesenteric masses such as carcinoma of the colon or stomach may lie immediately adjacent to the liver but feel as if they are of hepatic origin. The typical appearance of a gastrointestinal mass with an echogenic center and an echo-free rim is described in Chapter 15.

Pancreatic Pseudocyst

Pancreatic pseudocysts can originate in most areas of the abdomen and may migrate to the RUQ (see Chapter 7).

Renal Masses

Very large renal tumors or severe hydronephrosis may appear as RUQ masses. Only their size differentiates them from other nonpalpable renal tumors (see Chapter 17).

Adrenal Gland

A mass located above the right kidney may arise from the liver, adrenal, or retroperitoneal tissue. A fat line separates the retroperitoneum from the peritoneum (Fig. 9-3A,B). This line is displaced posteriorly by intraperitoneal masses such as hepatic lesions and anteriorly by masses originating in the retroperitoneum.

Any right upper quadrant mass of questionable origin necessitates a search for a normal separate adrenal gland to prove that the adrenal is not involved (see Chapter 32).

Abdominal Wall

Make sure that the mass is not in the abdominal wall. Occasionally lipomas and other superficial masses can be mistaken for intra-abdominal structures.

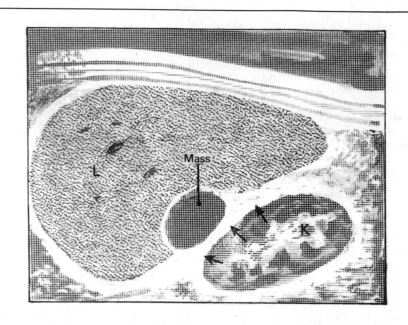

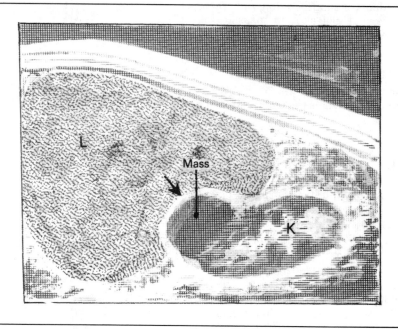

FIGURE 9-3. The retroperitoneal fat line anterior to the kidney and posterior to the liver (arrows) shows whether a mass is intra- or retroperitoneal. The line is displaced posteriorly, A, by intraperitoneal lesions, and anteriorly, B, by retroperitoneal masses.

PITFALLS

1. The *axis of the right kidney* is variable and occasionally the lower pole may be tilted anteriorly, making it palpable even though there is no mass present (Fig. 9-4).

2. *Riedel's lobe* is a normal variant of liver shape in which an unusually large right lobe of the liver causes a false impression of hepatomegaly (Fig. 9-5); however, the left lobe is very small.

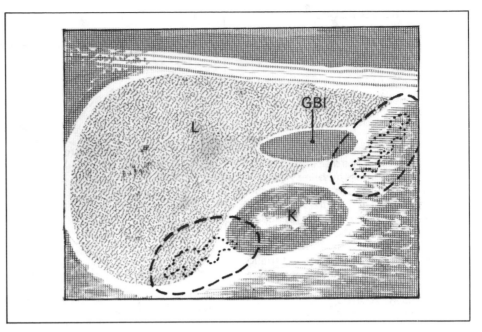

FIGURE 9-4. A kidney with a lower pole tilted forward may be palpable and may be clinically mistaken for a pathologic mass.

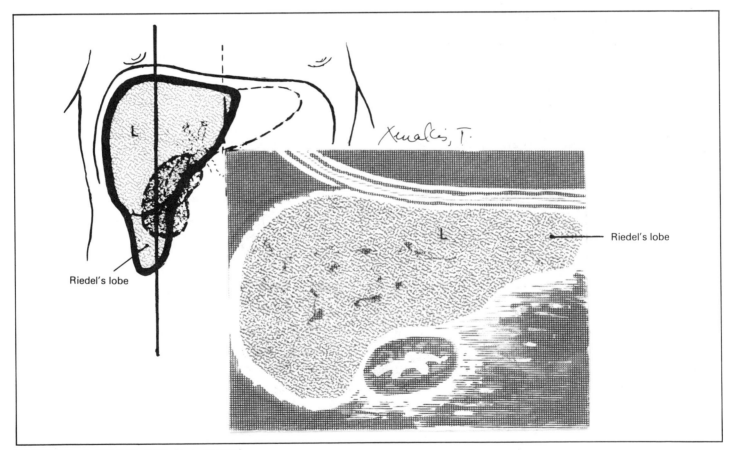

FIGURE 9-5. A Riedel's lobe is a normal variant in which the right lobe of the liver is larger and the left lobe is smaller than usual. The overall liver size is within normal limits.

WHERE ELSE TO LOOK

1. The discovery of a solid mass in the RUQ should prompt a search for metastatic lesions in the rest of the abdomen.

2. If the mass turns out to be a dilated hydronephrotic kidney, try to identify the cause of the obstruction in the pelvis or along the course of the ureter (Fig. 9-6).

3. If the mass is a greatly dilated gallbladder, look for the site and nature of the obstruction of the biliary tree. Be sure to evaluate the pancreatic head.

4. If the liver is abnormal in texture, look for splenomegaly and evidence of portal hypertension.

5. If mesenteric nodes are found, look for splenomegaly and evidence of malignancy in other areas of the abdomen.

SELECTED READING

Gore, R. M., Callen, P. W., and Filly, R. A. Displaced retroperitoneal fat: Sonographic guide to right upper quadrant mass localization. *Radiology* 142:701–705, 1982.

Gosink, B. B. and Leymaster, C. E. Ultrasonic determination of hepatomegaly. *J. Clin. Ultrasound* 9:37–41, 1981.

Harvey, A. M. et al. *The Principles and Practice of Medicine* (20th ed.). New York: Appleton-Century-Crofts, 1976.

Kurtz, A. B., Rubin, C. S., and Goldberg, B. B. Ultrasound and computed tomography of the liver. *CRC Crit. Rev. Radiol.* 18:279–317, 1982.

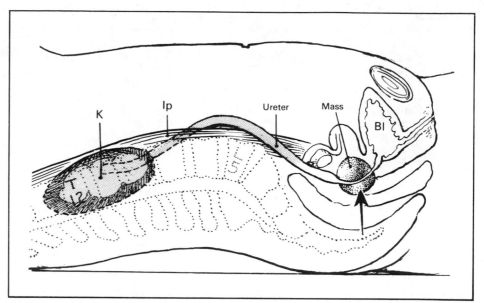

FIGURE 9-6. If the kidney is obstructed, look along the course of the ureter to detect the cause of obstruction, for example, a pelvic mass.

10. RIGHT UPPER QUADRANT PAIN

NANCY A. SMITH

SONOGRAM ABBREVIATIONS

Ao Aorta

GBl Gallbladder

IVC Inferior vena cava

K Kidney

L Liver

RPv Right portal vein

S Spine

KEY WORDS

Acute Abdomen. Sudden onset of abdominal pain. Causes include appendicitis, perforated peptic ulcer, strangulated hernia, acute cholecystitis, pancreatitis, and renal colic.

Adenomyomatosis. Condition causing right upper quadrant pain in which small polypoid masses arise from the gallbladder wall.

Cholangitis. Inflammation of a bile duct.

Cholecystitis. Inflammation of the gallbladder. *Acute*—usually caused by gallbladder outlet obstruction. *Chronic*—inflammation persisting over a longer period.

Choledochojejunostomy. Surgical procedure in which the bile duct is anastomosed to jejunum; food and air may reflux into the bile ducts.

Choledocholithiasis. Gallstone in a bile duct.

Cholelithiasis. Gallstones in the gallbladder or biliary tree.

Cholesterosis. Variant of adenomyomatosis in which cholesterol polyps arise from the gallbladder wall.

Hartmann's Pouch. Portion of the gallbladder that lies nearest the cystic duct where stones often collect.

Phrygian Cap. Variant gallbladder shape in which the fundus of the gallbladder is tilted and has a partial septum.

Roux-en-Y Procedure. Anastomosis of the common bile duct to the jejunum with consequent reflux of air into the biliary system.

Sphincterotomy. Procedure in which the sphincter of Oddi is widened surgically. Gas will reflux into the bile ducts.

THE CLINICAL PROBLEM

Right upper quadrant pain, either chronic or acute, may be caused by disease in the gallbladder, liver, porta hepatis, pancreas, right kidney, adrenal, lung, or diaphragmatic pleura. Differential diagnosis is sometimes difficult and often requires the use of many modalities, including the history and physical examination, laboratory tests, diagnostic radiology, and ultrasound. Important physical signs and symptoms include the presence or absence of jaundice, acute pain, fever, and vomiting, among others.

Because of the proximity of the gallbladder and pancreas to the right hemidiaphragm, patients with cholecystitis and pancreatitis sometimes experience referred pain in the right shoulder area. Pain may be referred into the right upper quadrant (RUQ) from inflammation of the diaphragmatic pleura. However, the finding of an unsuspected pleural effusion by sonography may shift the focus of the work-up to the chest. Pyelonephritis and renal stones as well as liver tumor or abscess may present as RUQ pain (see Chapter 18).

When RUQ pain is acute, rapid and accurate diagnosis on an emergency basis may be crucial. Many of the internal disasters that precipitate an acute abdomen, such as acute cholecystitis, renal colic, and secondary hydronephrosis and pancreatitis, are readily detectable sonographically. However, others, such as ruptured appendix and perforated ulcer, are not.

ANATOMY
Gallbladder

The gallbladder is situated on the inferior aspect of the liver, medial and anterior to the kidney and lateral and anterior to the inferior vena cava. It is more or less ovoid in shape and varies in size. The gallbladder may contain a kink, known as the junctional fold, close to the neck. It is divided into the fundus (the distal tip area), the body, and the neck (Hartmann's pouch is the area nearest the cystic duct). An echogenic line, the main lobar fissure (see Fig. 10-7A), leads from the gallbladder to the bifurcation of the right portal vein. This is a sonographic landmark for the gallbladder.

TECHNIQUE
Patient Preparation

Gallbladder studies should be performed when the patient is fasting. Water, which does not make the gallbladder contract, is permitted.

Supine Position

The gallbladder is first examined with the patient in a supine position using a real-time system such as a mechanical sector scanner. Real-time is preferable to static scanning because a more rapid and complete survey is possible. Try to obtain a long axis view by varying the obliquity of the transducer until the maximum length of the gallbladder is seen.

Right Side Up Decubitus Position

It is mandatory to obtain views in the decubitus (right side up), or erect position because stones may be missed if only supine views are obtained. The right side up decubitus position allows the liver to act as an acoustic window for visualization of the gallbladder. Additional techniques are required to identify gallstones and are described in the next section on pathology.

Local Tenderness

Make an effort to identify the source of local tenderness. Such information is very helpful to the sonologist and the clinician.

PATHOLOGY
Gallstones

Gallstones are seen with acute and chronic cholecystitis but may be found in symptom-free patients as well. They may have six different sonographic appearances.

GALLSTONE WITH SHADOWING

See Figure 10-1A. A stone surrounded by bile appears as a dense echogenic structure within fluid. If a stone is over 2 to 3 mm in size, the density of the stone will absorb and reflect sound, so that a column of acoustic shadowing is seen posterior to the gallstone.

FIGURE 10-1. Acoustic shadowing. A. Acoustic shadowing behind two gallstones. B. Because the stone is small, shadowing is not seen. The stone should not be mistaken for a polyp; it falls into the dependent fundus on the decubitus view.

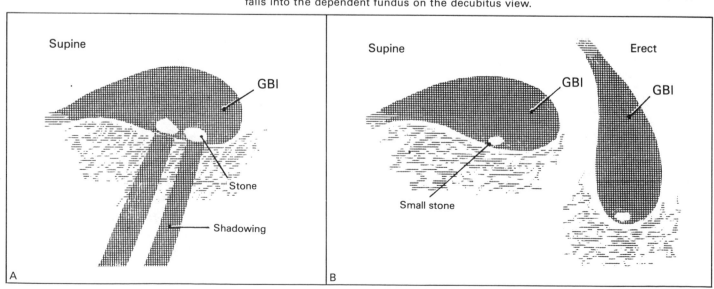

GALLSTONES WITHOUT SHADOWING

See Figure 10-1B. Small stones may not be associated with acoustic shadowing using standard transducers. If an echogenic focus (a possible stone) can be shown to move when the patient is repositioned, for example, in the left lateral decubitus or erect position, the lesion is probably a stone; if the focus does not move, the echoes probably represent a polyp or a septum.

GRAVEL

If there are many small stones present, they will layer out in the most dependent portion of the gallbladder. It is impossible to discern each separate stone; an irregular pattern of echoes is displayed along the posterior aspect of the gallbladder. Shadowing may or may not be seen. Gravel will layer out immediately along the dependent wall of a gallbladder in the decubitus position.

GALLBLADDER FILLED WITH STONES

Sometimes when the gallbladder contains many stones, no echo-free bile can be seen around them. The stones appear as a group of dense echoes with acoustic shadowing located near the liver edge but within the liver on all views. Because this looks suspiciously like a gas-filled duodenum, it can represent a diagnostic problem (Fig. 10-2A,B), and special techniques are required:

1. Make sure another candidate for gallbladder is not visible somewhere else in the abdomen.
2. A change in position may cause stones to settle in the dependent portion of the gallbladder and a thin layer of bile to appear across the top (Fig. 10-2B).

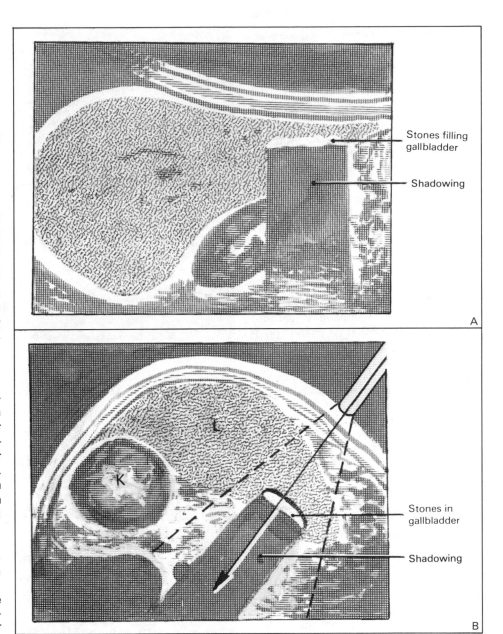

Stones filling gallbladder

Shadowing

Stones in gallbladder

Shadowing

FIGURE 10-2. Acoustic shadowing. A. Clear, well-defined shadowing is evidence that this is a gallbladder full of stones and not gas shadowing from adjacent bowel. The shadowing arises within the liver contour. B. If a gallbladder full of stones is examined on a decubitus view, a thin layer of bile may appear to support the diagnosis of gallstones.

3. Have the patient drink water; peristalsis will be seen if the suspect area is duodenum.

4. Evaluate the acoustic shadow. Air causes shadowing that has a less well defined pattern than dense stones (Fig. 10-3). The borders of a shadowed area caused by stones are generally sharper and more clearly outlined than those caused by gas.

STONES AS A FLUID LEVEL

Occasionally stones float and will be seen as a fluid level within the gallbladder. The stones appear as an echogenic line.

ADHERENT STONES

Small adherent stones may appear as echoes in the gallbladder without shadowing. Those that do change position when the patient is put into the decubitus (right side up) or erect position are proved to be stones. If the echoes do not change position, the possibilities include adherent stones, gallbladder polyps, or a tumor.

Acute Cholecystitis

When a patient has acute RUQ pain and gallstones are found, acute cholecystitis must be considered. Sonographic findings that suggest acute cholecystitis include (1) gallstones and (2) acute pain over the gallbladder. If the patient's most tender area turns out to be exactly where the gallbladder is located, this information should be noted because it is clinically valuable. Pain may be the only finding suggestive of cholecystitis because this condition is not always accompanied by gallstones. Checking to see if a patient has local tenderness over the gallbladder should be part of a routine gallbladder or RUQ pain examination. If the gallbladder is palpable, it is usually obstructed.

WALL THICKENING

A rim of decreased echogenicity caused by gallbladder wall thickening (Fig. 10-4) may be present. This finding is not specific for acute cholecystitis. The "wall" should not be more than 3 mm thick.

PERIGALLBLADDER FLUID COLLECTION

Discrete fluid collections, which represent small abscesses, may be seen around the gallbladder. This is the most definitive evidence of acute cholecystitis.

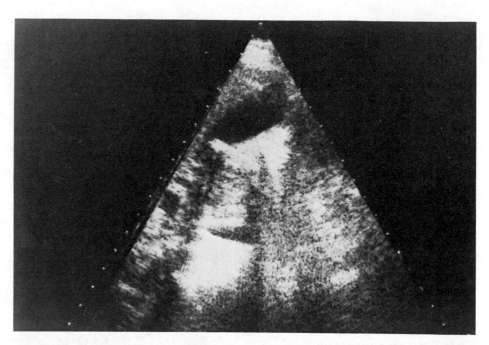

FIGURE 10-3. Sector scan of the gallbladder. An apparent echogenic lesion at the posterior aspect of the gallbladder suggests stones, but the shadowing is actually due to gas. Visualization of the gallbladder at a different phase of respiration showed that the lesion suggesting stones moved in relation to the gallbladder.

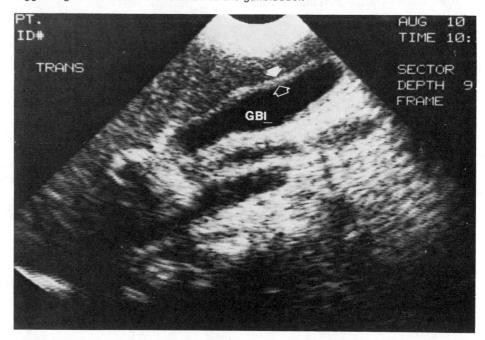

FIGURE 10-4. A thickened gallbladder wall (arrows), especially if it is accompanied by local tenderness, can indicate acute cholecystitis.

GAS IN THE GALLBLADDER

With "emphysematous" cholecystitis the gallbladder is filled with gas, which casts an acoustic shadow. The appearances are not dissimilar from those of a gallbladder filled with many stones, although the gas shadow will not be quite so "clean." The gallbladder will be acutely tender.

Intra- and Perihepatic Fluid Collections

Abscesses should be sought within the liver, in the right subhepatic space and under the diaphragm. They will generally be sonolucent with irregular borders, but internal echoes may occur. A collection of fluid on either side of the diaphragm is an important finding and should be easily shown on longitudinal scans through the liver. A pleural effusion appears as an echo-free, wedge-shaped area superior to the diaphragm (Fig. 10-5) on a longitudinal view. Trans-

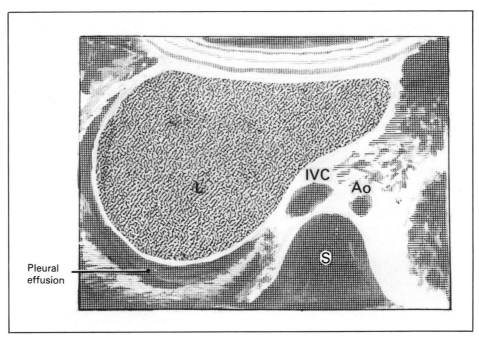

FIGURE 10-5. A transverse scan above the xiphoid shows a collection of pleural fluid above the diaphragm.

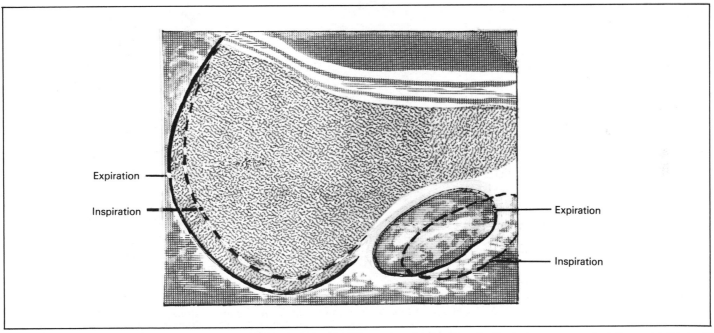

FIGURE 10-6. Inspiration and expiration longitudinal views exposed at the same time will demonstrate diaphragmatic movement.

versely there is an echo-free rim behind the diaphragm.

A subdiaphragmatic collection, which may be less well defined, is an area of decreased echogenicity inferior to the diaphragm. Real-time or superimposed inspiration-expiration static views can help evaluate the fluid collection's effect on the diaphragm, which may be immobilized by an abscess (Fig. 10-6).

Pyelonephritis

The tenderness may be localized to the kidney. The kidney itself can look normal even when acute inflammation (pyelonephritis) is present. There may be a focal swollen, relatively echopenic area of the kidney that represents an area of acute pyelonephritis. Renal calculi may be seen with hydronephrosis and can be the cause of right upper quadrant pain (see Chapter 17).

Pancreatitis

Although the patient complains of right-sided pain, the tenderness may be caused by pancreatitis. The pancreas will be swollen and more sonolucent than normal if pancreatitis is acute (see Chapter 7).

Adenomyomatosis and Carcinoma of the Gallbladder

These rare conditions cause the formation of echoes within the gallbladder and wall thickening. Carcinoma of the gallbladder is usually associated with gallstones. The whole gallbladder may be filled with echoes if gallbladder carcinoma is present.

PITFALLS

Artifact Versus Stone

Echogenic areas adjacent to the anterior wall of the gallbladder may be due to reverberation, and near the posterior wall of the gallbladder they may be due to the partial volume effect (see Chapter 17). To diminish these artifacts

1. Use a transducer with the correct focal zone frequency. A short focus, high frequency is usually correct.
2. A decubitus or erect view may increase the distance between the gallbladder and the transducer. This will eliminate near-field reverberation artifacts (Fig. 10-7).
3. Lowering the overall gain may decrease echogenicity, producing an artifact-free gallbladder. Remember that a good setting for viewing the gallbladder may not be appropriate for imaging other soft tissue organs.

Apparently Absent Gallbladder

When the gallbladder is small, it can be missed entirely. The main lobar fissure begins at the right portal vein bifurcation and runs directly to the gallbladder fossa, serving as a guide.

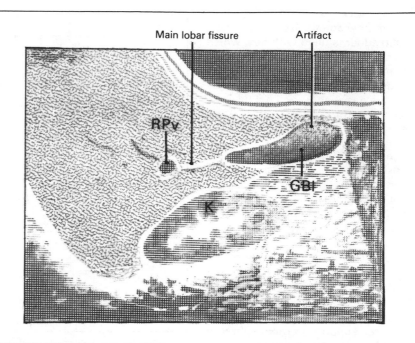

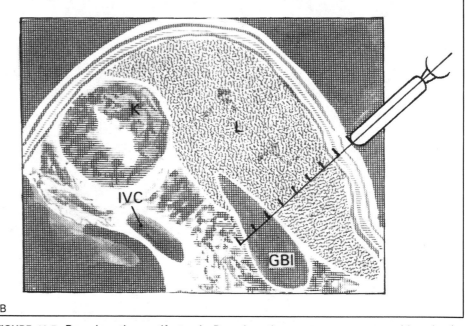

FIGURE 10-7. Reverberation artifacts. A. Reverberations are a common problem in the anterior aspect of the gallbladder (artifact). This gallbladder is easily located by following the main lobar fissure from the right portal vein to the gallbladder fossa. B. Increasing the gallbladder's distance from the transducer by turning the patient into a decubitus position will move the gallbladder wall into the focal zone of the transducer.

Polyp Versus Nonshadowing Stone

Acoustic shadowing can be enhanced by using a high frequency transducer, which places the stone in the correct focal zone. Overgaining can obscure shadowing.

Gallbladder Wall Thickening

Although wall thickening is suggestive of acute cholecystitis, other possible causes include (1) a recent meal, which causes subsequent gallbladder contraction, (2) ascites (Fig. 10-8), (3) hypoalbuminemia, (4) hepatitis, and (5) some chemotherapeutic drugs.

Food in the Gallbladder

Following a choledochojejunostomy or sphincterotomy, a communication between the gallbladder and the gut is created surgically, making it possible for food or gas to reflux into the gallbladder. There may even be acoustic shadowing owing to gas in the gallbladder or biliary tree.

Kink or Septum in the Gallbladder

Gallbladders often fold over on themselves or contain a septum, usually in the region where the neck and body meet (the junctional fold). If only a portion of the septum is seen on a single cut, it can resemble a gallstone or polyp in the dependent portion of the gallbladder (Fig. 10-9). A decubitus or erect view can straighten out a folded gallbladder and turn a suspected stone into a kink.

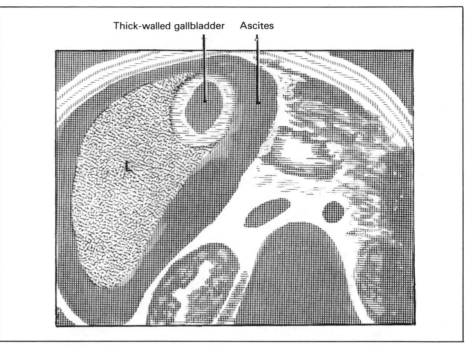

FIGURE 10-8. Ascites, even in very small quantities, can cause a thick gallbladder wall.

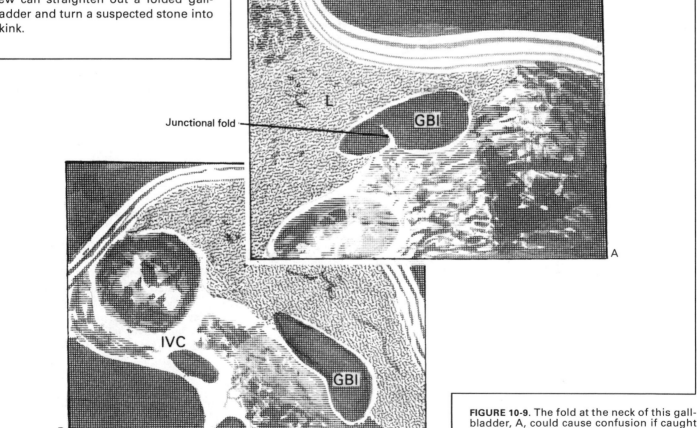

FIGURE 10-9. The fold at the neck of this gallbladder, A, could cause confusion if caught in a plane that demonstrated only a portion of it. The decubitus position, B, allowed the fundus to fall and the kink to straighten out.

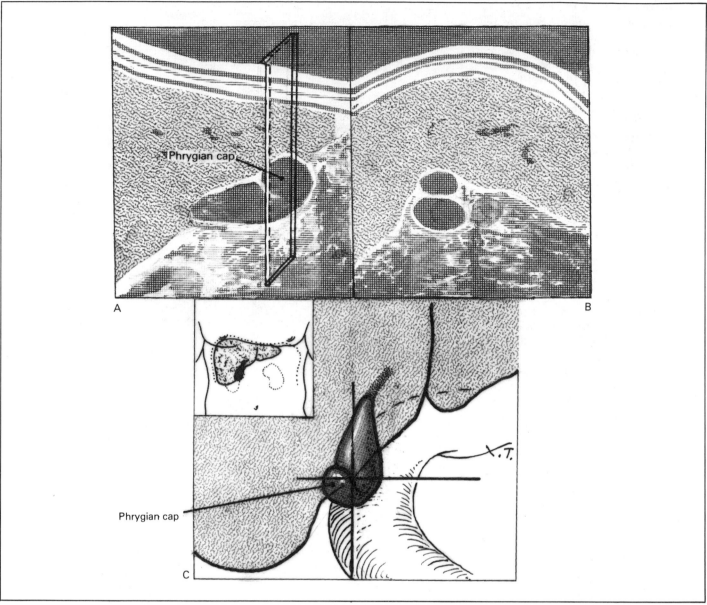

FIGURE 10-10. Phrygian cap deformity. This normal variant can produce a puzzling appearance, especially if scanned in the transverse plane shown in A and B. Long axis views should include the cap (C).

Phrygian Cap

Sometimes a septum develops in the fundus of the gallbladder, forming a "phrygian cap." This is a normal variant (Fig. 10-10).

Viscid Bile (Sludge)

Viscid bile usually causes low-level echoes in the dependent portion of the gallbladder akin to those seen with numerous small stones. The fluid level associated with viscid bile is usually not entirely horizontal. If the patient is placed in the erect or decubitus position, the fluid level takes many minutes to reaccumulate (Fig. 10-11A,B) whereas small stones almost immediately fall into a dependent site. Viscid bile is seen mainly in patients with obstructive jaundice, liver disease, hyperalimentation, or sepsis. A focal area of viscid bile can suggest a polyp or nonshadowing stone.

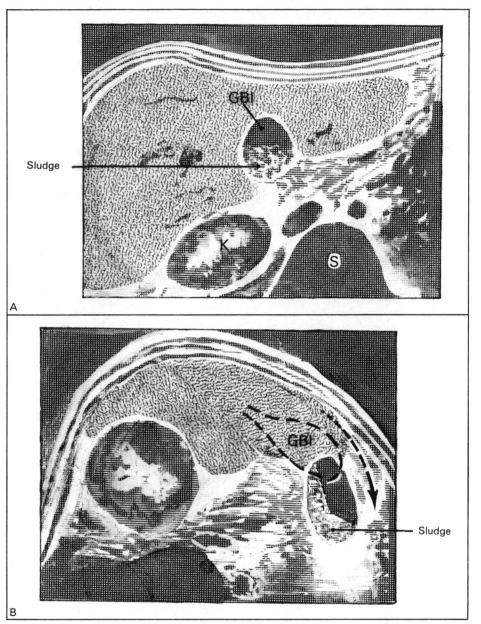

WHERE ELSE TO LOOK

If gallstones are found, look for dilatation of the biliary tree (see Chapter 11).

SELECTED READING

Crade, M. Comparison of Ultrasound and Oral Cholecystogram in the Diagnosis of Gallstones. In K. J. W. Taylor (Ed.), *Diagnostic Ultrasound in Gastrointestinal Disease* (Clinics in Diagnostic Ultrasound, Vol. 1). New York: Churchill Livingstone, 1979.

Rice, J., Sauerbrei, E. E., Semogas, P., et al. Sonographic appearance of adenomyomatosis of the gallbladder. *J. Clin. Ultrasound* 9:336–337, 1981.

Sanders, R. C. The significance of sonographic gallbladder wall thickening. *J. Clin. Ultrasound* 8:143–146, 1980.

Sommer, F. G., and Taylor, K. J. W. Differentiation of acoustic shadowing due to calculi and gas collections. *Radiology* 135:399–403, 1980.

FIGURE 10-11. Presence of sludge. A. Irregular echoes in the posterior aspect of the gallbladder, forming a poorly defined fluid level, suggest the presence of sludge. B. If the patient is placed in a decubitus position, the sludge does not reform a fluid-fluid level for many minutes.

11. JAUNDICE

NANCY A. SMITH
ROGER C. SANDERS

SONOGRAM ABBREVIATIONS

A	Ascites
Ao	Aorta
Ca	Celiac artery
CBD	Common bile duct
CD	Common duct
Co	Cornu
Du	Duodenum
GBl	Gallbladder
H	Heart
Hea	Hepatic artery
IMv	Inferior mesenteric vein
IVC	Inferior vena cava
K	Kidney
L	Liver
LPov	Left portal vein
P	Pancreas
PE	Pleural effusion
Pv	Portal vein
RPov	Right portal vein
S	Spine
SMa	Superior mesenteric artery
SMv	Superior mesenteric vein
Spa	Splenic artery
Spv	Splenic vein

KEY WORDS

Biliary Atresia. Condition in which the bile ducts become narrowed; affects infants a few months old.

Bilirubin. Yellowish pigment in bile formed by red cell breakdown. Causes jaundice if present in increased amounts and is elevated in all types of jaundice. Can be measured in the urine and serum. Direct elevation of bilirubin level is usually caused by obstructive jaundice.

Common Duct. Term used to describe the common hepatic and common bile ducts. Because the cystic duct junction is not seen ultrasonically, this term covers both structures.

Choledochal Cyst. A fusiform dilatation of the common duct that causes obstruction. This condition is usually found in children but may occur in adults also.

Cirrhosis. Diffuse disease of the liver with fibrosis. Causes portal hypertension.

Collaterals. Dilated veins that appear when portal hypertension is present. Seen in the region of the porta hepatis and pancreas.

Courvoisier's Sign. A right upper quadrant mass with painless jaundice implies that there is a carcinomatous mass in the head of the pancreas that is causing biliary duct obstruction. The palpable mass is due to an enlarged gallbladder.

Fatty Infiltration. Diffuse involvement of the liver with fat; associated with alcoholism, obesity, diabetes mellitus, steroid overadministration, jejeunoileal bypass, and malnutrition.

Glisson's Capsule. Layer of fibrous tissue that surrounds the bile ducts, hepatic arteries, and portal veins within the liver as they travel together; also surrounds the liver.

Glycogen Storage Disease. One of a number of congenital diseases in which abnormal materials are deposited within the liver.

Hepatitis. Inflammation of the liver due to viral infection transmitted by fecal-oral (type A) or hematogenous (type B) route. Disease may be acute or may become chronic after an acute episode.

Hepatocellular Disease. Disease affecting the liver parenchyma such as cirrhosis, fatty infiltration, or hepatitis.

Jaundice (Icterus). Yellow pigmentation of the skin due to excessive bilirubin accumulation. The severity of disease is best judged by the appearance of the sclerae (white of the eye).

Klatskin Tumor. A duct cancer at the bifurcation of the right and left hepatic ducts that can cause asymmetrical obstruction of the biliary tree.

Porta Hepatis. Portion of the liver in which the common bile duct, hepatic artery, and portal vein run alongside each other as they leave or enter the liver. Adenopathy often develops here.

Portal Hypertension. Increased portal venous pressure usually due to liver disease (e.g., cirrhosis); leads to dilatation of the portal vein with splenic and superior mesenteric vein enlargement, splenomegaly, and formation of collaterals. The condition can be caused by portal vein thrombosis.

Pruritus. Itching. It may be due to excess bilirubin and is found in patients with obstructive jaundice.

Serum Enzymes. SGOT (serum glutamic oxaloacetic transaminase), SGPT (serum glutamic pyruvic transaminase), LDH (lactic acid dehydrogenase), Alk. Phos. (alkaline phosphatase). These are liver enzymes released from damaged hepatic cells. They are elevated with both obstructed bile ducts and intrinsic liver disease. However, the alkaline phosphatase level is higher in obstruction, whereas the others are higher in intrinsic liver disease.

Sphincterotomy. Surgical procedure in which the common duct entrance into the duodenum is widened at the sphincter of Oddi.

Sphincter of Oddi. Opening of the common bile duct and pancreatic duct into the duodenum.

THE CLINICAL PROBLEM

There are three basic mechanisms by which jaundice occurs.

Red Blood Cell Destruction

Destruction of red blood cells occurs in hemolytic anemias when red cells are destroyed so rapidly that an elevated bilirubin results. The spleen, the principal site of red blood cell removal, may be enlarged.

Hepatocellular Disease

Reduced hepatic cell function leads to a build-up of bilirubin. Alcoholic liver disease is the commonest reason; it progresses from alcoholic hepatitis to fatty liver to cirrhosis. There are many other causes of hepatocellular disease such as congestive failure and infection.

Intrahepatic cholestasis is an arrest of bile excretion at a level above the bile ducts within the cells. It is treated with medical means, not surgery.

Obstruction of Intra- or Extrahepatic Ducts

The ducts dilate proximal to the site of obstruction. Unlike hemolytic anemia or hepatocellular disease, obstruction of the biliary system is treated surgically.

The major bile products whose serum levels are elevated when bile excretion is blocked are urine and serum bilirubin, serum cholesterol, and serum alkaline phosphatase. Biochemical tests for obstruction may be misleading.

Common causes of obstructed bile ducts include gallstones (choledocholithiasis) and tumors in the pancreas and bile ducts, such as Klatskin tumors. In the infant and small child two other important obstructive lesions occur. Biliary atresia, a condition in which the bile ducts narrow, is thought to result from infection. The narrowing occasionally occurs outside the liver, in which case operative anastomosis of the gut to the bile duct helps. In choledochal cyst a fusiform dilatation of the bile duct occurs, and the bile ducts are dilated above the "cyst." This condition may also be seen in older patients and is treated surgically.

ANATOMY

Several tubular structures that lie within the liver must be delineated if biliary obstruction is to be diagnosed (Fig. 11-1).

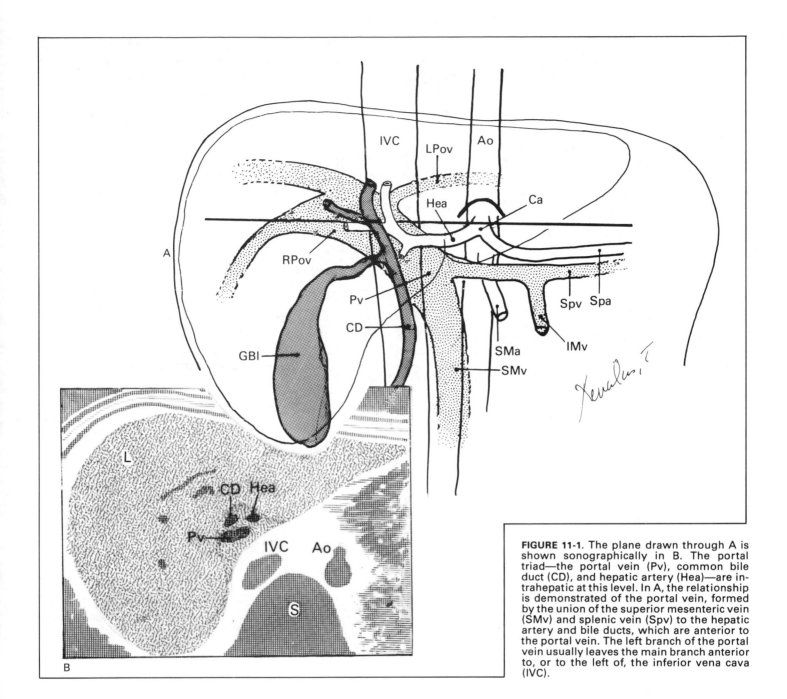

FIGURE 11-1. The plane drawn through A is shown sonographically in B. The portal triad—the portal vein (Pv), common bile duct (CD), and hepatic artery (Hea)—are intrahepatic at this level. In A, the relationship is demonstrated of the portal vein, formed by the union of the superior mesenteric vein (SMv) and splenic vein (Spv) to the hepatic artery and bile ducts, which are anterior to the portal vein. The left branch of the portal vein usually leaves the main branch anterior to, or to the left of, the inferior vena cava (IVC).

Biliary Tree

Normally, one can see only a small segment of the biliary tree within the liver—the common duct, a term used by ultrasonographers to describe the common hepatic duct and the common bile duct. The term *common duct* is a compromise based on the fact that the junction of the cystic duct, the dividing structure, and the common hepatic duct is not visible. Sonographically, the common duct lies just to the right of the hepatic artery, and both run anterior to the portal vein throughout their course in the porta hepatis (Figs. 11-1 and 11-2).

The peripheral biliary tree can occasionally be seen normally outside the porta hepatis area as very thin tubular structures lying anterior to portal veins. The walls of the bile ducts are echogenic, and they branch in a tortuous fashion.

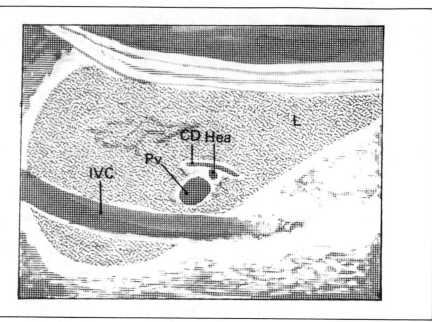

FIGURE 11-2. Supine longitudinal view. The common bile duct (CD) in the region of the porta hepatis lies anterior to the portal vein (Pv).

Portal Veins

The portal vein (Figs. 11-3 and 11-4) has to be distinguished from the common duct. It has echogenic walls and branches toward the diaphragm. The right branch bifurcates superior to the gallbladder. The left branch may appear as a line of echoes in the left lobe of the liver. Smaller branches are rarely seen.

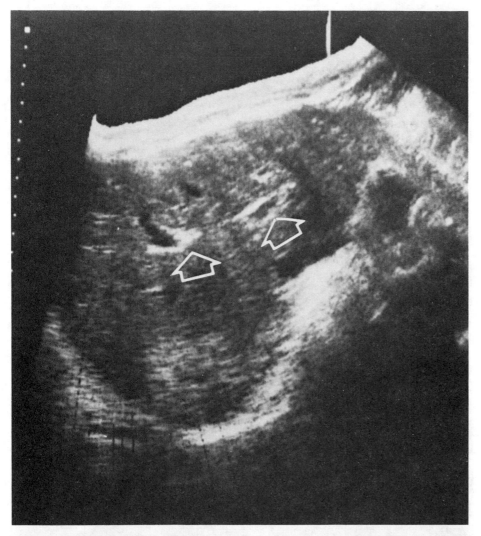

FIGURE 11-3. Right costal margin view showing segments of the portal veins within the liver (arrows). Note the echogenic outlines of the portal veins.

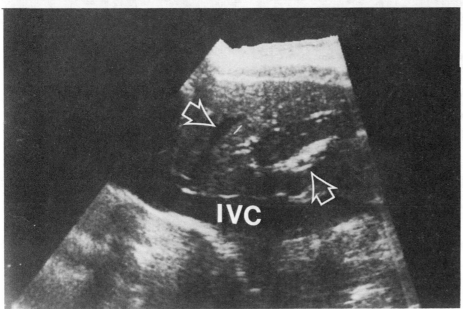

FIGURE 11-4. Longitudinal view showing the inferior vena cava (IVC), the middle hepatic vein (arrow), and the porta hepatis (open arrow).

Hepatic Veins

Hepatic veins (Figs. 11-5 and 11-6) are not often confused with bile ducts. They are not surrounded by an echogenic wall and branch in the direction of the feet. They can be traced to the inferior vena cava.

Hepatic Arteries

Hepatic arteries can be a source of confusion in the region of the porta hepatis, where they may reach 8 mm in diameter. They are pulsatile. The proper hepatic artery lies to the left of the common duct anterior to the portal vein and can be traced to the celiac axis. The right hepatic artery crosses between the common duct and the portal vein (Fig. 11-7). It may double back on itself (Fig. 11-8).

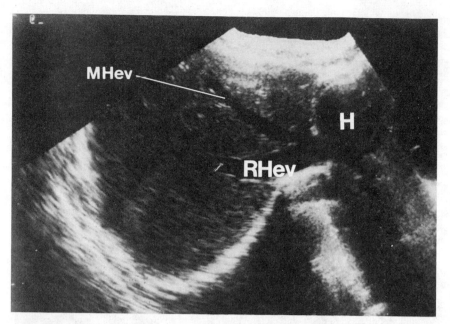

FIGURE 11-5. Right costal margin view showing the right (RHev) and middle hepatic veins (MHev) and the heart (H).

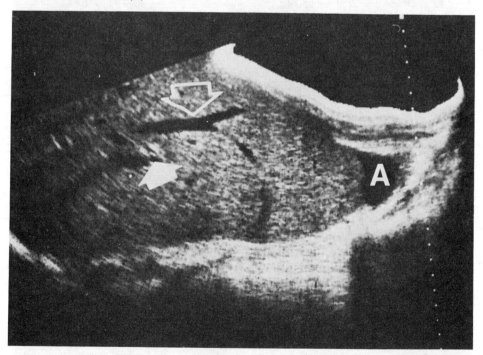

FIGURE 11-6. Longitudinal view showing the middle hepatic veins (open arrows), which bifurcate toward the feet. Note small portion of ascites, A, and the portal vein (arrow).

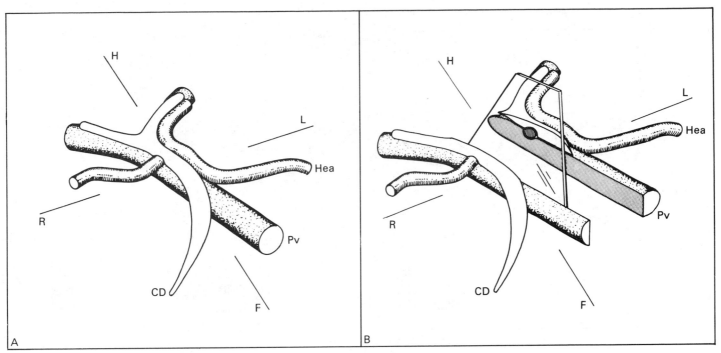

FIGURE 11-7. The relationship of the portal vein (Pv), the hepatic artery (Hea), and the common duct (CD) are demonstrated. Notice that the hepatic artery runs between the common duct and the portal vein and will be seen on a standard section through the porta hepatis. (Reprinted with permission from Berland, L. and Foley, D. Porta hepatis sonography discontinuation of bile ducts from artery with pulsed Doppler anatomic center. *AJR*, 138:833, 1982.)

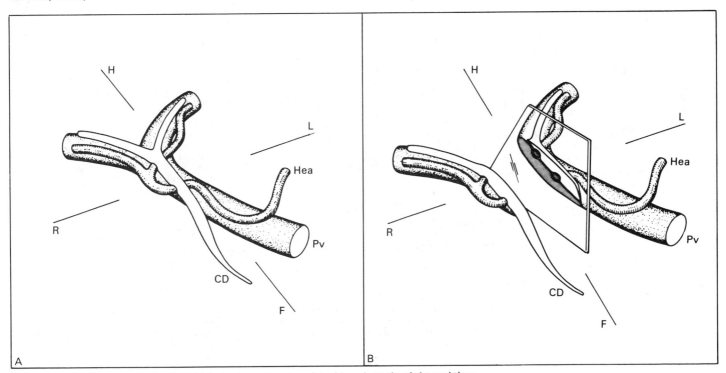

FIGURE 11-8. A variant situation in which the hepatic artery (Hea) bends to the right and then turns back to the left again. (Reprinted with permission from Berland, L. and Foley, D. Porta hepatis sonography discontinuation of bile ducts from artery with pulsed Doppler anatomic center. *AJR*, 138:833, 1982.)

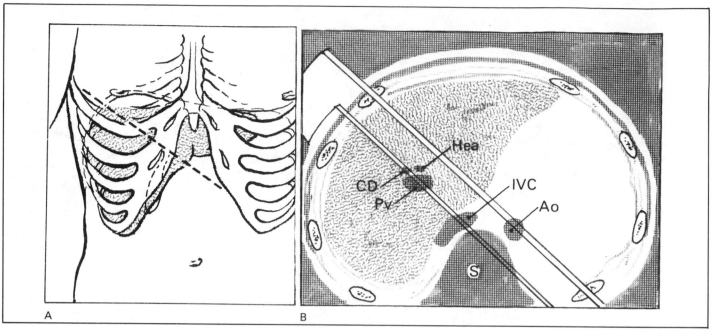

FIGURE 11-9. A,B. The two oblique views required to scan the long axis of the common duct are illustrated here. Not only is the path made oblique from a straight longitudinal plane, the scanning arm is angled in from the patient's side, throwing the ducts and portal vein into the same plane as the inferior vena cava (see also, Fig. 11-16).

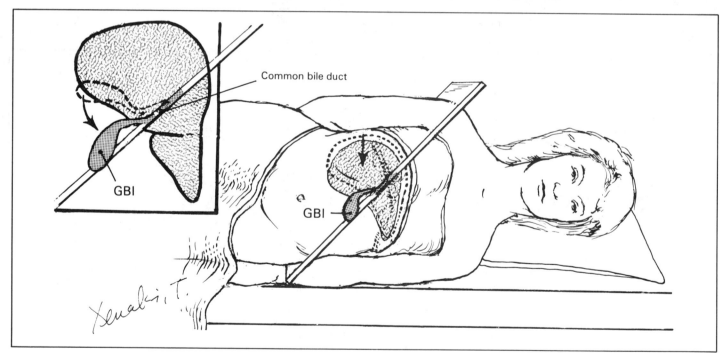

FIGURE 11-10. Appropriate position for obtaining the oblique-oblique view. A right-side-up decubitus allows the liver to fall medially, often providing easier access to the common duct. The gallbladder can be viewed at the same time for layering of stones.

TECHNIQUE

Oblique-Oblique View

The best view for demonstrating the common duct is a longitudinal oblique view with the transducer scanning along a plane perpendicular to the right costal margin and angled medially. This is referred to as an oblique-oblique view (Fig. 11-9). Turning the patient right side up as this oblique section is performed may help, because the liver drops below the costal margin and is more accessible to the transducer (Fig. 11-10).

Peripheral Ducts

Peripherally dilated ducts can be seen on standard transverse and longitudinal views of the liver (Fig. 11-11).

Head of the Pancreas

A transverse view through the head of the pancreas will show whether the common duct is dilated at that level (Fig. 11-12). Real-time longitudinal sections along the duct axis through the head of the pancreas are also important to show the duct at the level at which it is most likely to be obstructed.

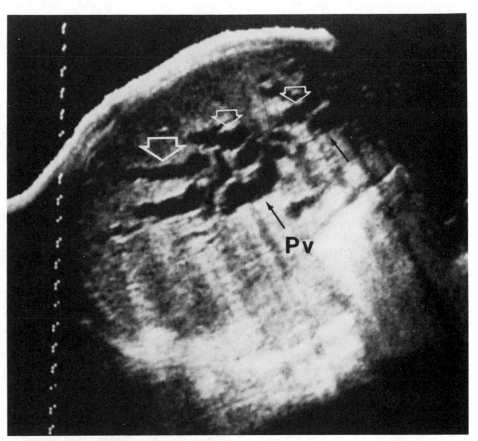

FIGURE 11-11. Peripheral dilated bile ducts are seen (white arrows) anterior to the portal vein (Pv) and branches (black arrows). Note the acoustic enhancement posterior to the ducts.

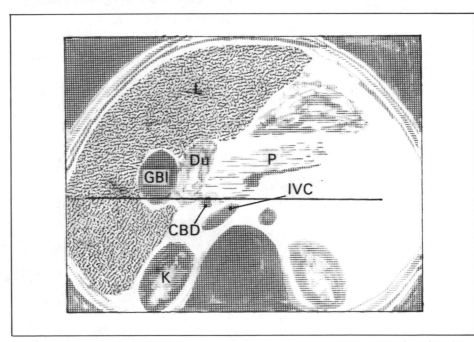

FIGURE 11-12. The transverse plane shown here should be a routine part of performing a jaundice study. The common bile duct (CBD) can be obstructed at this level even if the ducts are normal when seen intrahepatically. Masses occur in the inferior portion of the head of the pancreas, which can be hard to see on long-axis views of the pancreas.

PATHOLOGY

Diffuse Liver Disease

Diffuse parenchymal liver disease has a number of sonographic features, although one can rarely make a specific diagnosis. The following are the most typical patterns.

EARLY ALCOHOLIC LIVER DISEASE

Changes in shape indicate the presence of alcoholic liver disease. A large left lobe or a prominent caudate lobe heralds the development of textural abnormalities.

FATTY INFILTRATION

The liver, particularly the left lobe, will be enlarged with fatty infiltration. It will show a fine stippled echogenicity (Fig. 11-13). Visualization of the right hemidiaphragm (even with a low-frequency transducer) is difficult owing to increased acoustic attenuation. Comparing liver echogenicity to that of the right renal parenchyma helps to assess the degree of fatty infiltration.

ACUTE HEPATITIS

In acute hepatitis the portal vein borders are more prominent than usual. This is said to be a consequence of an overall decreased liver echogenicity.

CIRRHOSIS AND CHRONIC HEPATITIS

Changes similar to those typical of fatty infiltration are seen in these conditions, but the degree of sound attenuation will not be as great and the liver size will not be as large.

END-STAGE CIRRHOSIS

In longstanding cirrhosis the liver is small and very echogenic (Fig. 11-14). It will have a nodular border and may be outlined by ascitic fluid. One portion of the liver may have a different echogenicity from the remainder and form a bulge. This represents a regenerating lobule.

INFILTRATIVE DISORDERS

Glycogen storage disease, for example, causes a diffuse increase in echogenicity throughout the liver and overall liver enlargement.

Hemolytic Anemia

In most types of hemolytic anemia the only sonographic changes are enlargement of the liver and spleen. If hemolytic anemia is caused by lymphoma, there may be nodal enlargement.

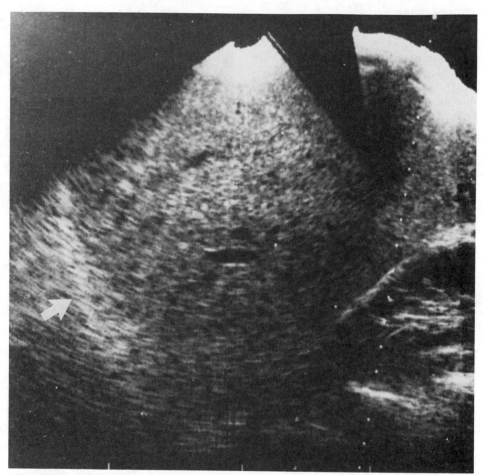

FIGURE 11-13. Fatty liver. The liver is enlarged and has a much coarser echogenic texture than normal and poor acoustic transmission. The diaphragm (arrow) can barely be seen.

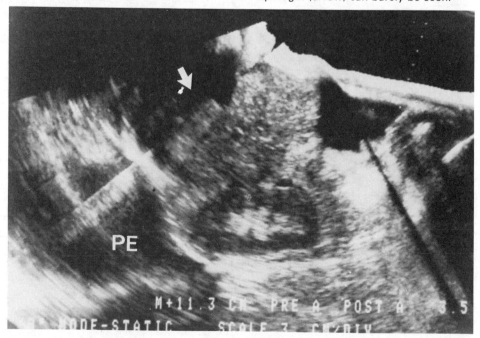

FIGURE 11-14. Cirrhotic liver. The liver is small, has a nobbly margin (arrow) and many increased internal echoes. Note pleural effusion (PE) and ascites surrounding the liver.

Biliary Obstruction

CRITERIA FOR DILATED DUCTS

Recognizing biliary obstruction by ultrasound is a matter of distinguishing the biliary ducts from the portal and hepatic veins and the hepatic arteries, and knowing what constitutes a normal duct size. Biliary ducts

1. Run *anterior* to the *portal veins.*
2. When dilated, a distinctive pattern is created that has been dubbed the *"double barrel shotgun"* or *"parallel channel"* sign (Fig. 11-11). Two tubular structures, the portal vein and the bile duct, are seen next to each other.
3. Unlike portal veins, bile ducts *branch repeatedly,* have irregular walls, and show acoustic enhancement (See Fig. 11-11). Suspicious tubular structures should be traced to their origins with real-time to ensure that they are part of the biliary system and not hepatic arteries.
4. The peripheral branches of the biliary tree, normally not seen, appear as branching tubes throughout the liver running alongside the portal veins (Fig. 11-11).
5. Unlike hepatic veins, bile ducts will not dilate with the Valsalva maneuver.

BILE DUCT MEASUREMENTS

The width of the common duct is usually measured at the point at which it crosses the portal vein in front of the inferior vena cava. If only the lumen of the duct is measured, the upper limit of normal is 6 mm. When measured from leading edge to leading edge, a measurement of up to 6 mm is usually considered normal in a patient who has not had a cholecystectomy (Fig. 11-15).

STONES IN BILE DUCTS

Occasionally stones can be seen in bile ducts. Only about 30% of those actually present are seen ultrasonically. An area of acoustic shadowing with an echogenic source represents a stone. The obstructing stone may not be seen, but other stones in the proximal dilated duct may be visible.

BILE DUCT TUMORS

Rarely, a tumor may be seen within a bile duct (a cholangiocarcinoma). This tumor often causes focal dilatation of a segment of the biliary tree (Fig. 11-16). Such focal dilatation can easily be missed if casual technique is used.

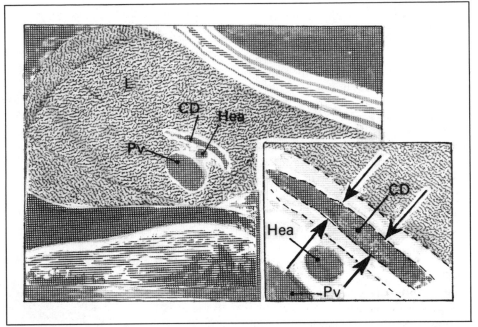

FIGURE 11-15. Oblique-oblique view. The width of the normal lumen of a common duct at this level is generally considered to be 6 mm. If the patient has had a cholecystectomy, the duct may measure up to 1 cm and still be considered nonpathologic. Rule of thumb—the width of the lumen of the duct here should approximate that of the hepatic artery.

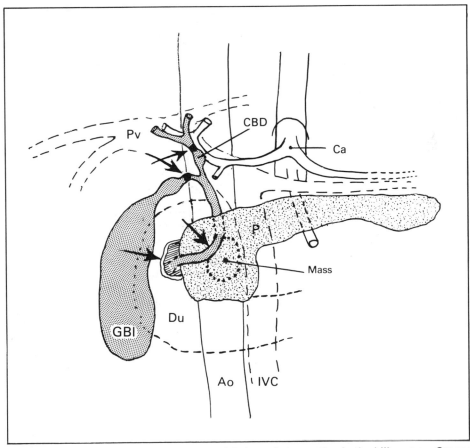

FIGURE 11-16. Arrows indicate some potential sites of obstruction in the biliary tree. Stones may lodge in these sites causing shadows that can be seen if scanned with the correct focal zone and gain. Another source of biliary obstruction is a mass in the head of the pancreas. The most superior arrow points to the usual site of Klatskin tumors (tumors of the biliary tree).

BILIARY ATRESIA

In biliary atresia, which occurs in children 3 to 6 months old, the bile ducts, even when dilated, are still very small and can just barely be seen. Even obstructed ducts are only 2 to 3 mm in diameter in this condition.

CHOLEDOCHAL CYSTS

These cysts are usually easy to see sonographically. With real-time one can see a cystic structure in the right upper quadrant inferior to the liver. Ducts will be seen entering this structure, and there will also be biliary duct dilatation elsewhere. The gallbladder will be visible separate from the cyst (Fig. 11-17).

PITFALLS

Pseudo-bile Duct Obstruction

PORTAL VEIN BIFURCATION

Superior to the gallbladder the right portal vein bifurcates into two large branches. For a short distance they run parallel to each other and mimic the appearance of a dilated bile duct and portal vein.

HEPATIC ARTERY

The hepatic artery runs anterior to the portal vein in close proximity to the common bile duct. It occasionally reaches a size of over 6 mm and can be mistaken for a dilated duct. However, it is pulsatile and can be traced to the celiac axis.

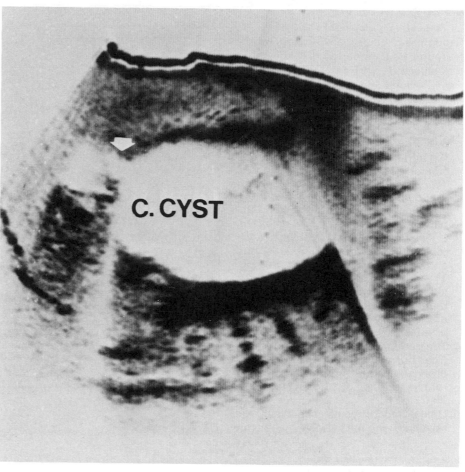

NECK OF GALLBLADDER

The neck of the gallbladder sometimes lies anterior to the common bile duct, and on some views it may appear to be separate from the body. It can thus be mistaken for a dilated duct.

Gas in the Biliary Tree Versus Stones

If there is free communication between the biliary tree and the gastrointestinal tract (e.g., following a sphincterotomy), gas can reflux into the biliary tree and cause pockets of acoustic shadowing that resemble stones.

FIGURE 11-17. Choledochal cyst. A dilated bile duct is seen entering this choledochal cyst (C. Cyst) on a longitudinal scan of the right upper quadrant. The dilated common duct can be seen (arrow).

Pseudo-Diffuse Liver Disease

By causing increased coarse echoes, a high-frequency transducer used with high gain can make the liver look as if it is abnormal due to diffuse liver disease. Comparison between the liver and kidney will show whether the increased echogenicity is genuine. The normal kidney parenchyma is slightly less echogenic than the liver.

WHERE ELSE TO LOOK

1. *Obstructed bile ducts.* It is essential to trace a dilated duct to the point of obstruction (Fig. 11-16). Often this obstruction is in the region of the pancreas. Mass lesions such as carcinoma of the pancreas, a pseudocyst, or focal pancreatitis are usually responsible. Occasionally, one is fortunate enough to see a stone within an obstructed duct. Rarely, obstructed ducts due to extrinsic pressure from nodes in the region of the porta hepatis may be demonstrated.

2. *Hepatocellular disease.* Diffuse textural changes within the liver are usually caused by alcoholic liver disease. When these changes are found, examine the other sites where alcoholism strikes—(1) the pancreas, which may show a pancreatic pseudocyst or pancreatitis, and (2) portal hypertension with splenomegaly, enlarged superior mesenteric and splenic veins, visible collaterals, and ascites.

3. *Hemolytic jaundice.* If the jaundice appears to result from hemolytic anemia with an enlarged liver and spleen, look for enlarged nodes, because there may be underlying leukemia or lymphoma.

SELECTED READING

Albarelli, J. N., and Springer, G. E. A technical approach to evaluating the jaundiced patient. *Semin. Ultrasound* 1:96, 1980.

Berland, L. L., Lawson, T. L., and Foley, W. D. Porta hepatis: Sonographic discrimination of bile ducts from arteries with pulsed Doppler with new anatomic criteria. *A.J.R.* 138:833–840, 1982.

Conrad, M. R., Linday, M. J., and Janes, J. O. Sonographic "parallel channel" sign of biliary tree enlargement in mild to moderate obstructive jaundice. *A.J.R.* 130:279–286, 1978.

Sarti, D. A., and Sample, W. F. (Eds.). Diagnostic Ultrasound: Text and Cases. Boston: G. K. Hall, 1979.

Taylor, K. J. W. Anatomy and Pathology of the Biliary Tree as Demonstrated by Ultrasound. In K. J. W. Taylor (Ed.), *Diagnostic Ultrasound in Gastrointestinal Disease* (Clinics in Diagnostic Ultrasound, Vol. 1). New York: Churchill Livingstone, 1979.

Taylor, K. J. W., Rosenfield, A. T., and Spira, H. M. Diagnostic accuracy of gray scale ultrasonography for the jaundiced patient: A report of 275 cases. *Arch. Intern. Med.* 139:60–63, 1979.

Zeman, R. K., Dorfman, G. S., Burrell, M. I., et al. Disparate dilatation of the intrahepatic and extrahepatic bile ducts in surgical jaundice. *Radiology* 138:129–136, 1981.

12. FEVER OF UNKNOWN ORIGIN (FUO)

Rule Out Abscesses or Occult Mass

NANCY A. SMITH

SONOGRAM ABBREVIATIONS

Ao	Aorta
Bl	Bladder
Ip	Iliopsoas muscle
IVC	Inferior vena cava
K	Kidney
L	Liver
LHev	Left hepatic vein
MHev	Middle hepatic vein
P	Pancreas
RAt	Right atrium
RHev	Right hepatic vein
S	Spine
Sp	Spleen
St	Stomach
Ut	Uterus

KEY WORDS

Anemia. Too few red blood cells. Causes include decreased blood cell formation, blood cell destruction, and bleeding.

Abscess. Localized collection of pus.

Cholangitis. Infection of the biliary tree.

Cystitis. Infection of the bladder.

Fever. A rise above the normal body temperature. Normal in most people is 98.4°F, 37°C.

Gutters (Paracolic). Areas in the flanks lateral to the colon where ascites and abscesses can form.

Hematocrit. The volume of erythrocytes packed by a centrifuge in a given volume of blood.

Hemorrhage, Hematoma. Collection of blood.

Hemolysis. Breakdown of red blood cells with release of hemoglobin into the plasma.

Immunosuppressed. Term describing a patient being treated with drugs that decrease the body's response to infection, for example, steroids or anticancer drugs.

Leukocyte. White blood cell; its primary function is to defend the body against infection.

Leukocytosis. An increase in the number of leukocytes.

Lymphadenopathy. Enlarged lymph nodes.

Leukopenia. An abnormally low leukocyte count.

Morison's Pouch. Space between the right kidney and the liver where ascites may lie or an abscess may develop.

Prostatitis. Infection of the prostate.

Pyogenic. Producing pus.

Pyrexia. Fever.

Sepsis. The presence of pathogenic microorganisms or their toxic products in the blood. The patient is usually febrile but may be hypothermic and in shock.

Staging. Demonstration of the areas that are involved in a malignancy. The more areas that are involved, the more severe the staging grade.

Subphrenic. Under the diaphragm.

Subpulmonic. Under the lung but above the diaphragm.

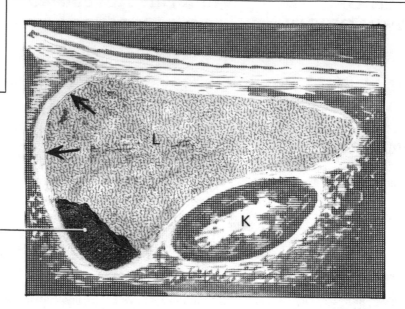

FIGURE 12-1. Right longitudinal section. Pleural effusions, subhepatic and perinephric collections, and subphrenic abscesses may immobilize the diaphragm (arrow). To show immobilization, perform real-time views on inspiration and expiration. A subphrenic abscess is shown.

Subdiaphragmatic collection

THE CLINICAL PROBLEM

Fever is a common manifestation of a great many illnesses and often arises from an easily identifiable source such as a postoperative wound infection. However, the cause is not always so well defined. Sonography is useful in detecting many of the less obvious causes of fever. Before commencing a study in a patient with fever of unknown origin (FUO), the history and laboratory data in the patient's chart should be searched for evidence suggesting any of the possibilities mentioned above (Key Word section). Understanding the patient's history will help the sonographer concentrate on the most appropriate areas.

Abscesses

Wound infection in the postoperative patient is a common problem. The accompanying symptoms may be masked by the administration of antibiotics and analgesics. Infections usually start approximately on the fifth postoperative day and develop into an abscess approximately on the tenth postoperative day. The following areas, which are common sites of abscesses, should be examined: the right and left subphrenic, subhepatic, perinephric, pelvic, the lesser sac, intrahepatic, intranephric, and psoas areas, and the region of the incision. Infection may originate in a site remote from the region where the abscess eventually settles.

Organ Inflammation

Infection may progress to actual abscess formation or may be limited to organ inflammation. Conditions such as hepatitis, pyelonephritis, cholecystitis, cholangitis, pancreatitis, cystitis, or prostatitis may give rise to fever that produces no localizing signs but has positive sonographic features.

Tumors

Some tumors, especially hypernephroma, lymphoma, and hepatoma, cause fever and leukocytosis that are similar to those characteristic of infections.

Bleeds

Hematoma formation may result in fever. Hematomas usually follow anticoagulant therapy or are related to either surgical injury or trauma. Common sites include the regions of the kidney, spleen, and liver and around incisions.

ANATOMY

See the relevant chapters for each organ.

TECHNIQUE

Routine Views

A routine should be followed when searching for the origin of FUO or examining a patient without localizing signs.

1. Start by examining the patient in a supine position. Scan along the inferior vena cava and aorta to make sure nodes are not present.
2. On longitudinal sections examine the liver, right diaphragm (Fig. 12-1), right kidney, subhepatic space (Fig. 6-15), and gallbladder area. A real-time sector scanner speeds the search and is effective, but to document liver size and present the information in a logical orientation, take some static scans. Make sure that the diaphragm moves and that no pleural effusions are present.
3. With the bladder full look in the pelvis for ascites, nodes, or a pelvic abscess. Be sure to include the iliopsoas muscles; these may contain an abscess or hematoma or may be surrounded by nodes. If the patient is male, check the prostate and seminal vesicles (see Chapter 19). If the patient is female, check the uterus and ovaries (see Chapter 23).
4. Using a transverse approach, look in the lesser sac area around the pancreas and in the "paracolic gutters" (see Fig. 6-15). Once nodes around the vessels are ruled out, transverse scans throughout the rest of the abdomen and the pelvis may be done at larger increments (i.e., 2 to 3 cm).
5. Turn the patient left side up and look in the region of the left hemidiaphragm (see Chapter 13). Deep inspiration helps to bring the diaphragm down to a level where it can be seen. Look at the spleen, the left kidney, and the perinephric area, including the psoas muscles (see Chapter 21). All are possible sites for abscesses. A left side up view can also show evidence of nodes between the aorta and the kidney. A pleural effusion may be evident above the diaphragm and may be the source of the infection.
6. In a postoperative patient, examine the incision area. If the incision is not closed, place a sterile plastic bag around the transducer as described in Chapter 42. Use sterile mineral oil. To avoid causing pain, sector around the wound instead of scanning too closely to it on the skin. A water-bath technique may help if the area is extremely sensitive.

7. The following special techniques may be valuable in difficult circumstances.
   a. *Diaphragm problems.* If you are not sure whether the fluid collection is above or below the diaphragm, sit the patient in an erect position. This may lower the diaphragm.
   Evaluate the mobility of the diaphragm. Superimpose an image taken with deep inspiration on one taken in expiration (see Chapter 38).
   b. *Small liver.* If the liver is small and high and the edge is obscured by gas, perform intercostal sector scans from a level superior to the liver edge. This places the beam more perpendicular to this interface. An alternative technique is to scan obliquely through the lateral aspect of the liver (see Fig. 6-15B).
   c. *Possible pelvic abscesses.* When a possible pelvic abscess is present, which could be located in the gut, examine the patient with real-time. If peristalsis is seen, the question is answered; however, because the sigmoid colon is often inactive, a water enema will need to be performed to prove that a lesion is not gut if no peristalsis is seen. Only enough water is inserted to cause flow through or around the questionable mass. In spite of the patient's objections, a full bladder should be maintained to serve as an acoustic window.

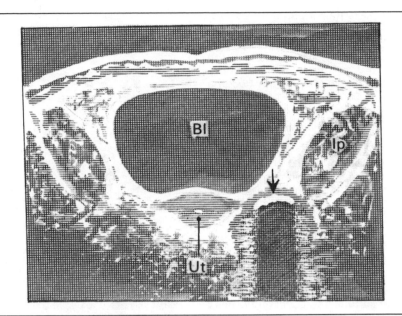

FIGURE 12-2. A transverse view of the female pelvis with a left-sided tubo-ovarian abscess. The abscess contains air, which rises to the top and casts a strong acoustic shadow.

PATHOLOGY

Abscesses

1. Abscesses tend to collect in spaces around organs and may displace structures or render them immobile (see Chapter 6, Fig. 6-15). Common sites are

   Subphrenic (Fig. 12-1)
   Subhepatic
   Perinephric
   Pelvic (Fig. 12-2)
   Intrahepatic (Fig 12-3)
   Intrarenal
   Around incisions

2. Abscesses usually appear to be predominantly fluid-filled and have thick irregular walls. There may be loculation. Some collections contain necrotic debris, which may float or settle in a dependent portion to create a fluid-fluid level. The amount of through transmission depends on the quantity and composition of the fluid.
3. When there is gas inside an abscess, shadowing varies with the amount and location of the gas (Fig. 12-2). Correlation with an abdominal radiograph is helpful. The contents of an abscess may resemble a dense mass.

4. Abscesses, often multiple, may also be found within organs such as the liver (Fig. 12-3) and the kidney. Less frequently, they are found in the spleen and the prostate. In alcoholics a pancreatic pseudocyst may become infected, forming a pancreatic abscess. Abscesses in the mesentery may resemble gut; local tenderness can help to identify them.

5. Aspiration of an abscess under ultrasonic control is of considerable help in clinical management because it allows identification of the responsible micro-organism and may permit curative drainage.

Inflammatory Changes

Most organs respond similarly to infection without abscess formation. In the involved area, the organ will be swollen and more sonolucent. Local tenderness will be present and should be noted by the sonographer.

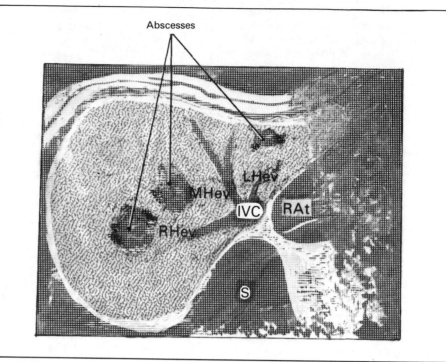

FIGURE 12-3. Multiple hepatic abscesses are seen in a right costal margin view of the liver.

Neoplasms

HEPATOMAS AND HYPERNEPHROMAS

Hepatomas and hypernephromas are common causes of fever and should be sought in the liver and kidney (See Chapters 9 and 17).

LYMPHOMA

An important cause of intermittent FUO, lymphomatous nodes are almost always echo-free. Common sites are (1) the para-aortic area, particularly in the region of the left renal hilum (Fig. 12-4); (2) the celiac axis, displacing the pancreas anteriorly and involving the porta hepatis; and (3) adjacent to the iliopsoas muscles in the pelvis. The spleen is usually enlarged and may be directly involved. Lymphomatous involvement of organs such as the kidney and liver may occur, appearing as echopenic areas in the parenchyma.

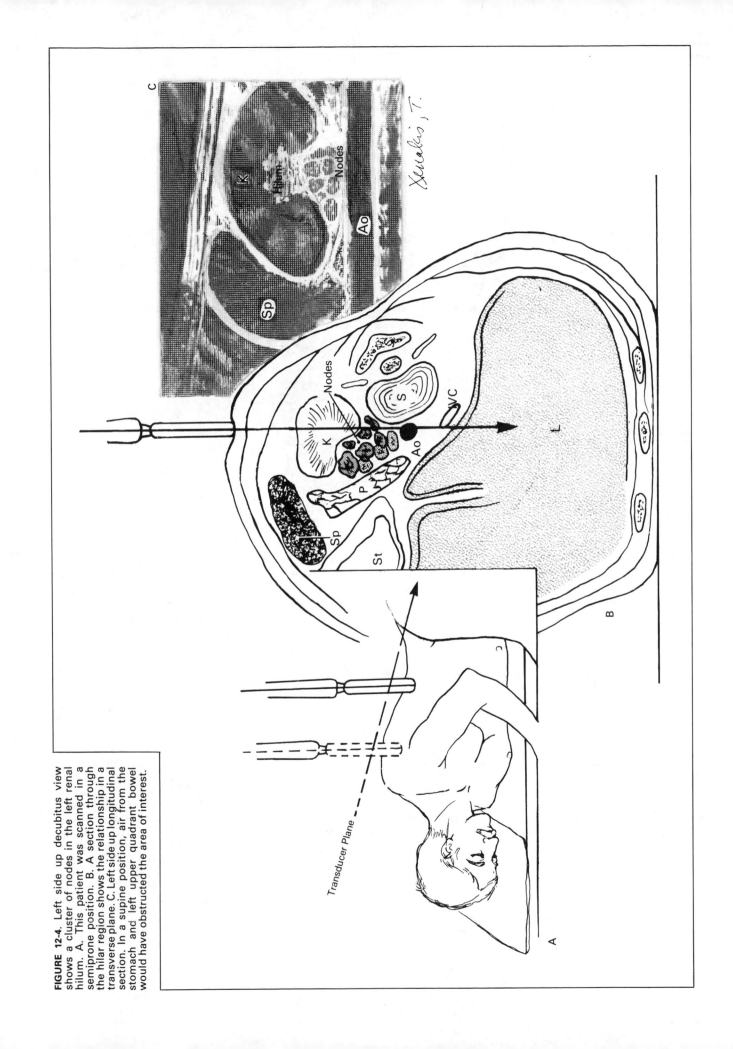

FIGURE 12-4. Left side up decubitus view shows a cluster of nodes in the left renal hilum. A. This patient was scanned in a semiprone position. B. A section through the hilar region shows the relationship in a transverse plane. C. Left side up longitudinal section. In a supine position, air from the stomach and left upper quadrant bowel would have obstructed the area of interest.

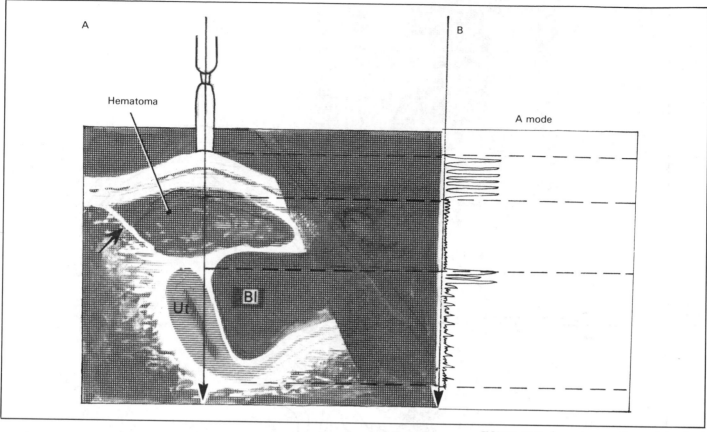

FIGURE 12-5. A post-operative pelvis. A. A hematoma in the abdominal wall is present. B. An A-mode scan through the hematoma and the uterus shows only low-level echoes.

Hematomas

Hematomas, whether occurring post-operatively or spontaneously, can cause fever (see Chapter 21). Hematomas undergo a confusing series of changes with time. They often are echogenic at first and then become echo-free during a period of days only to regain some echogenicity as they resolve. Hematomas tend to spread along fascial planes rather than bursting through tissues as occurs with abscesses (Fig. 12-5).

PITFALLS

Bowel Versus Abscess

To clarify the problem, examine the patient with real-time, perform a water enema, or give fluid by mouth. It may be necessary to have the patient return on another day; a real lesion will be unchanged during this time.

Ascites Versus Abscess

A localized area of ascites may be mistaken for an abscess. Place the patient in the erect or Trendelenburg position; ascites will shift, but an abscess will not.

TGC Artifacts

Poor use of time gain compensation control may give an impression of an echopenic area resembling inflammation or an abscess in an organ such as a transplanted kidney or spleen (see Chapter 20). The less echogenic area will extend beyond the organ in question if it is a technical artifact.

Fat Deposits

The preperitoneal fat anterior to the liver in obese people may resemble an abscess. However, this fat is symmetrical on either side of the midline and has well-defined borders.

Pleural Effusion Versus Subphrenic Collection

A pleural effusion may be mistaken for a subphrenic collection. Real-time observation of the diaphragm will distinguish subphrenic from subpulmonic lesions. Scanning the patient in the erect position may show the diaphragm more clearly, especially if there is an effusion that can be used as an acoustic window.

Reverberation Problems

Reverberations may create an apparent fluid collection deep in the pelvis behind the bladder. The following maneuvers may show the "collection" to be an artifact (see Chapter 45).

1. Jiggling the transducer will move the artifact with the transducer.
2. Scanning from a different direction may show that the suspect collection area is an artifact. This will change the distance between the transducer and the bladder border, thus eliminating or changing the reverberation.
3. Measuring the distance from the skin to the center of the collection may show that the supposed collection lies well behind the patient's back.

SELECTED READING

Harvey, A. M., et al. *The Principles and Practice of Medicine.* (20th ed.). New York: Appleton-Century-Crofts, 1976.

13. LEFT UPPER QUADRANT MASS

ROGER C. SANDERS

SONOGRAM ABBREVIATIONS

Ad Adrenal gland
Ao Aorta

D Diaphragm

IVC Inferior vena cava

K Kidney

L Liver

P Pancreas

R Ribs

Sp Spleen
St Stomach

KEY WORDS

Myeloproliferative Disorder. Term referring to chronic myeloid leukemia, myelofibrosis, and polycythemia vera—a spectrum of hematologic conditions associated with a large spleen. Sometimes one entity will change into another.

Pancreatic Pseudocyst. Fluid collection produced by the pancreas during acute pancreatitis.

Pheochromocytoma. A hormone-producing adrenal tumor.

Portal Hypertension. A rise in the pressure of the venous blood flowing into the liver through the portal venous system, causing an increase in the size of the portal, splenic, and superior mesenteric veins and of the spleen. If portal hypertension is severe, additional vessels known as collaterals develop around the pancreas.

Splenomegaly. Enlargement of the spleen.

Subphrenic Abscess. An abscess lying under the left or right diaphragm. Such abscesses commonly follow surgery in the area, for example, stomach surgery.

THE CLINICAL PROBLEM

Splenomegaly

The most frequent left upper quadrant mass is an enlarged spleen. Splenomegaly occurs in a wide variety of medical states.

1. *Infectious diseases* such as tuberculosis, malaria, infectious mononucleosis ("mono"), and subacute bacterial endocarditis (SBE) are often accompanied by an enlarged spleen. (The spleen is occasionally the site of an abscess, particularly with SBE or any other bacteremic state.)
2. *Myeloproliferative* disorders such as myelofibrosis may be characterized by splenomegaly.
3. Splenomegaly occurs when the veins draining the spleen are obstructed, as in *portal hypertension* or *splenic vein thrombosis.* Both pancreatic cancer and pancreatitis can cause splenic vein thrombosis.
4. *Metastases* may occur; however, the spleen is not often the site of neoplastic involvement.
5. *Lymphoma and leukemia* may involve the spleen directly or cause splenomegaly as a secondary phenomenon because blood production is disorganized.

Fluid-Filled Masses

A left upper quadrant fluid-filled mass is quite common and may be (1) a *renal mass* such as hydronephrosis or a large renal cyst, (2) a *splenic cyst,* (3) an *adrenal cyst,* or (4) a *pancreatic pseudocyst.*

Neoplasia

Neoplastic masses in the left upper quadrant include (1) *retroperitoneal sarcomas,* (2) *adrenal tumors,* which are usually small (e.g., metastases, pheochromocytoma) but occasionally become large, and (3) *pancreas and kidney cancers,* which can spread into the left upper quadrant and cause a palpable abdominal mass.

The surgical approach is dictated by the origin and nature of the mass. Cysts may be treated conservatively or by cyst puncture rather than by surgery.

Abscesses

The left subdiaphragmatic region is a common site for abscess collections, particularly in postoperative patients following removal of the spleen or stomach operations.

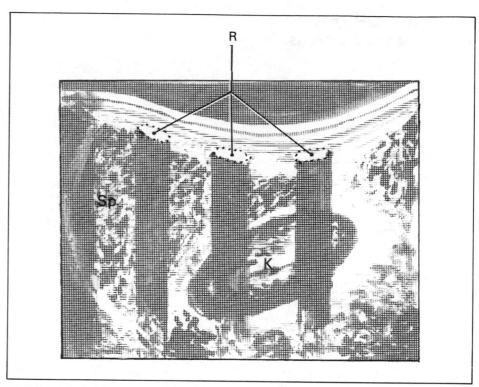

FIGURE 13-1. Left side up view of the spleen (Sp) and left kidney (K). Ribs (R) partially obscure the spleen and kidney.

ANATOMY

Spleen

The spleen is the predominant organ in the left upper quadrant. It lies immediately under the left hemidiaphragm and may be difficult to see because of gas in the neighboring lung and ribs. It lies superior to the left kidney and lateral to the adrenal gland and the tail of the pancreas. The left lobe of the liver is usually in contact with the spleen.

The splenic texture is even and less echogenic than that of the liver but more echogenic than the kidney. A high-level echo in the center of the spleen at its medial aspect represents the splenic hilum at the entrance of the splenic artery and vein.

TECHNIQUE

Left Side Up View

The left side up position (right lateral decubitus) is the preferred method for investigating the left upper quadrant (Fig. 13-1). Angling the transducer somewhat obliquely so that it passes between the ribs may be helpful. To identify your location, find the left kidney; the spleen will be above it. There should normally be nothing between the spleen and the left hemidiaphragm.

Transverse Supine View

Transverse supine sections taken with fluid in the stomach may be helpful in visualizing the spleen and the area around it.

Erect Position

Placing the patient in the erect position may allow a high, small spleen to fall into a site where it can be seen.

Real-Time

Real-time is invaluable in this area to obtain the correct axis between the ribs for best visualization of the spleen, kidney, and adrenal.

PATHOLOGY

Splenomegaly

In a supine view the spleen is enlarged when its anterior border lies in front of the aorta and the inferior vena cava, and it is at least as thick as a normal kidney (Fig. 13-2). On the left side up view the spleen is enlarged when it is more than twice the size of the kidney (providing the kidney is normal).

Though unusual, focal lesions may occur in the spleen. Abscesses usually have irregular borders and some internal echoes; they may show shadowing associated with gas. Metastatic lesions resemble those seen in the liver.

Splenic echogenicity may be altered when the spleen is enlarged. If it is less echogenic than usual, one should think of lymphoma; if more echogenic, consider myelofibrosis or infection.

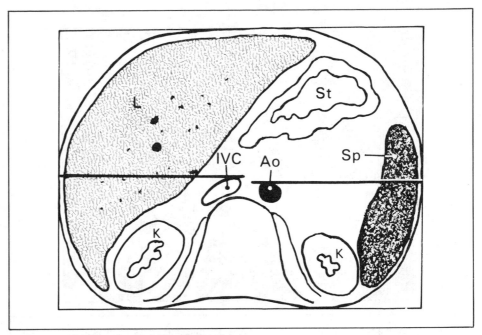

FIGURE 13-2. A spleen is considered enlarged on a supine view when its anterior border lies in front of a line at the level of the aorta (Ao) and inferior vena cava (IVC), and when it is approximately the same width as the kidney.

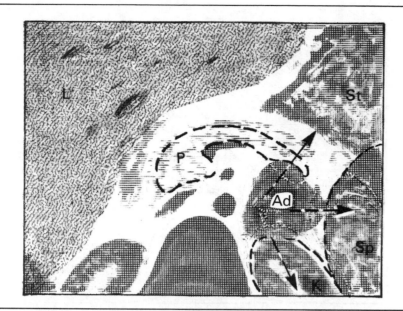

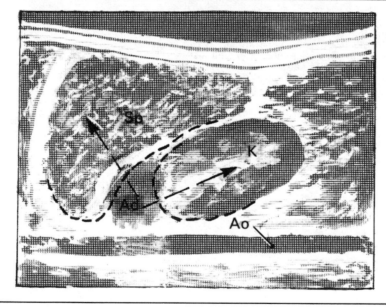

FIGURE 13-3. Adrenal mass. A. An adrenal mass (Ad) displaces the spleen laterally, the kidney posteriorly, and the pancreas (P) anteriorly. B. On a coronal view an adrenal mass will displace the kidney inferiorly, the spleen superiorly, and the aorta medially.

Cysts

If the cause of the left upper quadrant mass is a cyst, make sure you know the organ of origin.

1. *Splenic cysts* should have a rim of splenic parenchyma around them. An upright position may help to show the complete cyst. Splenic cysts may contain many internal echoes and septa.
2. *Renal cysts* will arise from the kidney, and there will be a claw-like portion of renal parenchyma surrounding the cyst. The kidney may become very large with hydronephrosis. Differentiation of hydronephrosis from a cyst is simple in most instances (see Chapter 16).
3. *Pancreatic pseudocysts* usually show some connection with the pancreas; they generally displace the spleen superiorly and the kidney inferiorly.
4. *Adrenal cysts* and masses displace the spleen anteriorly, the kidney inferiorly, and the pancreas anteriorly (Fig. 13-3A,B). Adrenal cysts may have a calcified border; if so, the rim of the mass lesion will be densely echogenic, and through transmission will not be seen.

Subphrenic Abscess

A fluid collection located in the splenic site following splenectomy or between the diaphragm and the spleen may represent a left subphrenic abscess. These abscesses are often difficult to see because this area is so inaccessible unless, as is common, there is a coincident pleural effusion.

Solid Mass

If the mass is solid, displacement of the adjacent organs will indicate its origin.

1. *Retroperitoneal sarcomas* will displace the kidney, spleen, and pancreas anteriorly.
2. *Pancreatic neoplasms* will lie superior to the kidney but will displace the spleen anteriorly.
3. *Renal neoplasms* will lie inferior to the spleen and pancreas.

Inverted Diaphragm

If the left diaphragm is inverted by a left pleural effusion, an apparent left upper quadrant cystic mass may develop. A longitudinal section will show the true site of the diaphragm and reveal that the cystic area—the pleural effusion—is intrathoracic (Fig. 13-4A,B).

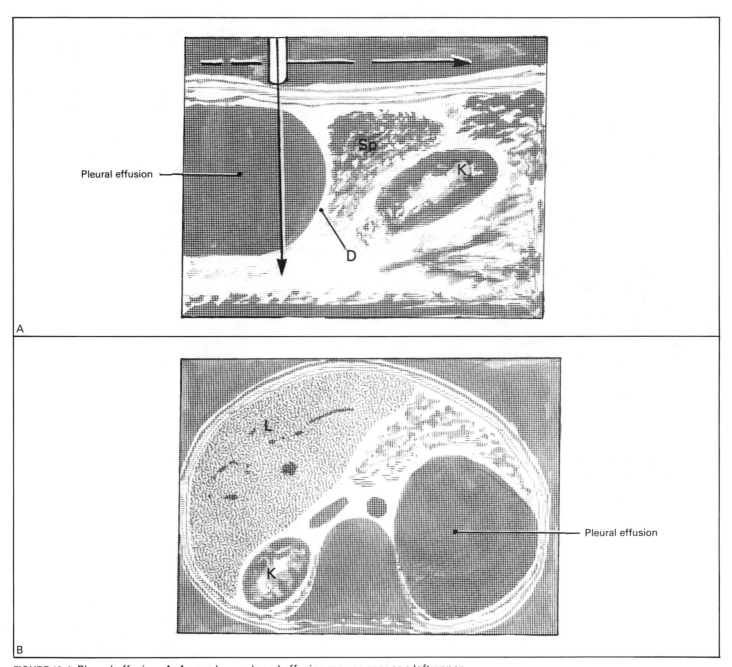

FIGURE 13-4. Pleural effusion. A. A very large pleural effusion may appear as a left upper quadrant mass. The diaphragm will be inverted, and the spleen and kidney will be displaced inferiorly. B. On a transverse view a large pleural effusion inverting the diaphragm can look like a large cyst.

PITFALLS

1. *Heart versus collection.* An enlarged heart may depress the left hemidiaphragm and appear to be an intraabdominal mass. Real-time will show pulsation and demonstrate the various chambers within the heart.

2. *Left lobe of the liver versus perisplenic collection.* The left lobe of the liver may extend superior to the spleen, especially if a partial hepatectomy has been performed. Trace the suspect mass into the normal liver.

3. *Stomach versus left upper quadrant collection.* The stomach may look like a left upper quadrant fluid collection. Give fluid by mouth, and peristalsis will be seen.

4. *Spleen versus effusion.* The spleen may resemble a pleural effusion if the sonographer is not careful to establish where the kidney lies, because a more or less horizontal diaphragm may not be imaged adequately.

5. *Splenic hilum.* An echogenic area, the hilum, at the site where the splenic vein and splenic artery enter the spleen, can be mistaken for a neoplasm. Real-time will show vessels in this area.

6. *Subphrenic versus subpulmonic collection.* It may be difficult to distinguish a subphrenic from a subpulmonic collection if the diaphragm is not easily seen. Real-time is helpful in making this distinction.

WHERE ELSE TO LOOK

1. If *splenomegaly* is present
   a. Examine the liver for evidence of diffuse liver disease and portal and splenic vein enlargement and collaterals with portal hypertension.
   b. Note whether nodes are present in association with splenomegaly and lymphoma.

2. If the mass appears to be a *pancreatic pseudocyst,* look for the stigma of alcoholism elsewhere and evidence of pancreatitis in the remainder of the pancreas.

3. If the cause of the left upper quadrant mass is *hydronephrosis,* look for the cause of obstruction in the pelvis along the course of the ureter.

SELECTED READING

Johnson, M. A., Cooperberg, P. L., Boisvert, J., et al. Spontaneous splenic rupture in infectious mononucleosis: Sonographic diagnosis and follow-up. *A.J.R.* 136: 111–114, 1981.

Mittelstaedt, C. A. Ultrasound of the spleen. *Semin. Ultrasound* 2:233–240, 1981.

14. PEDIATRIC MASS

ROGER C. SANDERS

SONOGRAM ABBREVIATIONS

K Kidney

L Liver

KEY WORDS

Aniridia. Congenital absence of a portion of the eye (the iris). Associated with Wilms' tumor.

Adrenal Hemorrhage. Hemorrhage into the adrenal gland occurring in the first few days of life and causing a large hematoma that is often mistaken for a kidney mass. It resolves spontaneously, often with development of calcification.

Beckwith-Weidemann Syndrome. Congenital anomaly in which many organs of the body, such as the tongue, are enlarged. Associated with Wilms' tumor.

Brat Board. An infant immobilization device. A child is strapped in the region of the chest and limbs to a board and cannot move. The abdomen can remain exposed.

Choledochal Cyst. Congenital focal dilatation of a segment of the biliary tree.

Enteric Duplication. Congenital duplication of the gut. The involved segment does not usually connect with the remainder of the bowel. Thus, this segment becomes filled with fluid and presents as a mass.

Hemihypertrophy. Congenital condition in which half of the body is larger than the other side. Associated with Wilms' tumor.

Hepatoblastoma. Liver tumor that is particularly common in small children.

Hydrops. The gallbladder is markedly enlarged and the cystic duct is functionally obstructed, although often nothing can be found at surgery. This self-limiting condition occurs in association with some childhood illnesses, for example, Kawasaki's syndrome, and following surgery.

Kawasaki's Syndrome. Mucocutaneous lymph node syndrome. This viral illness is associated with hydrops of the gallbladder and occurs in epidemics.

Meningocele. Cystic dilatation of the spinal canal at the site of a bony defect. May appear as an abdominal mass in the neonate when it protrudes anterior to the sacrum.

Mesenteric Cyst (omental cyst). Cyst filled with lymph found in the mesentery that presents as an asymptomatic abdominal mass.

Mesoblastic Nephroma. Rare tumor of the kidney occurring in neonates; it rarely metastasizes but needs immediate surgery.

Multicystic (Dysplastic) Kidney. Unilateral renal cystic disease that develops in utero, the commonest cause of a neonatal mass. May be found later in life as an incidental finding.

Neonate. Infant in the first 4 weeks of life.

Neuroblastoma. A tumor usually arising in the adrenals between birth and the age of 5; the child may have gait and eyesight problems ("dancing eyes and dancing feet") or metastatic bone lesions rather than an abdominal mass.

Precocious Puberty. Disease affecting small girls in which they start to menstruate and develop breasts. Often due to an ovarian tumor.

Pyloric Stenosis. A predominantly male disorder. The pylorus (the exit of the stomach) is narrowed and the wall is thickened. May cause vomiting in small children.

Rhabdomyosarcoma. Sarcomatous muscle tumor that occurs in childhood and has a particular affinity for the bladder and heart.

Teratoma. Mass composed of elements of most tissues in the body, notably skin, hair, bone, and especially teeth. May occur anywhere in the abdomen, but in the infant it is found predominantly in the sacrococcygeal area. Usually discovered at birth.

Stillbirth. Child born dead on delivery.

Ureterocele. Dilatation of the distal ureter as it inserts abnormally into the bladder. A "cobra-head" deformity develops owing to a stenosis.

Vacuum Immobilization Device. An infant immobilization device in which a plastic membrane, distended with air, surrounds and fixes the child, preventing movement.

Wilms' Tumor. Kidney tumor that generally occurs between the ages of 1 and 6, usually as an abdominal mass. Associated with hemihypertrophy, aniridia, and the Beckwith-Weidemann syndrome.

THE CLINICAL PROBLEM

The spectrum of masses in the neonate or small child is different from that in the adult.

Neonatal Masses

RENAL MASSES

The most common mass is a multicystic (dysplastic) kidney. Congenital hydronephrosis due to ureteropelvic junction obstruction is a close second. These two lesions, both fluid-filled, must be distinguished from a rare kidney tumor (mesoblastic nephroma). If the mass is fluid-filled, the child can be operated upon when older and healthier, but if it is a solid tumor, surgery should be performed immediately.

ADRENAL HEMORRHAGE

Adrenal hemorrhage, usually detected not at birth but a few days later, may be confused with a renal tumor. However, the sonographer should be able to tell that the mass is adrenal in location. Adrenal hematomas usually occur in children who have undergone a difficult delivery. Adrenal hematomas may be associated with unusual laboratory findings and hematocrit drop rather than with an abdominal mass.

OTHER MASSES

Other, rarer causes of neonatal abdominal masses are enteric duplication, ovarian cysts (which are surprisingly often found near the liver in neonates), mesenteric cysts, choledochal cysts (see Chapter 11), and teratomas. Teratomas are usually found deep in the pelvis in a sacrococcygeal location and often extend into the buttocks. Anterior sacral meningocele, a fluid-filled outpouching of the spinal canal, can be confused with a sacrococcygeal teratoma. Pyloric stenosis, a cause of "projectile vomiting" in predominantly male children a few months old, is caused by muscle thickening around the exit of the stomach.

Older Children

In the 1- to 5-year-old child the most common masses are again related to the kidney, with Wilms' tumor and neuroblastoma being most frequent. Rhabdomyosarcomas occur most commonly in the region of the bladder but may be found at any site in the abdomen. Hepatoma, hepatoblastoma, and other liver tumors are not that rare in this age group.

ANATOMY

Kidney

Because the cortex is more echogenic in infants than in adults, the renal pyramids in infants are prominent and may be mistaken for cysts (Fig. 14-1A). The perirenal and intrarenal fat is almost absent, so the sinus and capsular echoes are barely seen.

Biliary Tree

The bile ducts in small children are normally smaller than those in adults. Bile ducts are usually abnormal if they are visible in the first year of life.

Pancreas

The pancreas in children is much less echogenic than it is in adults; it has about the same echogenicity as the liver in young children. It slowly increases in echogenicity as the child becomes older. It is also relatively larger than in adults.

TECHNIQUE

Real-Time

Real-time is virtually essential in this age group. Use a high-frequency transducer so that the near field is well seen.

Immobilization

In the *neonate* the examination can usually be performed with restraint of the shoulders and legs by an adult so that the child falls asleep or at least lies quietly. With a *2- to 4-year-old* child cooperation can rarely be obtained, but distraction, for example, by playing with keys, may be helpful.

Older children should be shown the system before performing the examination so that they won't feel threatened by the equipment. Making a Polaroid image that is specifically labeled for the child may be very helpful. Asking the child to erase the image from the screen also induces cooperation.

If all else fails, perform the study while the child is screaming but is still relatively immobile before taking another breath.

Restraint Devices

Restraint devices may very occasionally be necessary in the 2- to 4-year-old. Vacuum-type systems or brat boards have been helpful if the relevant area is left exposed.

Sedation

Sedation may very rarely be necessary in a child who has had long-term hospitalization and distrusts anyone in a white uniform. Sublimaze and ketamine are useful sedative drugs.

Heating the Neonate

Remember that the neonate must be kept warm. A heating pad or heat lamp is desirable. Small infants should not be uncovered for more than 15 minutes.

PATHOLOGY

Multicystic (Dysplastic) Kidney

This lesion is a unilateral process unless the child is stillborn. Multiple cystic structures of varying size and shape with no evidence of renal pelvis or parenchyma are noted (Fig. 14-1B). Some cysts may be so small that they are visualized as echoes rather than as fluid-filled structures. These may be thought erroneously to be dense parenchyma.

Hydronephrosis

The appearance of hydronephrosis is the same in children as in adults, although the pelvis is usually more prominent and there may appear to be only a single cystic structure. The amount of parenchyma varies with the severity and duration of the condition. If the obstruction is at a low level, the ureter can be seen posterior to the bladder or in the region of the kidney, but usually hydronephrosis in this age group is caused by ureteropelvic junction obstruction. If the ureter can be seen, examine the bladder for a ureterocele (see Chapter 16). A ureterocele is a cystic structure within the posterior aspect of the bladder. If a ureterocele is present, it is commonly associated with a double collecting system with a hydronephrotic upper segment. The lower segment may look normal or may also be dilated owing to reflux.

Adrenal Hemorrhage

Adrenal hemorrhages are in most instances echogenic at first. Cystic areas rapidly develop, and within 2 to 3 weeks the mass will be entirely fluid-filled (Fig. 14-2). Eventually calcification will be apparent on plain radiographs. A steady shrinkage in size occurs as this progression takes place. Usually the condition is bilateral.

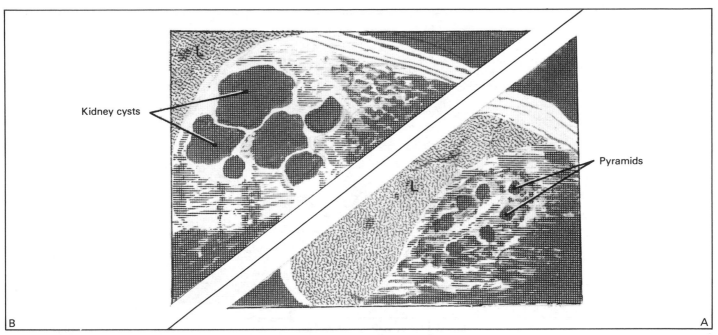

FIGURE 14-1. Renal "masses." A. Neonatal kidney, showing the relative absence of capsular and sinus echoes due to a normal paucity of fat. Note the prominence of the pyramids, which have been mistaken for cysts in this age group. B. Multicystic kidney. The kidney is replaced by cysts of varying sizes that do not communicate.

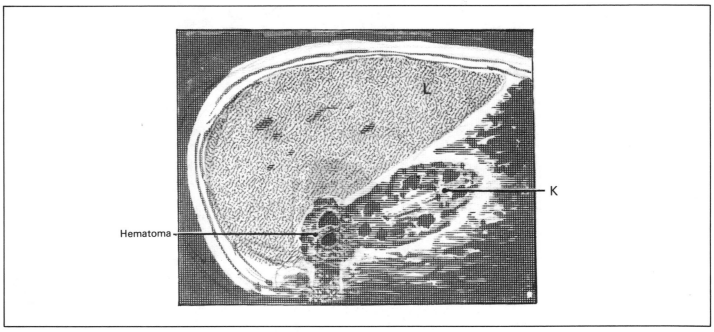

FIGURE 14-2. Adrenal hematoma. There is a mass superior to the kidney, which contains several echo-free areas.

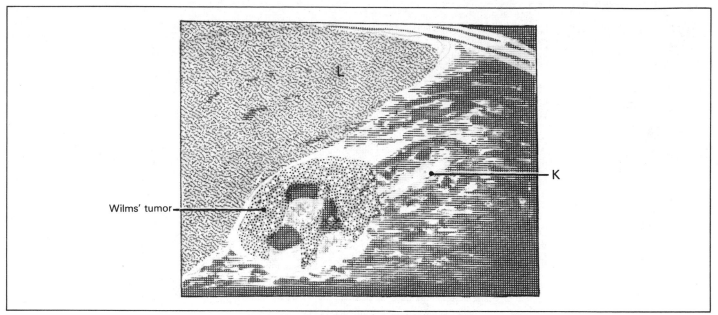

FIGURE 14-3. A Wilms' tumor has an even echogenicity apart from cystic areas that are thought to be due to areas of necrosis.

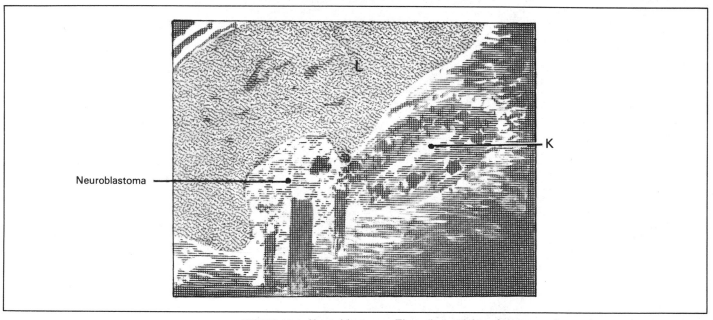

FIGURE 14-4. Neuroblastoma. The echogenicity of the mass is much more heterogeneous than it is in Wilms' tumor, and often shows some areas of calcification that cause acoustic shadowing.

Pyloric Stenosis

An epigastric mass will be present with an echogenic center and sonolucent walls, resembling the target sign of bowel wall thickening (see Chapter 15).

Wilms' Tumor

This malignant tumor occurs in the 1- to 6-year-old age group. The tumor is evenly echogenic at first but later develops sonolucent areas that are probably caused by areas of necrosis (Fig. 14-3). This cancer often causes secondary hydronephrosis. Although usually unilateral, Wilms' tumor is bilateral in 10% of cases. A more benign but rare variant (mesoblastic nephroma) is seen in the first year of life. The echo pattern is more variable, and the tumor may be partially cystic.

Neuroblastoma

This malignant tumor generally occurs in the age group from birth to 5 years old. Although neuroblastoma usually originates in the adrenal gland, it can arise elsewhere; for example, it may be paraspinous. The echogenic texture is much more heterogeneous than a Wilms' tumor, with areas of acoustic shadowing due to calcification (Fig. 14-4). Extension of the cancer beyond the midline is common and affects the staging. Involvement of the major arteries, which precludes operation, should be clearly demonstrated ultrasonically.

Enteric Duplication

An enteric duplication is a rare congenital lesion. It is either a fluid-filled structure in the mesentery or a mass filled with the usual contents of gut with acoustic shadowing. Most of those recognized ultrasonically are fluid-filled.

Mesenteric Cyst

This large, asymptomatic fluid-filled mass in the mesentery may be multilocular but is otherwise echo-free.

Teratoma

This tumor may contain any of the body's structural elements. Often teratomas contain bone with acoustic shadowing or hair, which may result in an evenly echogenic structure possibly with a fluid-fluid level. They are usually located in the pelvis or arise from the presacral region. However, teratomas can be seen anywhere in the abdomen, particularly in the region of the adrenals. These tumors may rarely be entirely fluid-filled.

Meningocele

Meningoceles, which occur in a location similar to that of teratomas, anterior to the sacrum, are entirely fluid-filled. Correlation with a sacral radiograph may show associated bony changes.

Ovarian Cysts

Ovarian cysts in the neonate are highly variable in position and may occur in the upper abdomen. They usually contain septa and echogenic material. Normal ovaries in the neonate or infant are usually very small (under 1 cm in diameter). The uterus is also small. As in the adult, a full bladder is essential for assessment of ovarian size.

Rhabdomyosarcoma

This sarcomatous lesion tends to affect the posterior wall of the bladder and can cause adenopathy anywhere in the abdomen.

Hepatoma and Hepatoblastoma

Liver tumors in small children are usually single and have a variable sonographic appearance, some being echopenic and some echogenic. Occasional tumors have large cystic components. The site of these tumors must be defined with respect to the hepatic veins, because they can be resected if they lie solely within one lobe of the liver (see Chapter 8).

Lymphoma

Lymphoma occurs in children and appears similar to adenopathy in adults.

Pancreatitis

Pancreatitis is not uncommon in children. It has the same features as in adults. The pancreas enlarges and becomes more sonolucent than normal for the pediatric age group. Pancreatic pseudocysts may occur. Pancreatitis is usually caused by trauma or occurs congenitally.

PITFALLS

1. *Adrenal hemorrhage versus tumor.* Do not mistake adrenal hemorrhage for a neoplastic mass. Following the patient for a few days with serial sonograms will show a change in the configuration of the mass with development of cystic areas.
2. *Cyst versus pyramids in kidney.* Do not mistake normal pyramids in the neonate for cystic disease.
3. *Pseudopancreatitis.* Because the pancreas is normally less echogenic in children than in adults, be cautious about making a diagnosis of pancreatitis unless the pancreas appears enlarged.

WHERE ELSE TO LOOK

1. If a *Wilms' tumor* is possible, examine
   a. The second kidney, because this neoplasm may be bilateral.
   b. The inferior vena cava and renal vein for clot or tumor.
   c. The liver for metastases.
   d. The para-aortic area for nodal enlargement.
2. If *neuroblastoma* is likely, look for midline spread. It alters the staging.
3. If *hydronephrosis* is discovered, examine the pelvis to see if the cause of obstruction is visible—for example, a ureterocele.
4. If a *bladder mass* is found, look elsewhere in the abdomen for evidence of rhabdomyosarcoma.

SELECTED READING

Haller, J. O., and Schkolnik, A. (Eds.). *Ultrasound in Pediatrics* (Clinics in Diagnostic Ultrasound Series). New York: Churchill Livingstone, 1981.

Haller, J. O., and Schneider, M. *Pediatric Ultrasound.* Chicago: Year Book, 1980.

Kangarloo, H., and Sample, W. F. *Ultrasound of the Pediatric Abdomen and Pelvis: A Correlative Imaging Approach.* Chicago: Year Book, 1980.

SONOGRAM ABBREVIATIONS

Ab	Abscess
Ao	Aorta
Bl	Bladder
Ca	Celiac artery
GBl	Gallbladder
Ia	Iliac artery
Ip	Iliopsoas muscle
IVC	Inferior vena cava
K	Kidney
L	Liver
N	Nodes
P	Pancreas
Pl	Placenta
Ps	Psoas muscle
QL	Quadratus lumborum muscle
RA	Rectus abdominis muscle
SMa	Superior mesenteric artery
Sp	Spleen

KEY WORDS

Adenopathy. Multiple enlarged lymph nodes in many locations.

Aneurysm. Dilatation of an artery, usually the abdominal aorta. Aneurysms may be true, if they have an intact wall, or false, if the wall has ruptured and only clot prevents hemorrhage into neighboring tissues.

Ascites. (1) *Exudative.* Free fluid in the peritoneum associated with malignancy or infection; may contain internal echoes. (2) *Transudative.* Free fluid in the peritoneum containing little or no protein and associated with heart, kidney, or liver failure.

Bifurcation. The abdominal aorta divides into the iliac arteries at the bifurcation, which is located approximately at the level of the umbilicus.

Crohn's Disease. Inflammatory bowel disease often accompanied by abscesses and associated with bowel wall thickening.

Dissecting Aneurysm. The wall of the aorta is composed of three parts—intima, media, and adventitia. In a dissecting aneurysm the intima separates from the media, so blood can flow through two channels on either side of the intima. The blood usually re-enters the aorta at a lower level.

Gutter. Area lateral to the ascending and descending colon where fluid may accumulate ("paracolic gutter").

Haustral Markings. Normal segmentation of the wall seen in the colon.

Hernia. Protrusion of gut through the abdominal wall muscle into a subcutaneous location. Dangerous because it can lead to obstruction if the bowel is blocked as it passes through the narrow opening. Hernias may be (1) *Ventral.* Usually midline and associated with previous surgery. (2) *Spigelian.* Lie lateral to the rectus muscles. (3) *Femoral or Inguinal.* Develop in the groin.

Ischemic Colitis. Bowel with a very poor blood supply—it has a thickened wall.

Intussusception. Obstructed bowel coiled on itself. Seen particularly in children. The walls are thickened.

Lymphoma. Malignancy that mainly affects the lymph nodes, spleen, or liver. It has various subgroups (e.,g., Hodgkin's, histiocytic, and lymphoblastic lymphoma).

Mesenteric Sheath (Transverse Mesocolon). A structure within which lie the superior mesenteric artery and the superior mesenteric vein and to which the mesentery that supports the bowel is attached.

Rectus Muscles. Muscles in the anterior midabdomen that are often the site of hemorrhage. The muscles are paired, one on either side of the midline, and extend the length of the abdomen.

"Sandwich" sign. Nodes in the mesentery characteristically form on either side of the mesenteric sheath in two large groups and have an appearance similar to a sandwich.

Valvulae Conniventes. Normal segmentation of the small bowel.

THE CLINICAL PROBLEM

Many of the masses that apparently lie in the midabdomen arise in the pelvis or upper abdomen and extend into the midabdomen (e.g., splenomegaly, fibroid uterus, pancreatic pseudocyst). Masses of truly midabdominal origin are related to structures in this area, that is, the abdominal wall, the aorta, the gut, and nodes. Air in the gut frequently interferes with sonographic visualization, but fortunately, if a mass is present, the mass itself usually provides an acoustic window and displaces gut.

Aortic Aneurysm

Aortic aneurysms are best looked for with ultrasound because it reveals the true internal and external dimensions of the aneurysm. An aortogram will show only the blood-filled lumen, not the clot-filled area. Surgeons will appreciate information about how the aneurysm is related to the major aortic branches such as the renal, mesenteric, and iliac arteries because it helps them choose the appropriate graft shape. An aneurysm that is leaking, forming a false aneurysm, is an acute emergency. The walls of a false aneurysm are formed by clot and may give way abruptly.

Nodes

Initial and follow-up assessment is helpful in dealing with nodal enlargement around the aorta and celiac axis. Such adenopathy is most commonly caused by lymphoma but may be caused by metastatic nodes from a primary cancer elsewhere. Ultrasound is preferable to lymphography because it shows nodes in locations that cannot be reached by lymphography such as in the mesentery or around the celiac axis. Detection of minimal nodal enlargement in lymphoma is worthwhile. Planning radiotherapy and chemotherapy for these patients depends on staging, which is based on the extent of lymphomatous spread.

Lymphoma is staged as follows:

Stage I. Disease limited to one anatomic region.
Stage II. Disease involving two or more anatomic regions on the same side of the diaphragm.
Stage III. Disease on both sides of the diaphragm involving lymph nodes or spleen.
Stage IV. Extranodal involvement such as bone marrow, lung, or liver.

Gut Masses

Masses that arise from gut may be sufficiently large to be palpated by the clinician and may have a typical sonographic appearance.

Ascites

Often the whole abdomen appears enlarged, and the clinical question is whether or not ascites is present. This is a relatively easy sonographic decision; obese people with much subcutaneous fat may be thought clinically to have ascites when none is actually present. Ultrasonic discovery of ascites is important because aspiration of the ascitic fluid often guides patient management. Causes of ascites include congestive heart failure, liver disease such as cirrhosis or nephrotic syndrome, infections such as tuberculosis and pyogenic peritonitis, malignancy, and blood, for example, from a ruptured aneurysm or trauma.

Bowel Obstruction

Another important cause of overall abdominal distention is intestinal obstruction or paralytic ileus. In these conditions, the gut is very distended. Dilated gut usually contains a mixture of air and fluid, and not much can be seen with ultrasound. If the bowel is entirely filled with fluid and no air is present, the sonogram can help by showing that the bowel is dilated—a finding that may not be appreciated on a plain radiograph. Sonography is particularly helpful if the obstruction is localized to a small segment of bowel.

Abdominal Wall Masses

The nature and presence of masses in the abdominal wall can be usefully clarified by ultrasound. Abscesses may develop in the abdominal wall, whereas a hematocrit drop may be due to a bleed into the rectus muscle.

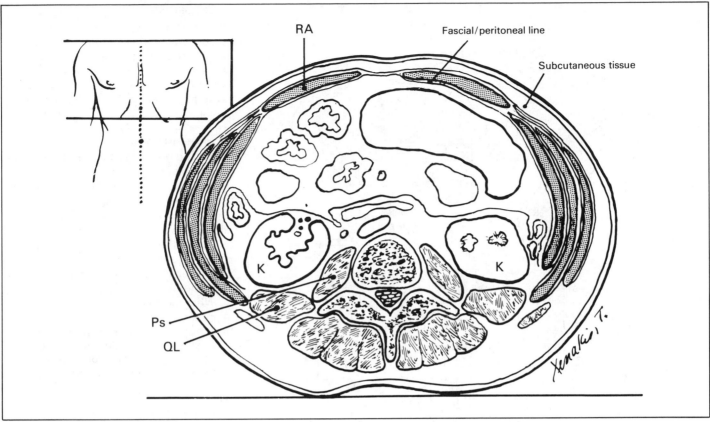

FIGURE 15-1. The rectus muscles (RA) lie on either side of the midline, anteriorly deep to the subcutaneous tissues.

ANATOMY

Aorta

As long as the abdomen does not contain much gas, the aorta and the inferior vena cava can be traced as far as the level of the bifurcation. The SMA, celiac axis, and renal arteries arise from the aorta. There is normally no gap between the spine and the aorta. The iliac arteries cannot usually be seen below the level of the sacral promontory because they are hidden by bowel gas.

Bowel

Most of the time normal bowel is not recognizable because of gas. However, cross-sectional views through normal empty bowel show an echogenic center with a thin echo-free wall (see Fig. 6-14A).

Psoas Muscle

The psoas muscles can be seen on either side of the spine and may be large in muscular individuals (Fig. 15-1). The psoas join with the iliacus muscles, which coat the anterior aspect of the iliac crest, just above the true pelvis.

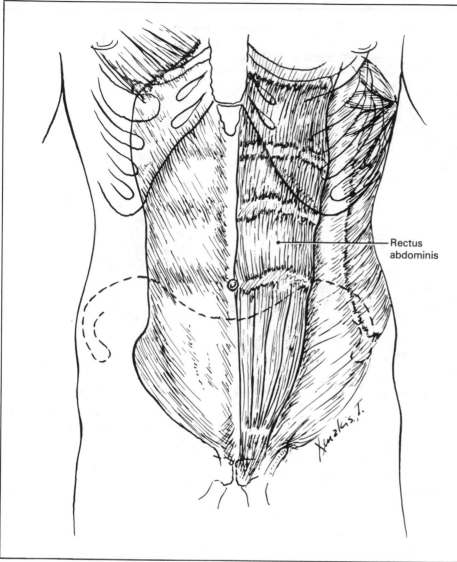

Rectus
abdominis

FIGURE 15-2. Diagram showing the location of the rectus abdominal muscles.

TECHNIQUE

Palpation

After feeling the abdominal mass, examine the same area with ultrasound. It should be immediately apparent whether the mass is superficial in the abdominal wall or is located at a deeper level.

Documentation

Once the mass has been found, obtain pictures that demonstrate the relationship of the abdominal wall, the organs, and the vessels to the mass.

Features of a mass at any site that should be documented are:

1. How it relates to other organs
2. Whether its borders are rough or smooth
3. Whether it is mobile
4. Its size
5. Its consistency in comparison with a known fluid-filled structure such as the gallbladder or bladder (i.e., whether it is cystic or solid).

Aorta

If the mass is clearly aortic in origin, perform longitudinal sections along the aorta, attempting to show both the normal aorta and the aneurysmal segment and to define where the major vessels lie in relation to the aneurysm. When there is considerable gas lying over the aorta, pressure with a linear array or static scan transducer may displace the gas and perhaps allow visualization. Should pressure prove unsuccessful, placing the patient in the left or right decubitus position will allow partial visualization of the aorta in the area of the kidney, although the region of the bifurcation is not usually visible unless the liver is enlarged (see Chapter 12).

Abdominal Wall

The abdominal wall may be the site of an abdominal mass. Hence, the various layers of the abdominal wall should be identified anterior to the peritoneal line (Figs. 15-1 and 15-2). The subcutaneous tissues contain mainly fat and are distinct from the muscular layers.

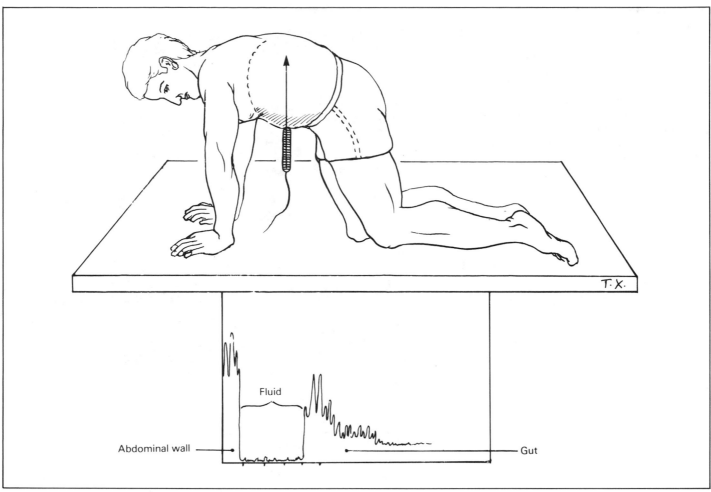

Mesenteric Masses

If the mass is anterior to the aorta within the mesentery, try to show its relationship to the superior mesenteric vein and artery, which lie in the "mesenteric sheath."

A left or right side up view looking through the spleen or liver may be needed to see the para-aortic nodes when gas obscures them in a supine position (see Chapter 12).

Real-time may be necessary to decide whether a possible node in the mesentery is gut or node.

Ascites

If the clinical problem is the presence or absence of ascites and it is not immediately obvious that there is fluid surrounding the bowel, examine the pelvis, the subhepatic space, and the paracolic gutters with the patient in a supine position.

If a very small amount of fluid is suspected and the patient is relatively mobile, place the patient in a knee-elbow position and put an A-mode transducer under the belly. The presence of an echo-free subcutaneous space indicates fluid (Fig. 15-3).

If fluid appears to be loculated in one area such as the subhepatic space place the patient in the Trendelenburg or erect position and note whether the fluid remains in the same position. If it does not shift, an abscess or hematoma should be suspected.

FIGURE 15-3. Diagram showing technique used to discover small quantities of ascitic fluid with A-mode. The A-mode display is shown below.

PATHOLOGY

Aneurysm

Aneurysms are pulsatile dilatations of the aorta. Most are found in the midabdomen just above the bifurcation (Fig. 15-4A,B). Midline aneurysms may bulge in either direction, although they generally bulge to the left. It may be hard to align the aneurysm with the aorta so that both the aneurysm and the normal aorta are shown in a single section (Fig. 15-5).

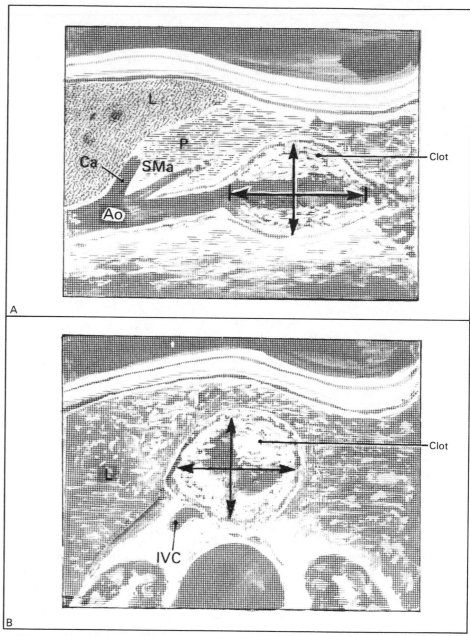

FIGURE 15-4A,B. Abdominal aneurysms are measured to the edge of the wall (arrows). Because they often contain clot there may be a relatively small patent lumen.

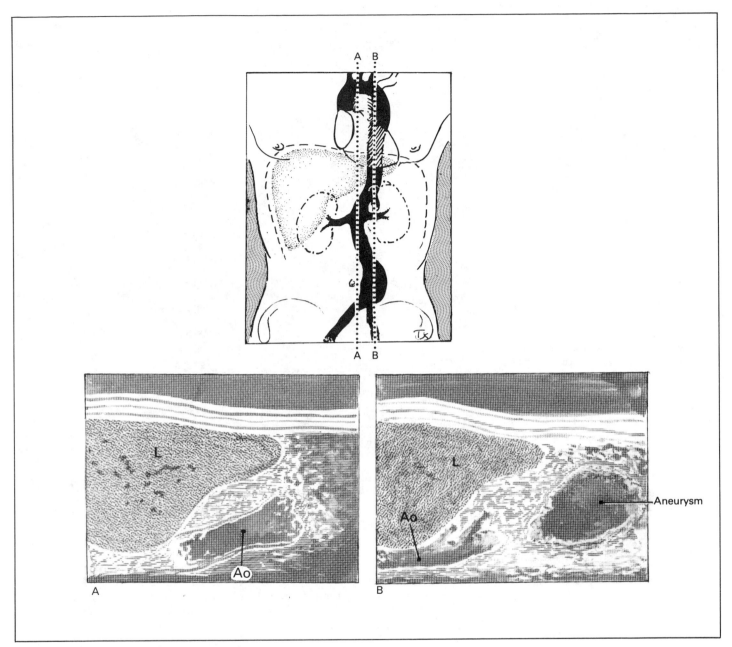

FIGURE 15-5A,B. Because the aneurysmal aorta is often tortuous, complete longitudinal sections through the aorta and the aneurysm may be technically impossible. Line A is drawn through the aorta, where it swings to the right; line B extends through the portion of the aorta where the major vessels arise.

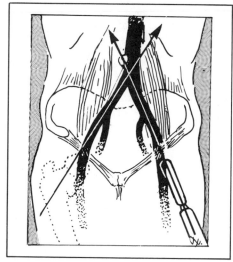

FIGURE 15-6. Attempt to show the iliac arteries by finding the bifurcation of the aorta and the femoral arteries in the groin by palpation. Align the transducer along this axis.

FEATURES TO LOOK FOR IN ANEURYSMS

ILIAC ARTERIES. Lower abdominal aneurysms often involve the iliac arteries. Attempt to show involvement of the iliac arteries by performing an oblique section between the umbilicus and the palpated femoral artery in the groin (Fig. 15-6).

CLOT. Clot may be present within the aneurysm. Make sure that reverberation artifacts are not mistaken for an aneurysm clot.

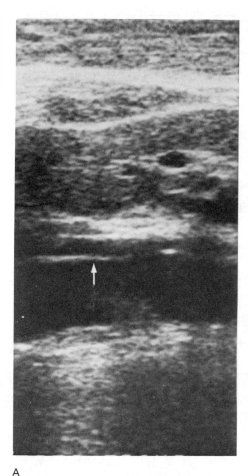

A

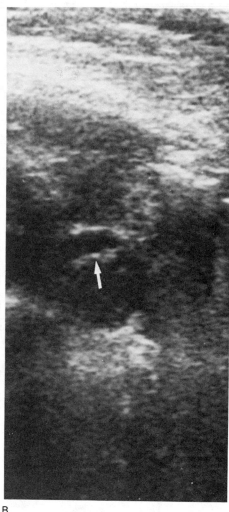

B

FIGURE 15-7A,B. Longitudinal and transverse sonographic views of a dissecting aneurysm. Note the line from the intima that represents one border of the dissection (arrow).

INVOLVEMENT OF MAJOR VESSELS. Some aneurysms of the upper abdominal aorta may involve the celiac axis and the superior mesenteric and renal arteries. Make special efforts to image these vessels because surgical management is altered if there is such involvement. The principal renal arteries are almost always located at the level of the superior mesenteric artery.

DISSECTION. Dissection of an aneurysm is a rare finding in the abdomen. The sonogram will show a line along the middle of the aneurysm that pulsates (Fig. 15-7).

LEAKING ANEURYSM. A fluid collection will be seen alongside the aorta, usually to the left of the spine anterior to the kidney. Another common location is at the junction of a graft and the patient's own aorta or iliac artery.

GRAFTS. Grafts can be recognized by the presence of linear parallel echoes within the aorta and iliac vessels. Frequently the grafts are placed within aneurysms, and the aneurysm is left in place. A baseline study following the operation is helpful because any subsequent changes in graft configuration can be detected.

FALSE ANEURYSMS. False aneurysms are aneurysms that do not have a wall but are surrounded by clot. They are usually masses with a large amount of echogenic material within them and a relatively small patent lumen.

Lymphadenopathy

Most nodes are lobulated, echo-free masses. There are several potential locations for nodes.

PARA-AORTIC NOTES

Such nodes can be lobulated (Fig. 15-8A) or smooth-bordered (Fig. 15-8B). These nodes may surround the aorta so intimately that the wall of the aorta may be invisible (Fig. 15-8B). The aorta is often displaced anteriorly, and the inferior vena cava is almost always displaced anteriorly. Nodes may be seen between the aorta and the inferior vena cava. A common pattern is a node that lies posterior to the inferior vena cava and anterior to the aorta. Nodes between the aorta and the left kidney are frequent.

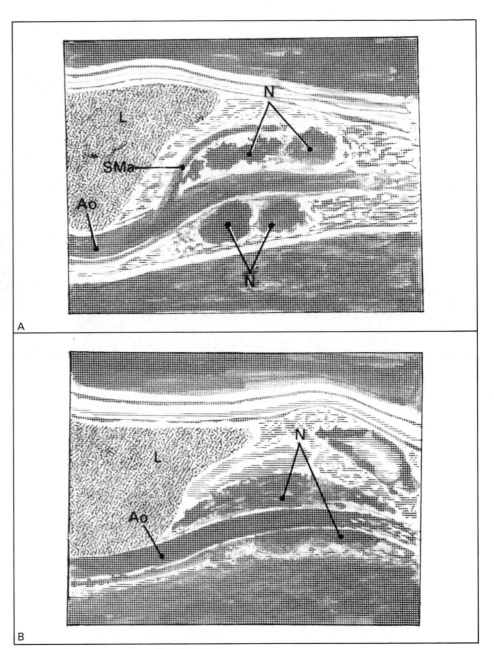

FIGURE 15-8. Para-aortic nodes. A. Lobulated nodes displace the aorta anteriorly and lie between the aorta (Ao) and the superior mesenteric artery (SMa). B. Smooth-bordered nodes silhouetting the aorta make it hard to see the border between the aorta and the nodes. Such a group of nodes may be mistaken for an aneurysm.

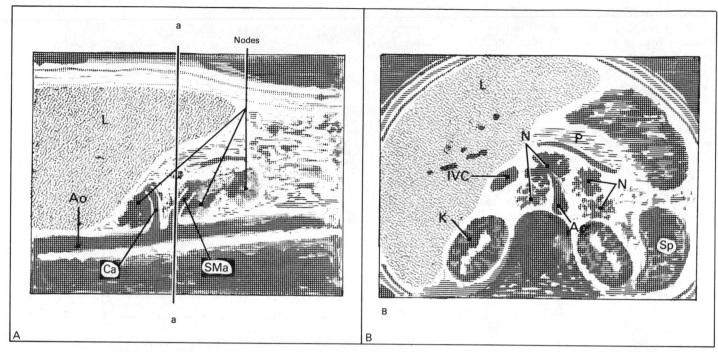

FIGURE 15-9A,B. Nodes straightening and surrounding the celiac axis (Ca) and the superior mesenteric artery (SMa).

CELIAC AXIS NODES

These nodes are sometimes termed porta hepatis nodes because they extend into the porta hepatis. The main bulk of the nodes lies around the celiac axis posterior and superior to the pancreas. They surround and straighten the celiac axis (Fig. 15-9A,B). The pancreas is displaced anteriorly by such nodes.

MESENTERIC NODES

Nodes in the mesentery are characteristically placed longitudinally anterior and posterior to the superior mesenteric artery and vein and the mesenteric sheath to form the so-called sandwich sign (Fig. 15-10). Nodes in the mesentery may be mistaken for gut. They have an ovoid shape and are usually echo-free.

PELVIC NODES

These nodes coat the lateral walls of the pelvis along the iliopsoas muscles in the region of the vessels. They may compress the bladder (Fig. 15-11).

INGUINAL NODES

These nodes are not large but are easily felt. They lie adjacent to the inguinal ligament in the groin.

NODES INVOLVING ORGANS

Any organ can be involved. The nodal mass is usually sonolucent and may be mistaken for a cyst if careful assessment of the degree of through transmission is not made.

Fluid-Filled Loops of Bowel

Bowel loops filled with fluid rather than air are well seen. They form tubular structures and tend to lie in groups (see Fig. 6-14). It is sometimes possible to see the detailed structure of the gut wall (i.e., the valvulae conniventes or the haustral markings). Only a few segments of the dilated bowel loops may be visible because other portions are air-filled.

A real-time examination is worthwhile because if there is no movement within the dilated loop of bowel, paralytic ileus or longstanding obstruction is present. Peristaltic movement indicates a mechanical obstruction.

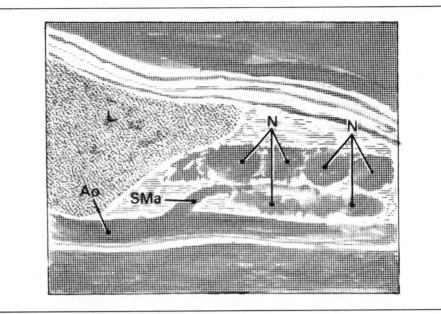

FIGURE 15-10. The sandwich sign. Nodes lie anterior and posterior to the superior mesenteric artery (SMa) and the mesenteric sheath in the mesentery.

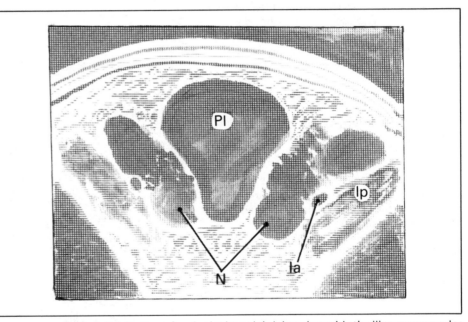

FIGURE 15-11. Typical distribution of nodes in the pelvis lying alongside the iliopsoas muscles (Ip) compressing the bladder.

Gut Mass

A palpable mass may originate from the bowel and may show the target or bull's eye sign. In the pathologic segment of bowel, there is a mass consisting of an echogenic center surrounded by a thick sonolucent rim, which is more than 1 cm wide (Fig. 15-12). This appearance is generally due to a carcinoma of the stomach or colon. Other causes include a variety of other non-neoplastic conditions in which there is bowel wall thickening such as Crohn's disease, ischemic colitis, and intussusception.

Other Mesenteric Masses

Intramesenteric masses within the peritoneum can usually be distinguished from retroperitoneal masses by the absence of distortion of the psoas muscles, kidneys, or quadratus lumborum muscles. Mesenteric masses can be moved from side to side on palpation. The fat line that runs in front of the retroperitoneal tissues will not be displaced anteriorly by the mass. Other than nodes, most intramesenteric masses are relatively benign including mesenteric cysts—large, fluid-filled asymptomatic masses that contain septa and are seen mainly in children, and lipomas—large asymptomatic masses that are evenly echogenic.

Ascites

If there is gross ascites, bowel loops surrounded by fluid will be seen. Small amounts of fluid accumulate first in the (1) subhepatic space along the posterior-inferior border of the liver, (2) in the pelvic cul-de-sac, and (3) in the right paracolic gutter where scanning from a lateral approach is desirable.

It is important to decide whether the ascites is free or loculated. If any segments of bowel are separated from each other or are tethered to the abdominal wall, loculation is present and suggests malignancy or infection (Fig. 15-13).

Internal echoes in fluid suggest infection or malignancy. If infection has occurred in the past, a cobweb-like appearance may be seen within the fluid.

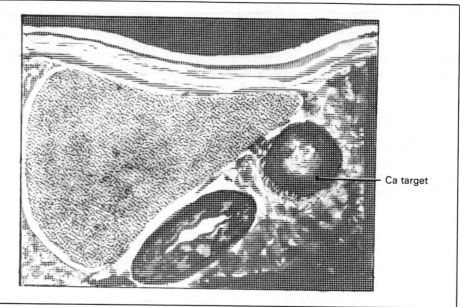

FIGURE 15-12. Target sign of intestinal wall thickening. If the wall is more than 1 cm thick, it is abnormal.

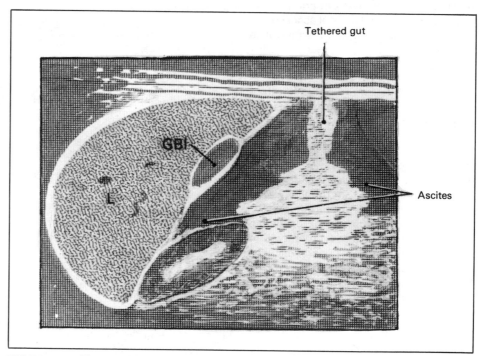

FIGURE 15-13. The usual sites for ascites accumulation are the subhepatic space and the cul-de-sac. In loculated ascites the bowel is tethered to the abdominal wall.

Abdominal Wall Problems

Masses that lie in the abdominal wall are usually easily recognized as superficial by palpation. They remain easily palpable when the patient lifts his head. Gain settings should be set to concentrate on this superficial area.

RECTUS SHEATH HEMATOMA

A rectus sheath hematoma causes enlargement of one of the rectus sheath muscles in the abdominal wall. The other muscle is usually uninvolved (Fig. 15-14).

ABSCESSES

Abscesses do not respect tissue spaces and may involve both the rectus sheath and the area superficial to the muscles (Fig. 15-15).

NEOPLASM

Neoplastic deposits also involve muscle, subcutaneous tissue, and intramesenteric areas but are better demarcated and usually have a more even internal echo than abscesses.

LIPOMA

These benign masses often occur in the abdominal wall and cause an echogenic structure that is seen in the subcutaneous tissues.

HERNIA

An intermittently palpable abdominal mass may be caused by a hernia. Ventral hernias are often associated with a previous incision and are found in the midline. Spigelian hernias are found more laterally. Femoral and inguinal hernias are found in the groin. At the site of a hernia, there will be an interruption of the peritoneal line between the muscles and the contents of the abdomen. It is common to see an area of acoustic shadowing associated with such a mass because the bowel within the hernia contains gas. Such hernias may be intermittent and will become obvious with a change in the patient's position.

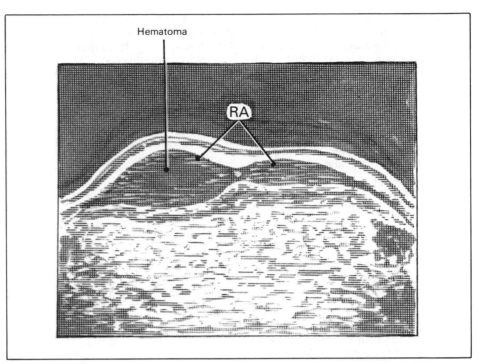

FIGURE 15-14. Widening of the right rectus abdominus muscles due to a hematoma.

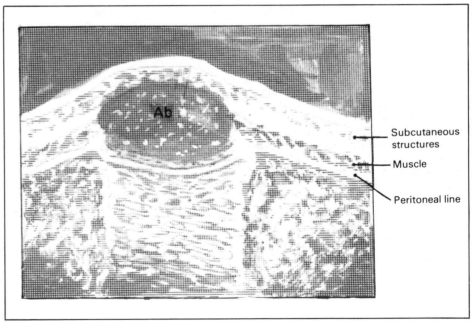

FIGURE 15-15. Abdominal wall abscess (Ab). The abscess has expanded and broken through the tissue planes.

PITFALLS

1. *Abdominal fat.* In obese people the sonolucent area beneath the peritoneum that is due to fat may be confused with ascites but will not be gravity-dependent.

2. *Ovarian cyst.* Ovarian cysts can be huge and may occupy most of the abdomen. They may be confused clinically with ascites because serous fluid will be obtained when a peritoneal tap is performed. The sonographic appearances are quite different because cauliflower-shaped loops of bowel will not be seen within the supposed ascites.

3. *Nodes versus aneurysm.* Para-aortic nodes may be easily confused with an aortic aneurysm. Real-time examination can be helpful, and on transverse sections the shape of the nodes is usually not that of an aneurysm. The overall configuration of adenopathy is lobulated, and the nodes extend laterally over the psoas muscles. An aortic aneurysm will be more or less round.

4. *Dilated bowel loops versus nodes.* Nodes can resemble dilated loops of fluid-filled bowel. Real-time will show evidence of peristalsis in some instances, and a water enema will clarify some problems in the pelvic region. In other cases a further examination on another day may be required to make sure that there has been no change in shape and that the suspect nodes do not represent bowel.

5. *Retrocaval pseudolesions due to mirror artifact.* A mirror-like technical artifact can create an apparent group of nodes posterior to the inferior vena cava on a supine view.

6. *Ascites versus peritoneal dialysis.* When ascites is found, make sure that the patient has not had fluid introduced at the time of peritoneal dialysis for renal failure.

WHERE ELSE TO LOOK

1. *Nodes.* If nodes are found, search for splenomegaly. It supports the diagnosis of lymphoma.

2. *Loculated ascites.* If evidence of loculation of ascites is seen, it is worth looking for evidence of peritoneal metastases adherent to the abdominal wall.

3. *Ascites.* Examine the inferior vena cava and hepatic veins to see if they are unduly dilated as is usual in congestive failure. Study the liver size and shape for any evidence of cirrhosis.

4. *Aneurysm.* If an aneurysm is present, examine the kidneys for secondary hydronephrosis. Try to follow the iliac arteries because they may also be aneurysmal.

SELECTED READING

Callen, P. W., and Marks, W. M. Lymphomatous masses simulating cysts by ultrasonography. *J. Can. Assoc. Radiol.* 30:244–246, 1979.

Carroll, B. A. Ultrasound of lymphoma. *Semin. Ultrasound* 3:114–122, 1982.

Carroll, B. A., and Ta, H. N. The ultrasonic appearance of extranodal abdominal lymphoma. *Radiology* 136:419–425, 1980.

Gooding, G. A. W. Aneurysms of the abdominal aorta, iliac, and femoral arteries. *Semin. Ultrasound* 3:170–179, 1982.

Harter, L. P., Gross, B. H., Callen, P. W., et al. Ultrasonic evaluation of abdominal aortic thrombus. *J. Ultrasound Med.* 1:315–318, 1982.

Lyons, E. A., and Barki, Y. *Ultrasound in the Evaluation of the Pulsatile Epigastric Mass* (Clinics in Diagnostic Ultrasound Series). New York: Churchill Livingstone, 1981.

Mueller, P. R., Ferrucci, J. T., and Harbin, W. P. Appearance of lyphomatous involvement of the mesentery by ultrasonography and body computed tomography: The "sandwich sign." *Radiology* 134:467–473, 1980.

Schnur, M. J., Hoffman, J. C., and Koenigsberg, M. Gray-scale ultrasonic demonstration of peripancreatic adenopathy. *J. Ultrasound Med.* 1:139–143, 1982.

Yeh, H. C., and Rabinowitz, J. G. Ultrasonography of gastrointestinal tract. *Semin. Ultrasound* 3:331, 1982.

16. RENAL FAILURE

SUSAN M. GUIDI
ROGER C. SANDERS

SONOGRAM ABBREVIATIONS

IVC Inferior vena cava

K Kidney

L Liver

Ps Psoas muscle

R Rib
RRv Right renal vein

S Spine
Sp Spleen

KEY WORDS

Anuria. No urine production.

Acute Tubular Necrosis (ATN). Acute renal shutdown following an episode of low blood pressure (hypotension). Spontaneous and fairly rapid recovery is usual, but the condition can be fatal.

Benign Prostatic Hypertrophy (BPH). In older men the prostate is enlarged and replaced by glandular tissue. A large prostate may obstruct the urethra.

Caliectasis. Dilatation of a kidney calyx.

Central Echo Complex (CEC, Sinus Echo Complex). The group of central echoes in the middle of the kidney that are caused by fat.

Column of Bertin. A normal renal variant in which there is enlargement of a portion of the cortex between two pyramids. Can mimic a tumor on pyelography.

Cortex. More peripheral segment of the kidney tissue. Surrounds medulla and sinus echoes.

Dehydration. If a patient does not drink enough fluid, the skin becomes lax and the eyes sunken. Hydronephrosis may be present but may be missed sonographically because the kidneys are not producing much urine.

Dialysis. Technique for removing waste products from the blood when the kidneys do not work properly. (1) *Hemodialysis.* Used in long-term renal failure. The patient's blood is circulated through tubes outside the body, which allow the exchange of fluids and removal of unwanted substances. (2) *Peritoneal dialysis.* A tube is inserted into the abdomen. Fluid containing a number of body constituents is run into the peritoneum, where it exchanges with waste products. This technique is used when renal failure is transient. A sonogram shows evidence of apparent ascites.

Glomerulonephritis. Medical condition with acute and chronic forms in which the kidneys function poorly owing to inflammation. Usually it is a self-limiting condition if acute, but if chronic, it may require long-term treatment with dialysis or transplantation.

Hydronephrosis. Dilatation of the kidney collecting system due to obstruction at the level of the ureter, bladder, or urethra.

Infundibulum (Major Calyx). A tube connecting the pelvis to the calyx.

Medulla. Portion of the kidney adjacent to the calyx; also known as a pyramid. It is less echogenic than the cortex.

Nephrostomy. Tube inserted through the skin into the kidney to drain an obstructed kidney.

Nephrotic Syndrome. Type of medical renal failure, often due to renal vein thrombosis, in which excess protein is excreted by the kidney.

Pyelonephritis (Chronic). Repeated infections destroy the kidneys, which become small with some parenchymal areas narrowed by scar formation.

Pyonephrosis. Hydronephrotic collecting system filled with pus.

Pyramids. See *Medulla* (above).

Serum Creatinine. Waste product that accumulates in the blood when the kidneys are malfunctioning. Levels above approximately 1.0 are abnormal.

Serum Urea Nitrogen (SUN), Blood Urea Nitrogen (BUN). Waste products that accumulate in the blood when the kidneys are malfunctioning. Levels above approximately 40 are abnormal.

Sinus Echo Complex. See *Central Echo Complex* (above).

Staghorn Calculus. Large stone located in the center of the kidney.

Ureterectasis. Dilatation of a ureter.

Ureterocele. Congenital partial obstruction of the ureter at the place where it enters the bladder. A cobra-headed deformity of the lower ureter is seen on pyelography.

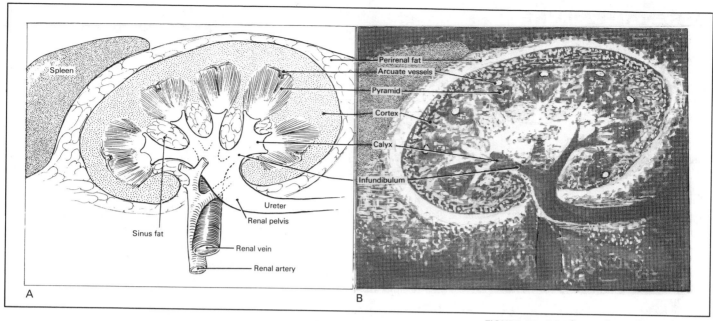

A   B

THE CLINICAL PROBLEM

"Renal failure" occurs when the kidneys are unable to remove waste products from the bloodstream. Waste products used as a measure of the severity of renal failure include the serum creatinine level and the SUN level.

The onset of renal failure is often insidious. The patient may have the condition for months before seeking medical attention with anemia, nausea, vomiting, and headaches. Renal failure may be the result of either kidney disease or lower genitourinary tract disease within the ureter, bladder, or urethra with obstruction of urine excretion.

Medical Renal Disease

Kidney disease can be either an *acute process* or a *chronic* and irreversible one, which is treatable only by dialysis or transplant. In potentially reversible, short-term renal failure (such as ATN or acute glomerulonephritis), the kidneys are normal or large in size. In patients with longstanding renal failure (such as chronic glomerulonephritis or chronic pyelonephritis), the kidneys are small.

Hydronephrosis

By far the most important diagnosis to exclude in patients with renal failure is hydronephrosis. With renal failure both kidneys are likely to be obstructed unless the patient has some other renal disease coincident with obstruction. If obstruction is the sole cause of renal failure, the level of the obstructive site is probably in the bladder or urethra because bilateral ureteral obstruction is not common. Once renal obstruction has been documented, a drainage procedure such as bladder catheterization, nephrostomy, or prostatectomy is urgently required to relieve obstruction. If a drainage procedure is not performed and obstruction persists, kidney function will be permanently impaired. Sonography has largely replaced retrograde pyelography as the screening procedure of choice for hydronephrosis in renal failure.

FIGURE 16-1A,B. Coronal section of left kidney showing major structures. The echogenic area at the center of the kidney is due to renal sinus fat. The pyramids are less echogenic areas adjacent to the sinus. The cortex is slightly more echogenic, and the capsule (perirenal fat) is an echogenic line.

ANATOMY

Length

The normal kidney as measured by ultrasound is between 8 and 13 cm in length in the adult (radiographic measurements are magnified by a factor of 1.3). At birth the kidney is about 4.5 cm in length.

Sinus and Capsular Echoes

The kidney is surrounded by a well-defined echogenic line representing the capsule in the adult (Fig. 16-1). This line may be difficult to see in the infant owing to the sparse amount of perinephric fat. At the center of the kidney are dense echoes (the central sinus echo or sinus echo complex) due to renal sinus fat (Fig. 16-1). In the infant or emaciated patient these echoes may be virtually absent.

Parenchyma

The renal parenchyma has two components. The centrally located pyramids, or medulla, are surrounded on three sides by the peripherally located cortex. The medullary zone or pyramid is slightly less echogenic than the cortex (Fig. 16-1A,B). In infants or thin people a differentiation of medulla from cortex may be very obvious, but in other normal adults this separation may be undetectable.

Column of Bertin

The cortex that usually surrounds and separates the pyramids may be unduly large as a normal variant, in which case it is termed a column of Bertin.

Vascular Anatomy

See Figures 16-1 and 16-3.

RENAL VEINS

These large veins connect the inferior vena cava with the kidneys and lie anterior to the renal arteries. The left renal vein has a long course and passes between the superior mesenteric artery and the aorta.

RENAL ARTERIES

Posteriorly located, the renal arteries may be multiple and too small to visualize but are sometimes seen (Fig. 16-1).

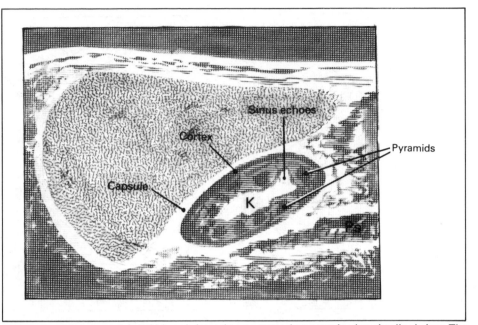

FIGURE 16-2. The normal right kidney is best demonstrated on a supine longitudinal view. The sinus echoes are surrounded by less echogenic pyramids than the neighboring cortex.

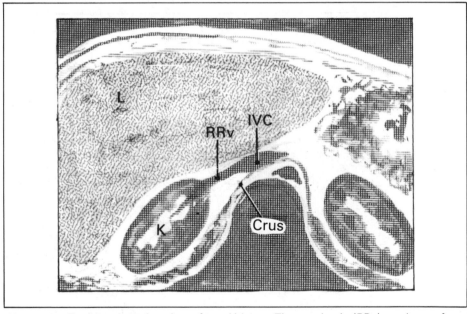

FIGURE 16-3. Transverse supine view of two kidneys. The renal vein (RRv) can be confused with the crus of the diaphragm, but it can be followed into the kidney and can be seen to connect with the inferior vena cava.

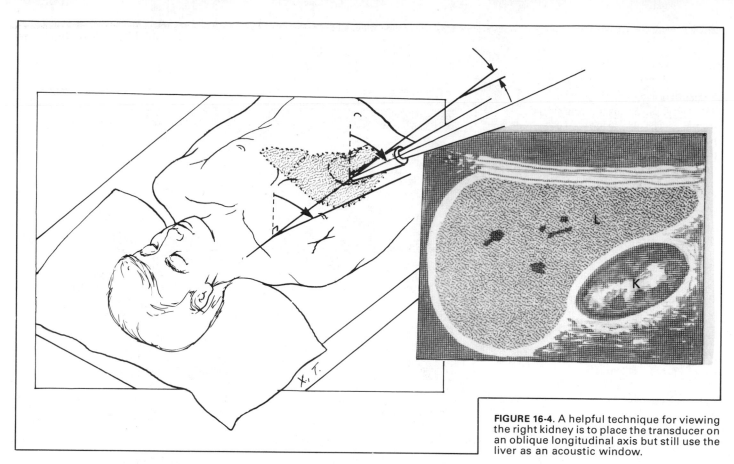

FIGURE 16-4. A helpful technique for viewing the right kidney is to place the transducer on an oblique longitudinal axis but still use the liver as an acoustic window.

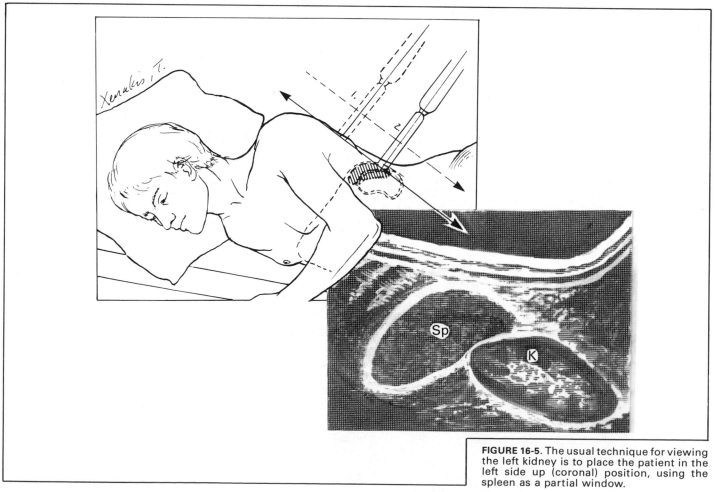

FIGURE 16-5. The usual technique for viewing the left kidney is to place the patient in the left side up (coronal) position, using the spleen as a partial window.

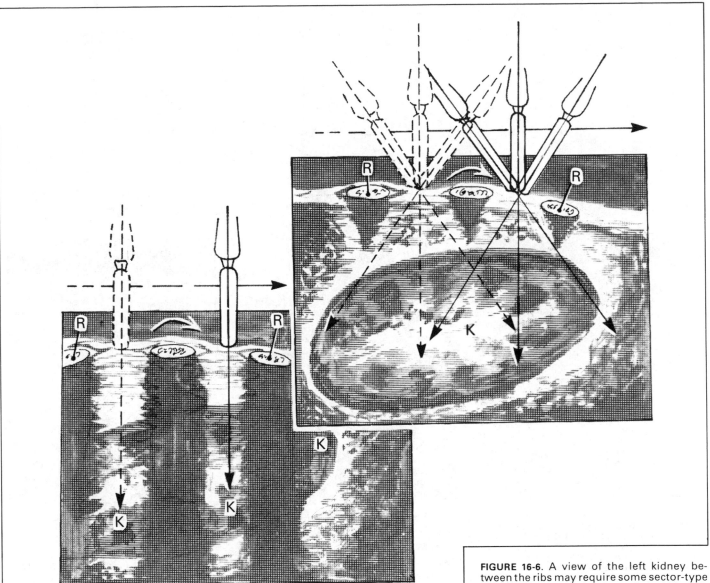

FIGURE 16-6. A view of the left kidney between the ribs may require some sector-type motion. If sectoring is not used, the kidney is obscured by bone in the ribs.

TECHNIQUE

Right Kidney

The right kidney is best seen in the supine position through the liver (Fig. 16-2). Angle the transducer obliquely if the liver is small (Fig. 16-4). Local lateral sector sections may be desirable.

Left Kidney

The left kidney is best seen in the left side up position with the patient leaning slightly forward (coronal view). Although the spleen is used as an acoustic window, it is not a very good one because it is usually small. Placing a pillow under the patient can improve the size of the acoustic window between the iliac crest and the ribs (Fig. 16-5).

Alternative Positions

1. Erect or prone views may be required for either kidney in patients with high livers or small spleens.
2. Suspended maximal inspiration is necessary at times for visualization of the upper pole.
3. Intercostal views are sometimes most helpful (Fig. 16-6).

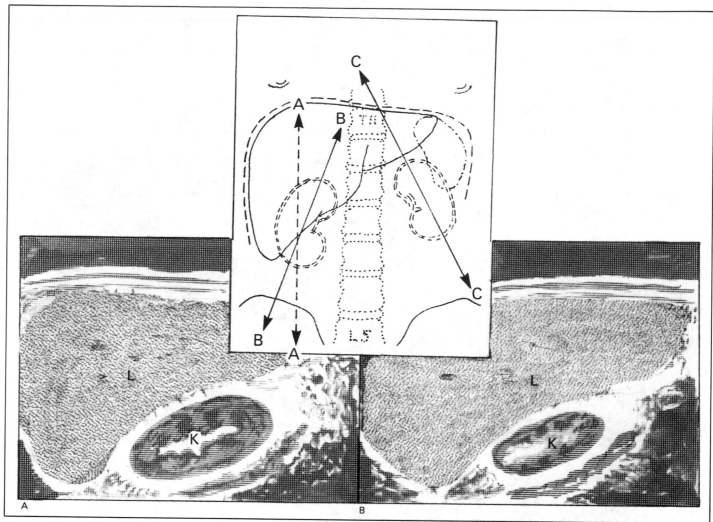

FIGURE 16-7. Renal length. The longest renal length (lines B and C) should be obtained. A length taken along a standard longitudinal view of the kidney, (line A) is too short. The kidneys usually have a slightly oblique axis.

Length

Make sure you have found the longest length of the kidney by trying various oblique views to see which yields the largest value (Fig. 16-7).

Portable Studies

Renal failure often has to be investigated on an emergency basis with a portable unit. Either a linear array or a mechanical sector scanner is a satisfactory means of excluding the possibility of hydronephrosis. Real-time is helpful because it readily shows that the cystic spaces interconnect that form the hydronephrotic kidney.

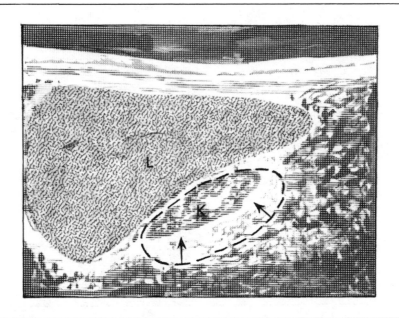

FIGURE 16-8. A small, shrunken, misshapen kidney (arrows) is usually a long-term consequence of chronic pyelonephritis. The dotted lines indicate the original kidney size.

PATHOLOGY

Acute Medical Renal Disease

1. The kidneys are normal in length or enlarged.
2. There is generally increased parenchymal echogenicity compared with the liver (the normal ratio of echogenicity is kidney < spleen < liver < pancreas). The degree of parenchymal echogenicity can be graded as follows:

Grade I. The renal parenchymal echogenicity equals that of the liver.

Grade II. The renal parenchymal echogenicity is greater than that of the liver.

Grade III. The echogenicity of the renal parenchyma is equal to the renal sinus echoes.

Small End-Stage Kidney

1. Both kidneys are small, 5 to 8 cm in length, but renal sinus echoes are visible.
2. The amount of renal parenchyma is usually shrunken. Focal loss of parenchyma indicates chronic pyelonephritis or a renal infarct (Fig. 16-8).
3. The renal parenchyma may show evidence of increased echogenicity.

Infantile Polycystic Kidney

This condition causes bilateral enlarged kidneys. One or two small cysts may be seen. Most of the cysts are too small to be resolved as cystic spaces but are large enough to cause echoes. Increased echoes due to hepatic fibrosis may be noted in the liver parenchyma.

Vascular Disease

RENAL ARTERY OCCLUSION

Bilateral renal artery occlusion can be a cause of renal failure. We have not convincingly demonstrated an occluded artery sonographically. An infarcted kidney enlarges at first but later shrinks in size. Focal infarcts are echopenic at first but may later become echogenic.

RENAL VEIN THROMBOSIS

Renal vein thrombosis can cause renal failure and the nephrotic syndrome. The inferior vena cava may contain internal echoes due to clot. On rare occasions clot within the renal vein has been documented. In such a case the kidneys will be enlarged with multiple echoes in the sinus and medullary areas.

Hydronephrosis

1. The sinus echoes surround a fluid-filled center because the calyces, infundibula, and pelvis are dilated. Usually the renal pelvis is more distended than the calyces. The calyces and infundibula can be traced to the pelvis with real-time (Fig. 16-9A,B,C). The calyces may be so effaced that only a single large sac is seen. However, multiple cystic structures due to dilated calyces may dominate the sonographic picture.

2. The amount of renal parenchyma may be thinned depending on the severity and duration of hydronephrosis.

3. The ureter can sometimes be traced toward the pelvis or seen behind the bladder, indicating that the obstruction is not at the uteropelvic junction.

FIGURE 16-9A,B,C. Varying degrees of dilatation of the renal pelvis due to hydronephrosis. Note the decreased parenchyma as hydronephrosis becomes more severe. The renal parenchyma may shrink to such an extent that only septa are seen between dilated calyces. Note the dominant renal pelvic cystic area in C.

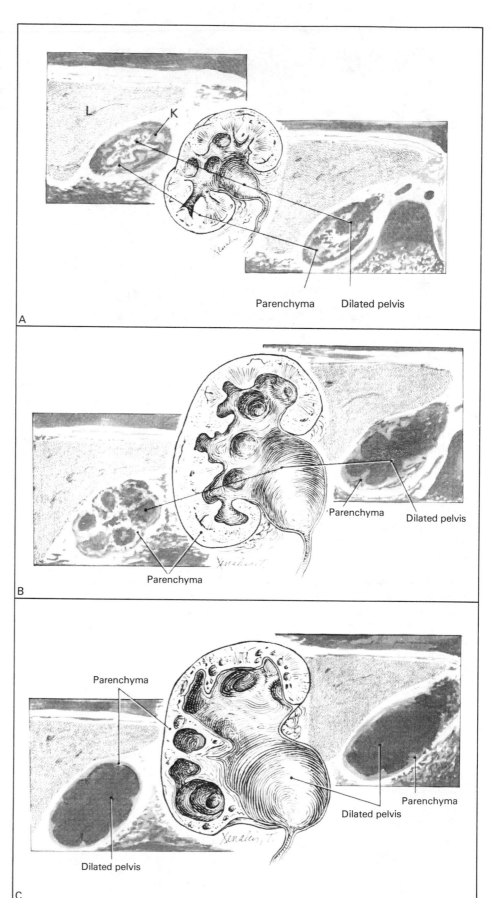

Parenchyma Dilated pelvis

A

Parenchyma Dilated pelvis

Parenchyma

B

Parenchyma

Parenchyma

Dilated pelvis

Dilated pelvis

C

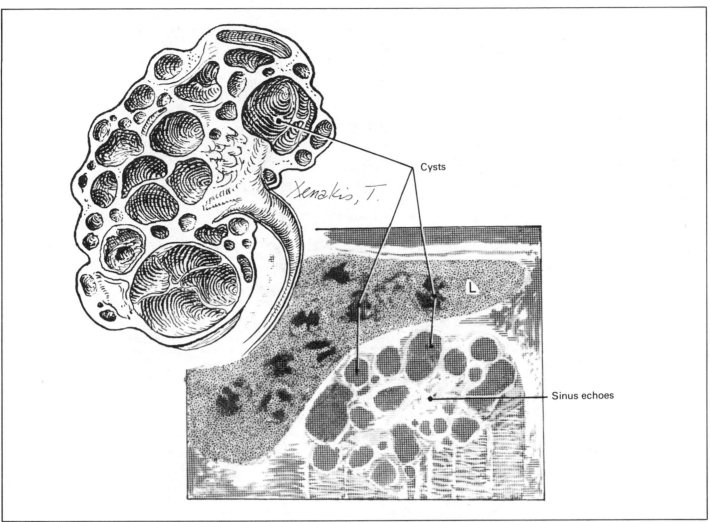

FIGURE 16-10. Adult polycystic disease causes the kidneys to enlarge and develop cysts of differing shapes and sizes. The liver is involved in polycystic disease in 40% of cases.

Adult Polycystic Kidney

1. Both kidneys are involved sonographically and are very large (15 to 18 cm) by the time a patient has renal failure. Multiple cysts with lobulated irregular margins and variable size are present throughout the kidney (Fig. 16-10).

2. The central sinus echo complex may be visible although markedly distorted.

3. In areas where no cysts are sonographically apparent, the renal parenchyma will be more echogenic than usual due to cysts that are too small to be demonstrated with current equipment.

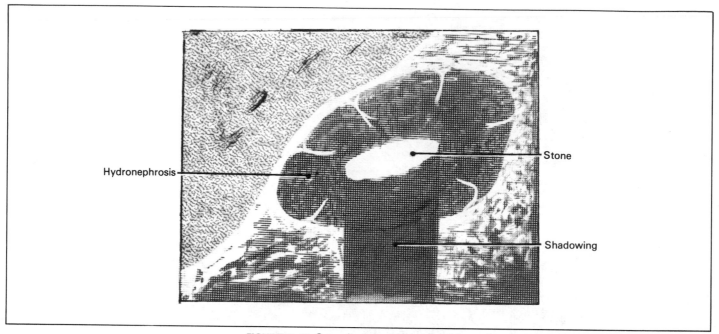

FIGURE 16-11. Gross hydronephrosis with large "staghorn" stone in the center. The staghorn could be mistaken for the renal pelvis, but note the shadowing.

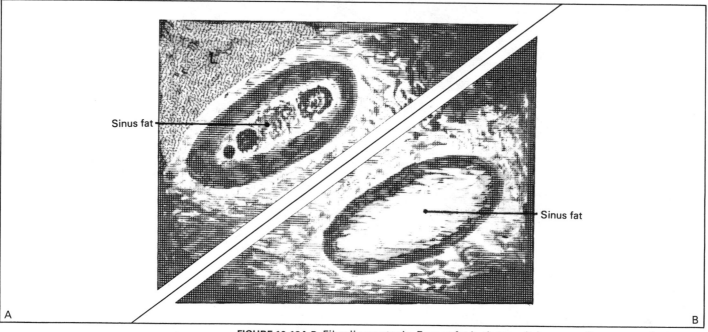

FIGURE 16-12A,B. Fibrolipomatosis. Excess fat in the renal sinus usually causes enlargement of the echogenic center of the kidney; on occasion it may look less echogenic, as in A. The less echogenic appearances can be mistaken for hydronephrosis or transitional cell cancer.

PITFALLS

1. *Pseudohydronephrosis*
   a. Make sure that the bladder is empty before hydronephrosis is diagnosed definitively. In children and in patients with renal transplants, a full bladder can provoke apparent hydronephrosis, which disappears when the bladder is empty.
   b. Try to ensure that apparent hydronephrosis is not caused by a parapelvic cyst. In general, parapelvic cysts do not have a dense echogenic margin as do dilated calyces.
   c. An extrarenal pelvis may mimic hydronephrosis because it is a large cystic structure at the renal hilum. Dilated infundibula may also be seen normally, but connecting calyces will be delicately cupped (if they can be seen).
2. *Possible missed hydronephrosis*
   a. Be cautious about excluding hydronephrosis in the presence of renal calculi, which may obscure dilated calyces.
   b. Make sure that the patient is not considerably dehydrated with lax skin and sunken eyes. Dehydration can mask hydronephrosis.
3. *Calculi.* In the presence of severe hydronephrosis a staghorn calculus can be confused with a normal renal pelvis but will show evidence of shadowing (Fig. 16-11).
4. *Splayed sinus echoes.* Do not overlook relatively mild separation of the renal sinus echoes. The correlation between the severity of hydronephrosis and the degree of separation is not good. Separation of the sinus echoes may be (1) a normal variant due to an extrarenal pelvis, (2) due to a parapelvic cyst, (3) a consequence of overdistention of the bladder, or (4) due to reflux rather than renal obstruction.
5. *Renal parenchyma.* If you are assessing the degree of renal parenchymal echogenicity in comparison with the liver, make sure you think that the liver is normal. Patients with liver disease are prone to renal failure.
6. *Length.* Make sure that you have obtained the longest renal length. Careless technique can make the kidney appear shorter than it really is (Fig. 16-7A,B).
7. *Sinus fat.* The fat within the renal sinus (fibrolipomatosis) can have a confusing sonographic appearance, sometimes appearing more extensive than usual (Fig. 16-12A,B) and at other times appearing less echogenic than normal and mimicking hydronephrosis.

WHERE ELSE TO LOOK

The discovery of *hydronephrosis* should prompt an effort to identify the site of obstruction.

1. Look within the kidney and bladder for *renal calculi* (see Chapter 19). Look for an impacted stone at the ureterovesical junction that may be associated with edema of the bladder wall.
2. Look along the course of the ureter as well as in the pelvis for *masses*.
3. Examine the true pelvis to see if the bladder is distended. If it is, look for evidence of *bladder neoplasm* or *prostatic hypertrophy* (see Chapter 19).
4. Follow the course of the ureter behind the bladder; a *ureterocele* may be present.

SELECTED READING

Resnick, M., and Sanders, R. (Eds.). *Ultrasound in Urology.* Baltimore: Williams & Wilkins, 1979.

Rosenfeld, A. I., Taylor, K. J. W., Dembner, A. G., et al. Ultrasound of the renal sinus. *A.J.R.* 133:441, 1979.

17. POSSIBLE RENAL MASS

ROGER C. SANDERS

SONOGRAM ABBREVIATIONS

Ao Aorta

Bl Bladder

K Kidney

L Liver

Sp Spleen

KEY WORDS

Angiomyolipoma. Rare, benign, fatty tumor of the kidney associated with tuberous sclerosis; usually seen in middle-aged women.

Calyx (Calyces). A portion of the renal collecting system adjacent to the renal pyramid in which urine collects and which is connected to an infundibulum.

Calyceal Diverticulum. Postinflammatory fluid-filled structure adjacent to a pyramid.

Dromedary Hump. A bulge off the lateral margin of the left kidney—a normal variant.

Ectopic Ureterocele. The ureter inserts abnormally into the bladder, resulting in a balloon-shaped (cobra-headed) deformity of the bladder wall around the ureterovesical junction.

Fibrolipomatosis. Excess fat deposition in the center of the kidney; seen with aging.

Hydronephrosis. Dilatation of the pelvic collecting system due to obstruction.

Hypernephroma (Renal Cell Carcinoma, Von Clawitz Tumor). Interchangeable terms used for adenocarcinoma of the kidney.

Infundibulum. Funnel-shaped tube connecting the calyx to the renal pelvis. Also known as a major calyx.

Renal Pelvis. Sac into which the various infundibula drain. The pelvis drains into the ureter.

Transitional Cell Carcinoma. A tumor of the kidney, collecting system, ureter, or bladder lining cells that often recurs in another site in the genitourinary tract after removal.

Tuberous Sclerosis. A disease manifest by skin lesions, mental deficiency, and renal angiomyolipoma. Milder forms occur with only one manifestation.

Uric Acid Calculus. A renal stone that is invisible on plain radiographs.

THE CLINICAL PROBLEM

Although the intravenous pyelogram (IVP) remains the usual method of detecting renal masses, it does not effectively aid in deciding whether such a mass is fluid-filled (a cyst) or solid tissue—a decision that can be made with ultrasound. Cysts are managed by cyst puncture or benign neglect, whereas tumors need operation. If the patient is not in renal failure, do not perform a sonogram without first examining the IVP, if available, so you know exactly where to look for the abnormality.

ANATOMY

See Chapter 16.

TECHNIQUE

See Chapter 16. Real-time is helpful for examining the inferior vena cava and the renal vein to detect tumor involvement as well as for looking at stones. Some stones and their shadowing are only visible with real-time.

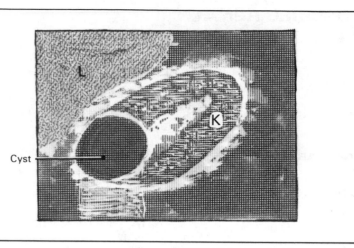

FIGURE 17-1. A cyst at the upper pole of the kidney shows good through transmission, smooth borders, and absence of internal echoes.

PATHOLOGY

Fluid-Filled Masses

RENAL CYSTS

Renal cysts (Fig. 17-1) are common in the elderly and are not too rare in younger people. They may be single or multiple. The sonographic features of a cyst are

1. Acoustic enhancement (good through transmission)
2. Usually a smooth spherical outline
3. Usually no internal echoes

Unusual cysts may have irregular walls and may contain low-level echoes in a dependent position owing to debris. Septa dividing a cyst into compartments may be seen (Fig. 17-2). Such septa prove that a cyst is fluid-filled but may be difficult to visualize completely and may be mistaken for a mural mass. Peripelvic cysts may be centrally located and hard to distinguish from a dilated pelvis or calyx (Fig. 17-4B).

POLYCYSTIC DISEASE

Renal cysts in patients with polycystic disease are usually multiple, have an irregular outline, and are of markedly varied size (Fig. 17-3A). The background parenchymal echogenicity is often increased in polycystic disease due to small cysts that are not large enough to be seen as fluid-filled structures but are large enough to cause echoes. Multiple simple cysts can occur but are fewer in number, more equal in size, and smoother in outline than the cysts seen in polycystic disease (Fig. 17-3B).

CALYCEAL ENLARGEMENT

Calyceal diverticula and locally obstructed calyces look like cysts but connect with the pelvocalyceal system. They are generally surrounded by an echogenic border owing to sinus fat.

SECOND COLLECTING SYSTEM

An upper pole, congenitally duplicated hydronephrotic collecting system may look like a cyst but will usually have a septum separating the calyces.

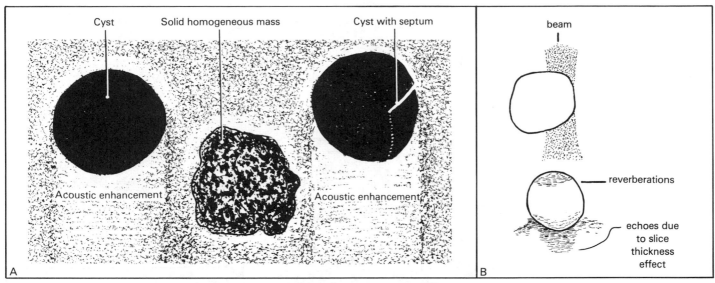

FIGURE 17-2. Cyst versus solid homogeneous mass. A. Diagram showing the difference between a cyst and a solid homogeneous mass. Through transmission beyond a solid homogeneous mass is limited, although there will be a back wall, and there are usually a few internal echoes. Septa are incompletely seen unless they are at right angles to the acoustic beam. B. Artifactual echoes due to reverberations and slice thickness effect.

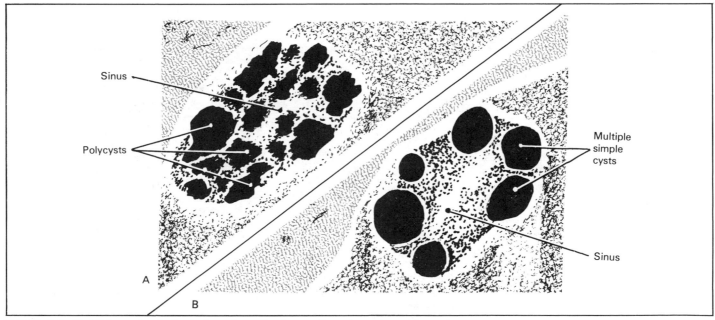

FIGURE 17-3. Multiple cysts. A. Cysts in polycystic disease have irregular walls and are variable in size. They distort the renal sinus echoes. B. Multiple simple cysts have smooth walls, are not nearly as numerous, and vary less in size.

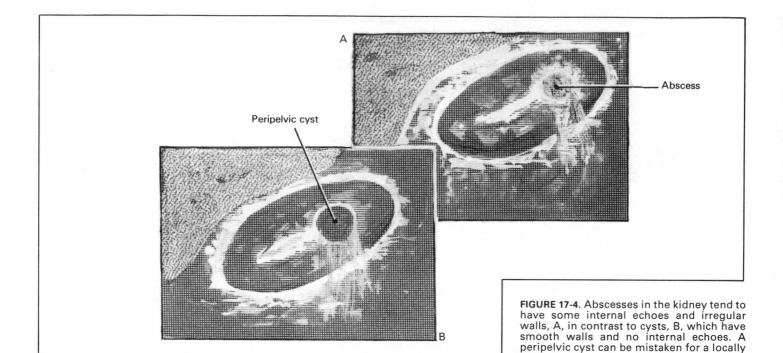

FIGURE 17-4. Abscesses in the kidney tend to have some internal echoes and irregular walls, A, in contrast to cysts, B, which have smooth walls and no internal echoes. A peripelvic cyst can be mistaken for a locally dilated calyx.

ABSCESS

Abscesses contain fluid but are rarely totally echo-free (Fig. 17-4A). They often contain a number of internal echoes and have an irregular border that looks something like a tumor.

HEMATOMA

Hematomas that occur following trauma have varied sonographic appearances. They may be entirely fluid-filled or may contain internal echoes of an irregular pattern.

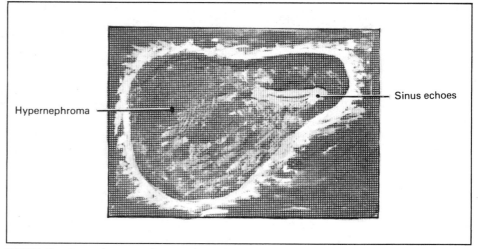

FIGURE 17-5. Large hypernephroma expanding the upper pole of the kidney. Notice that it is only slightly more echogenic than the renal parenchyma. Hypernephroma are frequently relatively hypoechoic but show poor through transmission.

Neoplastic Masses

TUMORS

These masses contain internal echoes, do not show good through transmission, and usually have an irregular border that expands the outline of the kidney. Most hypernephromas have the same or a little less echogenicity than the adjacent renal parenchyma (Fig. 17-5) but have one or two dense internal echoes in addition. Some are more echogenic than the remaining kidney.

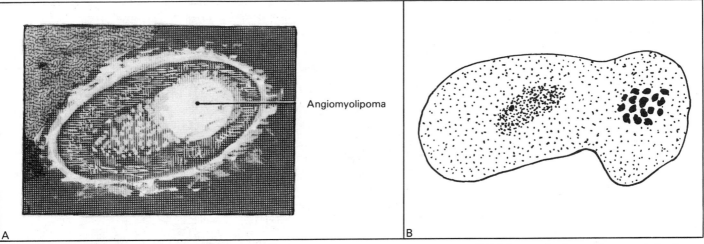

FIGURE 17-6. Angiomyolipoma at the lower pole of the kidney. Angiomyolipomas are almost always densely echogenic.

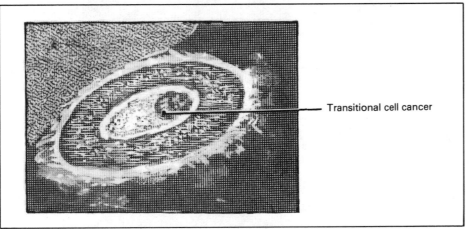

FIGURE 17-7. Transitional cell cancer involving the sinus of the kidney, causing a hypoechoic area.

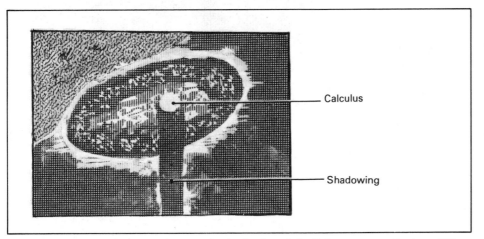

FIGURE 17-8. Renal calculus with acoustic shadowing. Calculi do not cause shadows if they are small (less than about 5 mm).

ANGIOMYOLIPOMA

A highly echogenic tumor should suggest an angiomyolipoma (Fig. 17-6), but may be a hypernephroma.

TUMORS IN CYSTS

Tumors may occur within cysts with focal irregularity of the cyst wall at one site. However, the iregularity may be due to a septum. A cyst with an irregular wall and internal echoes is usually subjected to cyst puncture or CT scan to rule out neoplasm.

TRANSITIONAL CELL TUMORS

Tumors such as transitional cell carcinoma (Fig. 17-7) do occur in the renal pelvis and are difficult to distinguish from fibrolipomatosis.

LYMPHOMA

If the suspect mass has no internal echoes but rather poor through transmission, an acoustically homogeneous tumor, typically lymphoma, should be considered.

FILLING DEFECTS IN RENAL PELVIS (CALCULI)

A small filling defect in the renal pelvis on IVP has a number of possible causes, including transitional cell cancer. Some are due to uric acid stones. Stones can be recognized on sonography by an acoustic shadow arising from the renal pelvis echoes (Fig. 17-8).

PITFALLS

1. *Normal variants versus pseudolesions.* Normal variants or congenital abnormalities may create the impression of a mass.

   a. An *enlarged spleen* or liver can compress the kidney, causing an apparently abnormal IVP appearance (Fig. 17-9).

   b. The left kidney often has a hump on its lateral aspect known as a *"dromedary"* hump (Fig. 17-10).

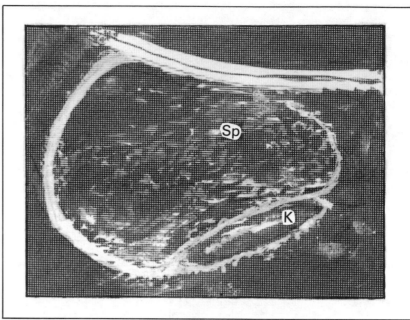

FIGURE 17-9. The left kidney is squashed by an enlarged spleen. Splenomegaly can cause an apparent renal mass on an intravenous pyelogram.

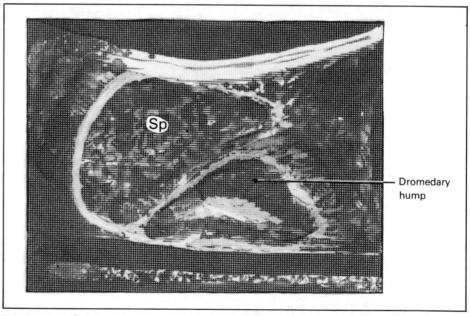

FIGURE 17-10. Bulge at the lateral border of the left kidney known as a dromedary hump, a normal variant.

c. A *bifid pelvocalyceal pattern* may suggest a central mass on the IVP. The intervening tissue between the two portions of the collecting system appears sonographically normal (Fig. 17-11).

d. A *pelvic kidney* has a normal appearance in an abnormal location (Fig. 17-12).

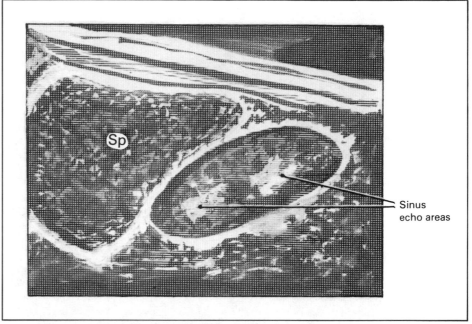

FIGURE 17-11. Bifid pelvicalyceal system; the sinus echoes are separated into two groups. A similar appearance is seen with a double collecting system.

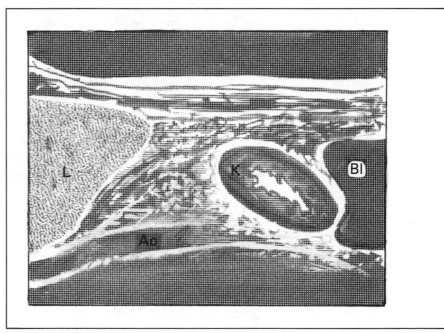

FIGURE 17-12. Pelvic kidney. A sonographically normal kidney is located in the pelvis.

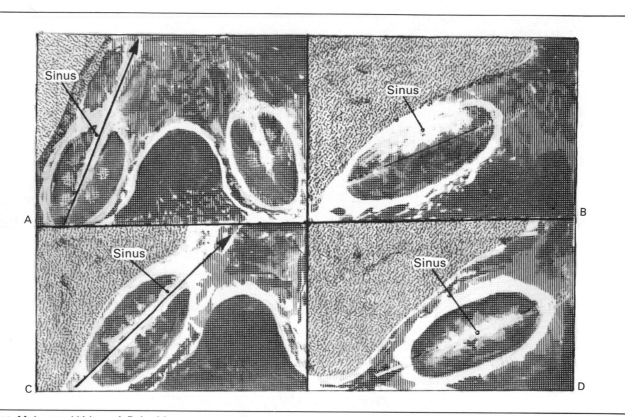

FIGURE 17-13. Malrotated kidney. A,B. In this variant the axis of the kidney is rotated so that the sinus echoes exit in an anterior direction. Compare with the normal findings in C and D.

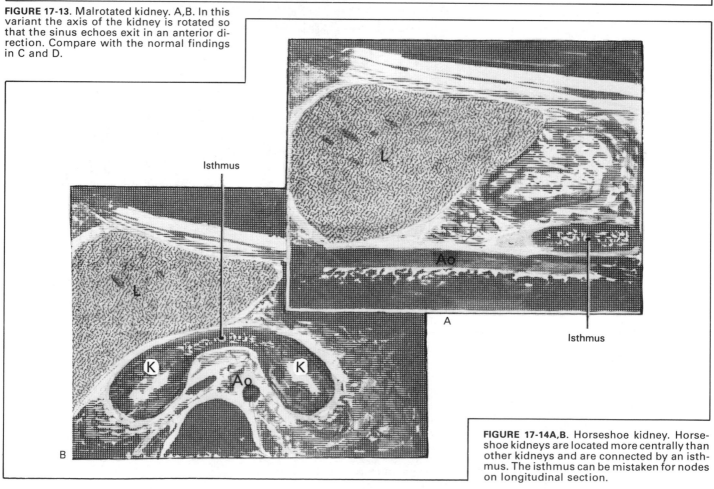

FIGURE 17-14A,B. Horseshoe kidney. Horseshoe kidneys are located more centrally than other kidneys and are connected by an isthmus. The isthmus can be mistaken for nodes on longitudinal section.

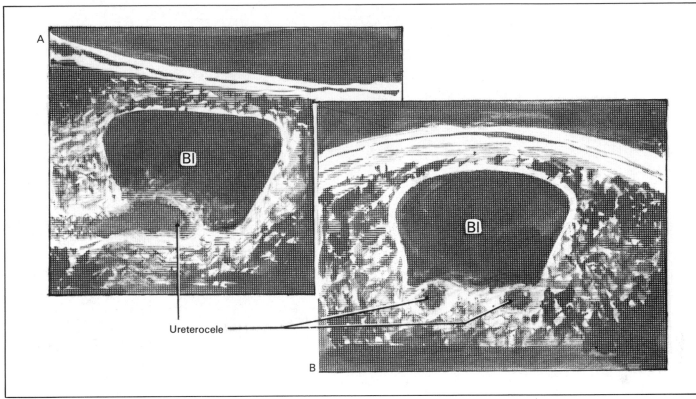

FIGURE 17-15A,B. An ectopic ureterocele, a cause of hydronephrosis and ureterectasis, is seen indenting the bladder (Bl). This is a congenital variant.

e. *Malrotated kidneys* often look abnormal on IVP but are normal, except for an unusual axis, on the sonogram (Fig. 17-13).

f. *Fibrolipomatosis,* excessive fatty infiltration of the renal pelvis, is often a consequence of aging. The sonographic appearances are variable and include (1) an enlarged central echogenic complex, (2) fat that may be relatively sonolucent, giving the impression of mass lesions, and (3) fat that may be densely echogenic (see Chapter 16).

g. *Horseshoe kidneys* are deceptive sonographically (Fig. 17-14A,B). The kidneys are medially placed and are often difficult to see on a supine view because of overlying gas. An isthmus of tissue connects the inferior portions of the segments of the horseshoe kidney. However, this feature can be difficult to demonstrate owing to the overlying bowel gas; if seen, it may be misdiagnosed as nodes or retroperitoneal fibrosis.

2. *Cyst versus neoplasm.* A cyst may be difficult to distinguish from a solid homogeneous mass (Fig. 17-2A). The use of A-mode or higher frequency transducers may more easily demonstrate good through transmission. The presence of a septum indicates

that the structure is fluid-filled. Look at the inner wall of the cyst in a supine, longitudinal, decubitus position so that wall irregularities can be clearly seen. Echoes on the transducer side of the cyst may be due to reverberations, and on the far side, to the "slice thickness" effect (Fig. 17-2B; see Chapter 45).

3. *"Blown" calyx versus cyst.* Remember to look at the IVP because a cystic lesion in the kidney might be a focally dilated portion of the renal collecting system.

4. *Tumor origins.* Subtle changes in the renal parenchyma that are indicative of tumor may be missed if a white background is used. It is easier to see parenchymal changes on a black background.

5. *Arcuate vessels.* The arcuate vessels may give rise to some subtle acoustic shadowing and mimic the appearance of a stone.

WHERE ELSE TO LOOK

1. With any *renal tumor,* examine the renal vein and the inferior vena cava for *tumor extension (clot).* Look for para-aortic nodes and for liver metastases.

2. With *polycystic disease* of the kidney, examine the liver, pancreas, and spleen for associated cysts. Forty percent of patients with polycystic disease have liver cysts.

3. With a more or less *echo-free mass,* think of *lymphoma* and look for evidence of *splenomegaly* and para-aortic *adenopathy.*

4. With a *tumor in the renal pelvis,* examine the bladder. There may be a synchronous *transitional cell tumor* there as well.

5. With *localized hydronephrosis* of the upper pole of the kidney, look in the bladder for an ectopic *ureterocele* into which the duplicated ureter inserts (Fig. 17-15A,B).

SELECTED READING

Resnick, M., and Sanders, R. (Eds.). *Ultrasound in Urology.* Baltimore: Williams & Wilkins, 1979.

Sanders, R. C. Kidneys. In B. B. Goldberg (Ed.), *Ultrasound in Cancer* (Clinics in Diagnostic Ultrasound Series, Vol. 6). New York: Churchill Livingstone, 1981.

18. KIDNEY NOT SEEN ON INTRAVENOUS PYELOGRAM

ROGER C. SANDERS

THE CLINICAL PROBLEM

If one kidney is poorly seen or not seen at all on the intravenous pyelogram (IVP), a number of possible explanations can be offered. Perhaps the commonest is hydronephrosis (previously discussed in Chapter 16). Other causes include multicystic dysplastic kidney (see Chapter 14) and small kidneys (see Chapter 16). A tumor may also be responsible for nonvisualization of the kidney on IVP if it is large enough to involve the whole kidney or has occluded the renal vein (see Chapter 17). This chapter will consider a few other rare problems that may cause unilateral nonvisualization of the kidney on IVP (end-stage kidney, renal vein thrombosis, renal artery occlusion, xanthogranulomatous pyelonephritis, and pyonephrosis).

ANATOMY AND TECHNIQUE

These topics have already been discussed in Chapter 16.

PATHOLOGY

Small End-Stage Kidney

As mentioned previously, the kidney in end-stage renal failure shrinks to about 6 cm in length before the patient experiences serious clinical problems. However, if only one kidney is small and diseased, (for example, in recurrent unilateral pyelonephritis), the kidney may be extremely small. In fact, the kidney may be almost impossible to visualize, yet the patient will be asymptomatic. Even when an end-stage kidney measures only 2 to 3 cm in length, an echogenic center and some renal parenchyma will still be visible. The parenchyma may show evidence of focal narrowing due to scars (see Fig. 16-8).

Renal Vascular Problems

RENAL ARTERY OCCLUSION (INFARCT, EMBOLUS)

If the arterial blood supply to the kidney is occluded, little immediate change takes place in the sonographic appearance. The kidney first swells and then slowly shrinks over a period of weeks or months. Thus a surprising dichotomy arises between the sonogram and the IVP. The IVP demonstrates nonvisualization, whereas for some time the sonogram looks almost normal.

RENAL VEIN THROMBOSIS

Renal vein thrombosis occurs in both acute and chronic forms. In the acute form the kidney swells, and the central sinus echoes usually become more prominent, although this is a variable phenomenon. Sometimes thrombosis can actually be visualized within the renal vein. In the chronic form, the kidney is small and somewhat echogenic.

Xanthogranulomatous Pyelonephritis

This rare infection is associated with renal calculi and hydronephrosis. A large staghorn calculus is usually present with secondary hydronephrosis and echogenic changes in the parenchyma. A rare focal form in which there is a mass lesion with increased echogenicity due to fat may occur.

Pyonephrosis

A unilateral hydronephrotic kidney filled with stagnant urine may become infected and filled with pus. This life-threatening condition can rapidly lead to death if it is not discovered and treated rapidly. Sometimes the kidney has an appearance that is indistinguishable from ordinary noninfected hydronephrosis. More often, low-level echoes will occur throughout the pus-filled renal pelvis. A fluid-fluid level may even develop. Percutaneous nephrostomy under ultrasonic control may be lifesaving.

PITFALLS

A very small end-stage kidney can easily be mistaken for the target sign seen with loops of bowel. Conversely, make sure that an apparently small kidney is not a relatively empty colon by examining it with real-time.

SELECTED READING

Sanders, R. C. Normal Ultrasonic Renal Anatomy. In M. Resnick and R. Sanders (Eds.), *Ultrasound in Urology.* Baltimore: Williams & Wilkins, 1979.

19. HEMATURIA, PROSTATE SIZE, AND PROSTATE ABNORMALITIES

ROGER C. SANDERS

SONOGRAM ABBREVIATIONS

Bl   Bladder

Ip   Iliopsoas muscle

L   Liver

Ob   Obturator muscle

Pr   Prostate gland

Sp   Symphysis pubis
SV   Seminal vesicle

Ur   Urethra

KEY WORDS

Benign Prostatic Hypertrophy (BPH). Enlargement of the glandular component of the prostate. The true prostate forms a shell around the enlarged gland.

Cystitis. Infection or inflammation of the wall of the bladder.

Nephrocalcinosis. Multiple small calculi deposited in the renal pyramids. Found in association with renal tubular acidosis and medullary sponge kidney.

Pyelonephritis. Infection of the kidney without abscess formation.

Seminal Vesicles. Paired organs located posterior to the bladder in which semen collects.

Trigone. Base of the bladder. Area between the insertion of the ureters and the urethra.

Urethra. Urinary outflow tract below the bladder.

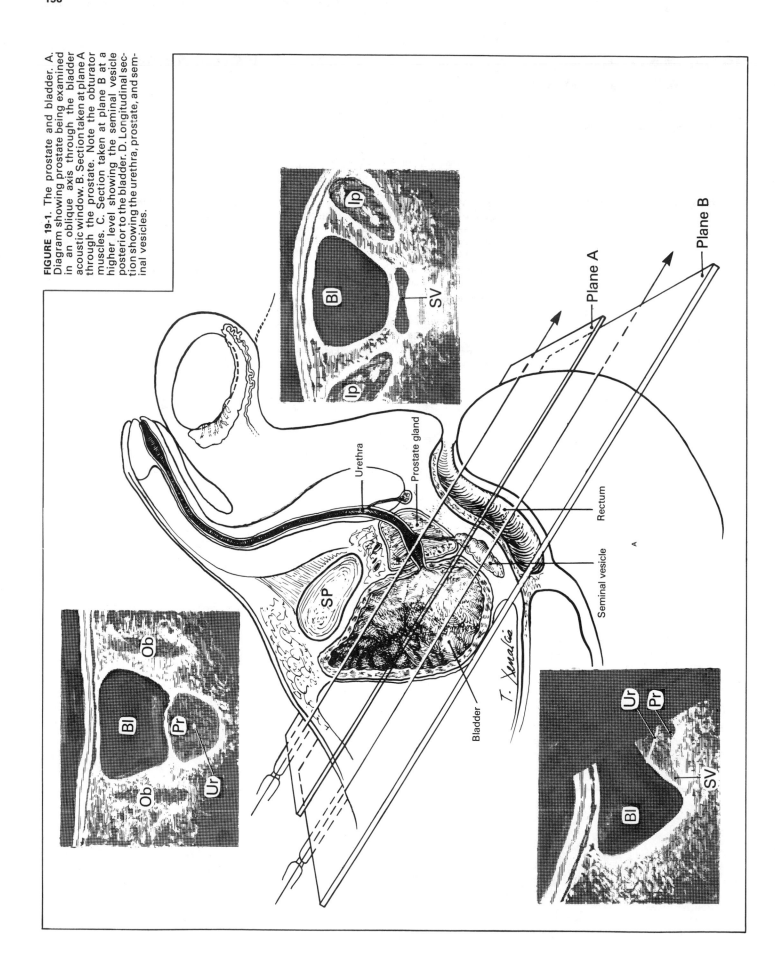

FIGURE 19-1. The prostate and bladder. A. Diagram showing prostate being examined in an oblique axis through the bladder acoustic window. B. Section taken at plane A through the prostate. Note the obturator muscles. C. Section taken at plane B at a higher level showing the seminal vesicle posterior to the bladder. D. Longitudinal section showing the urethra, prostate, and seminal vesicles.

Plane A

Plane B

Urethra

Prostate gland

Rectum

Seminal vesicle

Bladder

T. Xenakis

Ip

Bl

SV

Ip

Ob

Bl

Pr

Ob

Ur

Ur

Pr

Bl

SV

SP

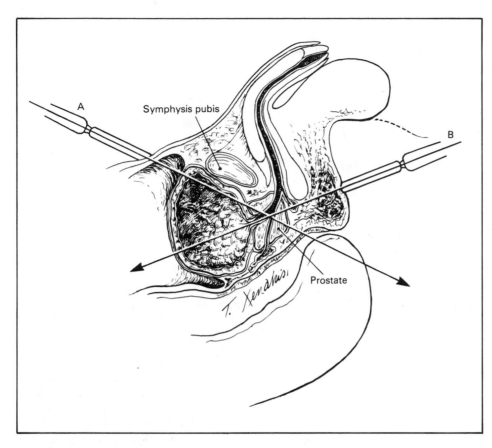

FIGURE 19-2. Diagram showing two approaches used to avoid the bone in the symphysis pubis when scanning the prostate. From an abdominal approach, A, the transducer is tilted toward the feet at an angle of 15° to 30°; the beam passes through the acoustic window of the bladder to the prostate. A second approach, B, uses the perineum as a window for viewing the prostate. The sonographer scans through a site posterior to the scrotum.

Bladder

The bladder can be examined only when it is distended. The transducer is pressed, if necessary somewhat vigorously, into a site just above the pubic symphysis and arched superiorly to show the upper portions of the bladder wall. The bladder normally has a smooth curved surface and is surrounded by an echogenic line that represents the wall. The anterior wall of the bladder can not be seen adequately owing to reverberations unless a water bath technique is used (Fig. 19-1).

Prostate

A similar technique is used to evaluate the prostate except that the transducer is arched inferiorly under the pubic symphysis. Transverse sections are performed at an angulation of about 15° toward the feet (Fig. 19-2).

PERINEAL APPROACH

Imaging the prostate from an abdominal approach may be difficult if the bladder cannot be filled adequately. A perineal approach can be used, scanning between the legs behind the scrotum. This will help to give a more complete view of the overall prostatic size (Fig. 19-2).

CATHETERIZATION

It may be necessary to insert a catheter to fill the bladder adequately. One cannot perform a satisfactory ultrasonic examination of the bladder and prostate without a full bladder. Care must be taken not to introduce air if the patient is catheterized.

REAL-TIME

A real-time transducer in the highest possible frequency should be used to examine for renal calculi because acoustic shadowing will be emphasized and stones are best seen with real-time.

THE CLINICAL PROBLEM

Hematuria is an important sign of genitourinary tract problems. The abnormality may be located within the kidneys, ureter, bladder, or urethra. Therefore, the segments of the genitourinary tract that can be visualized by ultrasound (i.e., the kidney, upper and lower portions of the ureter, bladder, and upper part of the urethra) should be examined. Although the intravenous pyelogram (IVP) is the primary method of evaluating hematuria, lesions can be found with ultrasound that are not visible on IVP. Because these are relatively minute abnormalities such as small calculi or small tumors, good scanning technique is essential.

ANATOMY
Bladder

The bladder has a muscular wall whose thickness can be discerned with ultrasound. It usually has a symmetrical shape and is more or less square on transverse section (Fig. 19-1). The base of the bladder where the ureters enter is known as the trigone.

Male

Posterior to the lower bladder lie the mustache-shaped seminal vesicles (Fig. 19-1). The prostate lies posterior to the symphysis pubis and inferior to the bladder and seminal vesicles. It is more or less round. Sometimes a line of echoes due to the urethra can be seen at its center.

Female

In the female the uterus and vagina lie postero-inferior to the bladder. The vagina and lower segment of the uterus are normally never separated from the bladder (see Chapter 22).

TECHNIQUE
Kidney

The sonographic examination of the kidney has been reviewed in Chapter 16.

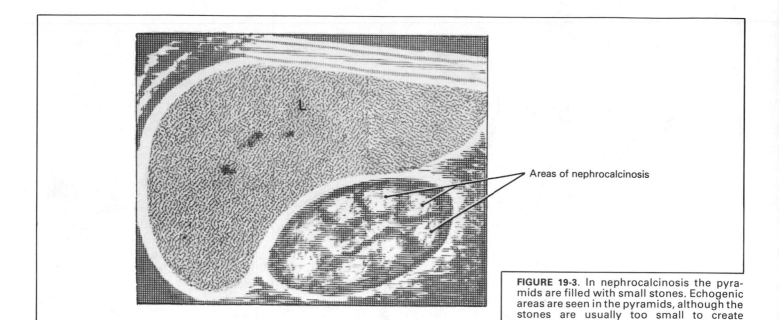

Areas of nephrocalcinosis

FIGURE 19-3. In nephrocalcinosis the pyramids are filled with small stones. Echogenic areas are seen in the pyramids, although the stones are usually too small to create shadows.

PATHOLOGY
Calculi
RENAL CALCULI

Ultrasound can be a more sensitive method of detecting calculi than IVP. Some calculi cannot be seen on IVP because they are not radiopaque or because they are concealed by gas or feces. If they are more than 5 or 6 mm in size, acoustic shadowing will be seen beyond a dense echo.

Smaller calculi appear as densely echogenic structures within the renal sinus echoes; decreasing the gain will make them stand out more against the background echogenicity of the renal sinus. In nephrocalcinosis the calculi are too small to cast shadows but are seen as echogenic areas where the pyramids normally lie (Fig. 19-3).

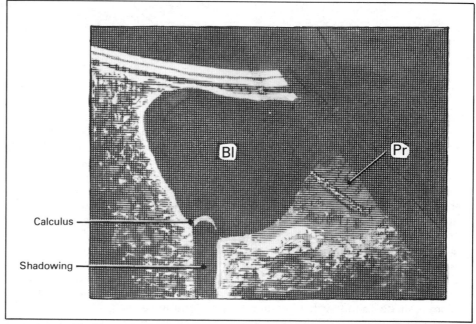

Bl

Pr

Calculus

Shadowing

FIGURE 19-4. Bladder calculi usually cause acoustic shadowing.

BLADDER CALCULI

Bladder calculi may be missed on IVP because they can be confused with phleboliths. They are particularly easy to see with ultrasound because they are surrounded by fluid (Fig. 19-4). Movement of a bladder calculus can be demonstrated by turning the patient into a sideways position.

Tumors

Tumors in the kidney and bladder may be seen first with ultrasound and may be responsible for hematuria. Tumor appearances in the kidney are described in Chapter 17. Tumors in the bladder are usually small, relatively echogenic structures adjacent to the bladder wall (Fig. 19-5). The extent of invasion of the bladder wall can be assessed with ultrasound. The echogenic line around the bladder is absent when a tumor has invaded the wall. The degree of bladder wall invasion affects the staging and therefore the therapy of a bladder tumor.

Infection

Infection can be responsible for hematuria. In the kidney the appearances will be those of an abscess or pyelonephritis (see Chapter 17). In the bladder, infection may cause generalized or local thickening of the bladder wall (cystitis). If localized, such thickening may be indistinguishable from thickening caused by a tumor. Infection may occur in association with a diverticulum. These are cystic buds arising from a bladder that is chronically obstructed (Fig. 19-6). The neck of a diverticulum is easy to see with ultrasound. To be sure which is the bladder and which is the diverticulum watch with real-time as the patient voids. The diverticulum will enlarge as the bladder contracts.

Traumatic Changes

Traumatic damage to any site in the genitouriary tract will produce hematuria. In the kidney evidence of trauma may be seen as either a localized area of altered echogenicity, which may be fluid-filled due to a blood clot, or a laceration of the kidney—the outline of the kidney will be distorted and a line through the kidney may be present indicating a kidney fracture. A perinephric hematoma will almost certainly be present at the site of the laceration. Bladder trauma will be revealed by the presence of a perivesical hematoma—a collection of blood lying outside the bladder. The actual site of a bladder wall tear will probably not be visible with ultrasound.

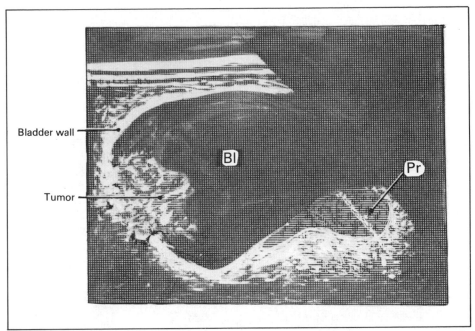

FIGURE 19-5. Tumors are echogenic areas within the bladder lumen. If they involve the bladder wall, the echogenic line around the bladder is disrupted.

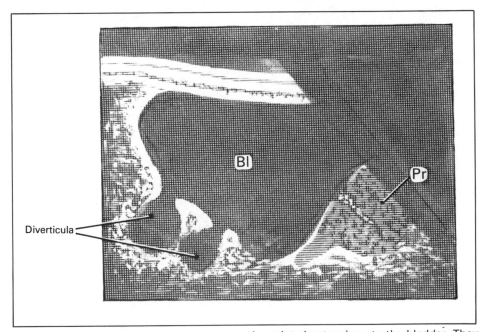

FIGURE 19-6. Bladder diverticula appear as pedunculated extensions to the bladder. They have relatively small necks.

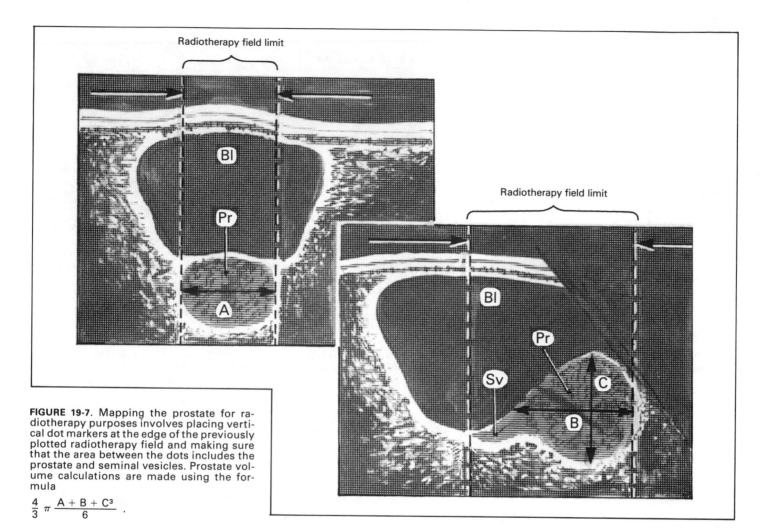

FIGURE 19-7. Mapping the prostate for radiotherapy purposes involves placing vertical dot markers at the edge of the previously plotted radiotherapy field and making sure that the area between the dots includes the prostate and seminal vesicles. Prostate volume calculations are made using the formula

$$\frac{4}{3} \pi \frac{A + B + C^3}{6} \quad .$$

Prostate

Prostatic hypertrophy may be responsible for hematuria. The engorged veins that run along the surface of an enlarged prostate bleed easily. Enlargement of the prostate is detected by impingement of a prostatic soft tissue mass on the bladder or by extension of the prostate toward the rectum (Fig. 19-7). It is still not possible to predict reliably the presence of carcinoma of the prostate, another cause of hematuria, by ultrasound. Altered echogenicity within the prostate may indicate prostatic calculi, a prostatic neoplasm, or benign prostatic hypertrophy. Prostatic volumes can be calculated by using the formula $\frac{4}{3} \pi r^3$ (as for a sphere, see Fig. 19-7).

PITFALLS

1. Do not mistake *air* in the kidney or bladder for *calculi*. Air will lie in the most superior aspect of the organ being examined and will remain there when positional changes are made.

2. Do not mistake *blood clot* for *tumor* within the bladder. Changing the patient's position will usually alter the blood clot configuration and position but will not make much change in a tumor.

WHERE ELSE TO LOOK

If the prostate is found to be enlarged or a mass is found in the bladder, examine the kidneys to be certain there is no secondary hydronephrosis.

SELECTED READING

Resnick, M., and Sanders, R. (Eds.). *Ultrasound in Urology.* Baltimore: Williams & Wilkins, 1979.

20. RENAL TRANSPLANT

SUSAN M. GUIDI
ROGER C. SANDERS

SONOGRAM ABBREVIATIONS

Bl   Bladder

K   Kidney

KEY WORDS

Anuria. Total absence of urine production.

Acute Tubular Necrosis (ATN). Acute renal "shutdown," usually due to abrupt lowering of blood pressure.

Creatinine. A waste product excreted in the urine. Values of more than 1.0 indicate that the patient is in renal failure.

Iliac Fossa. Area on either side of the lower part of the abdomen. Usual location of a transplant kidney.

Immunosuppression. Depression of host defenses.

Infarct. Occlusion of the blood supply to an organ.

Ischemia. Sudden decrease in blood supply. Prolonged ischemia results in an infarct.

Lymphocele. A collection of lymphatic fluid. Usually a postoperative complication.

Oliguria. Decreased urine production (less than 400 ml per day).

Rejection. Reaction of the body to the presence of a foreign kidney shown by production of antibodies against the transplant.

Steroids. Drugs similar to the hormones produced by the adrenal glands. Steroids lead to a decrease in immunologic response.

Urinoma. A collection of extravasated urine. Usually a postoperative complication.

THE CLINICAL PROBLEM

Within the last 20 years, renal transplantation has become the usual long-term treatment for chronic renal failure. Most of the many complications that follow renal transplantation can be usefully assessed by ultrasound. The most common indication for examination of a renal transplant by ultrasound is worsening renal failure. Possible explanations include hydronephrosis, rejection, acute tubular necrosis, and vascular problems such as a focal infarct or venous thrombosis. Renal transplant rejection, the usual cause of fever and increasing serum creatinine levels, has a typical ultrasonic appearance. Some of the other conditions, notably hydronephrosis, can be diagnosed by ultrasound. Because pyelography is rarely of value in renal transplants and hydronephrosis is especially distastrous in these patients, the contribution of ultrasound is pivotal.

Another common clinical problem in a renal transplant patient is postoperative fever, which may be due to an infected fluid collection. Possible collections that may develop following transplantation include abscess, hematoma, urinoma, and lymphocele. These collections are easily localized with ultrasound. Renal transplant patients cannot usually wait for a study. Because they are immunosuppressed serious infections may produce few signs, and infection may spread rapidly.

ANATOMY

A renal transplant is usually placed in the iliac fossa (Fig. 20-1). The ureter of the donor kidney is anastomosed to the bladder. Sometimes the patient's own kidneys (native kidneys) and ureters are left intact. The variability of each operative procedure may result in a kidney with a large renal pelvis or an unusual axis. A baseline ultrasonic examination in the immediate postoperative period is worthwhile so that a dilated sinus echo complex or an unusual renal axis or site is not mistaken for a postoperative complication.

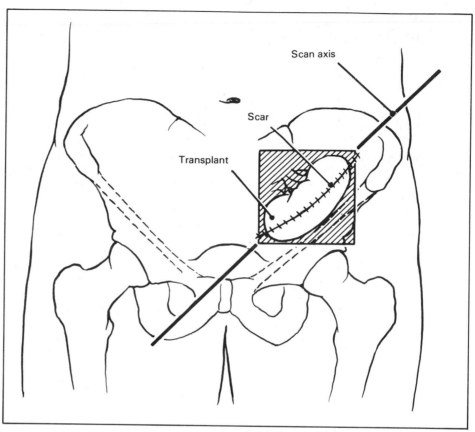

FIGURE 20-1. Diagram showing the usual placement site of the renal transplant. As a rule, the renal transplant is best shown by scans that are parallel to the scar. The transplant can be in either iliac fossa.

TECHNIQUE

Standard Scan

Perhaps the simplest way of obtaining reproducible sonograms is to perform sections along the axis of the scar and at right angles to the scar (Fig. 20-1). The longest height, width, and length of the kidney should be documented with the help of real-time so that the size changes due to rejection can be followed (Fig. 20-2).

Rejection

The sonographic diagnosis of rejection depends on subtle parenchymal changes. Therefore, the technique used should be identical on consecutive examinations. During the baseline study the time gain compensation curve and gain factors should be recorded.

Collection

A view that includes the renal pelvis of the kidney and the bladder (Fig. 20-3) should always be obtained because collections commonly lie in this region; without this view the sonologist may not be able to decide whether a "collection" is in fact the bladder.

Patients with Open Wounds

In patients with transplants, the field must be kept sterile because any sort of infection spreads rapidly in these immunosuppressed patients. Place the transducer in a sterile bag filled with gel and scan through the bag. The bag provides relatively little interference with the ultrasonic beam. Use sterile mineral oil around the wound. Real-time can also be used through a sterile bag.

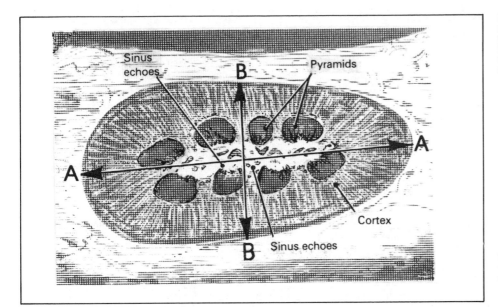

FIGURE 20-2. Diagram showing the usual measurements (A,B) obtained to see whether the size of the transplant is changing. The pyramids are seen well in most transplants. Both the pyramids and the renal sinus enlarge in rejection.

FIGURE 20-3A,B. Collections, generally hematomas, are common with renal transplants. Collection 1 is in the usual site of hematoma accumulation. Collection 2 is a site where urinomas or lymphoceles commonly occur. The axis along which the "sonogram" was performed is shown in A.

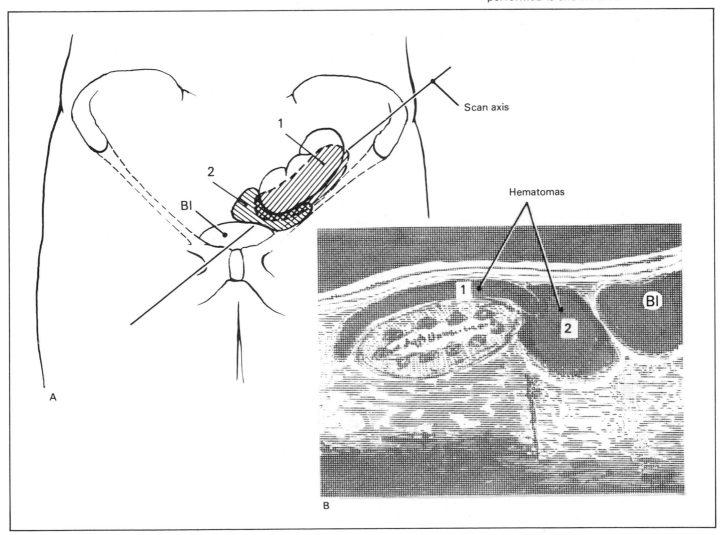

PATHOLOGY

Rejection

ACUTE REJECTION

Acute rejection occurring within the first few months after operation has a typical sonographic appearance. The kidney is enlarged in length, width, and height, the pyramids are larger and more sonolucent than usual, and the central sinus echo complex shows a decrease in both size and echogenicity. Volumetric changes in renal size can be followed by using the formula : length × width × height × 0.5233 (formula for a prolate ellipse, see Fig. 20-2).

CHRONIC REJECTION

In chronic rejection the renal parenchyma becomes more echogenic, but this change takes months to develop.

Acute Tubular Necrosis (ATN)

The condition most easily confused clinically with acute rejection is acute tubular necrosis due to hypotension and subsequent ischemia. In ATN some renal enlargement may also occur. However, the pyramids are not enlarged, and the sinus echoes are normal.

Obstruction

Acute renal obstruction occurring in the first few weeks after operation presents with signs and symptoms similar to those of rejection. The sonographic appearances of hydronephrosis have already been described (see Chapter 16). However, comparison with a baseline study may be crucial because a minimal change in the degree of apparent hydronephrosis that has occurred since the baseline study was made may indicate considerable obstruction. Views of the bladder both empty and full should be obtained because apparent transient hydronephrosis may be caused by overdistention of the bladder.

Vascular Problems

The vascular causes of transplant failure (renal vein thrombosis and renal artery occlusion) cannot be diagnosed by ultrasound alone. However, in conjunction with a nuclear medicine scan, such diagnoses may be suggested because absence of function on the nuclear scan will contrast sharply with apparently normal sonogram. In addition, focal areas of infarction (or infection) may result in a swollen sonolucent segment of the kidney.

Fever or Local Tenderness of Renal Transplant

Fever in the postoperative period following a transplant may be due to an abscess, hematoma, or, usually, rejection. Because such patients are treated with steroids, they are immunosuppressed, and local tenderness over a collection may be relatively trivial. Whenever hydronephrosis is found, a collection should be sought as its cause.

HEMATOMAS

Hematomas occur commonly after renal transplantation and are usually located either in the subcutaneous tissues or around the transplant. Hematomas often have a number of internal echoes and may indeed be so echogenic that they are hard to distinguish from neighboring structures. They are often aligned along the renal capsule. Their borders are usually quite well defined (Fig. 20-3).

ABSCESSES

Abscesses usually develop when a hematoma becomes infected. They are difficult to distinguish from hematomas by their sonographic appearance.

LYMPHOCELES

Lymphoceles usually occur some months after a renal transplant has been performed. They may contain septa but are generally echo-free. They are often located betwen the transplant and the bladder. Hydronephrosis due to obstruction by the lymphocele may develop.

URINOMAS

Urinomas are usually a consequence of extravasation due to ureterovesical junction obstruction. They are almost always echo-free and well defined.

As a rule, the presence of a collection is an indication for the performance of a percutaneous aspiration to discover the nature of the collection. Urinomas, however, can be diagnosed by a nuclear medicine study in a noninvasive fashion.

PITFALLS

1. *Pseudohydronephrosis*
   a. *Bladder overdistention.* An erroneous diagnosis of hydronephrosis may be made if the bladder is unduly full. Make sure that a postvoid view is obtained if hydronephrosis appears to be present. Sometimes the apparent hydronephrosis will disappear when the bladder is empty.
   b. *Baseline sinus distention.* An incorrect diagnosis of hydronephrosis may be made if a baseline study has not been performed because many transplanted kidneys show some apparent renal pelvic fullness.
2. *Rejection.* Rejection may be incorrectly diagnosed if different time gain compensation factors are used on follow-up examination. Try to use the same ultrasonic system and settings for consecutive examinations of a renal transplant.
3. *TGC problems.* Poor time gain compensation settings may give the appearance of a collection anterior to the kidney or even an anterior infarct if the time gain compensation is too steep (Fig. 20-4).
4. *Echogenic collections.* Hematomas and abscesses may be missed unless their occasional high echogenicity is kept in mind.
5. *Bladder versus collection.* Make sure that an apparent collection below the kidney is not the bladder; ask the patient to void or fill the bladder.

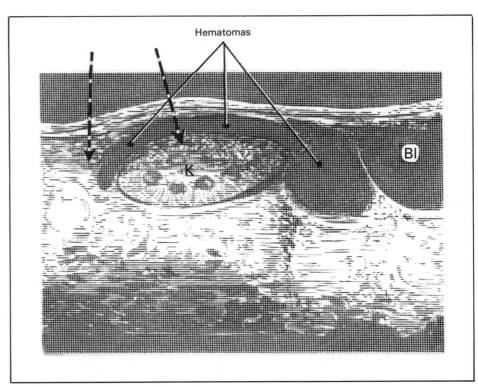

FIGURE 20-4. Unsatisfactory time gain compensation settings may prevent assessment of the anterior aspect of the kidney. This hematoma is hard to distinguish from the neighboring tissues because the TGC was too steep. Broken arrows indicate areas where a TGC artifact is apparent.

WHERE ELSE TO LOOK

If no collection has been found around the transplant kidney or bladder in a patient with a fever of unknown origin, look at the sites where the native kidneys used to lie (the nephrectomy sites). Abscesses may develop within these areas. Intrahepatic or perihepatic abscesses are also quite common. Occasionally, patients with renal transplants have pancreatitis due to steroid overadministration.

SELECTED READING

Hricak, H. Renal Medical Disorders: The Role of Sonography. In R. C. Sanders (Ed.), *Ultrasound Annual 1982.* New York: Raven Press, 1982.

Resnick, M., and Sanders, R. (Eds.). *Ultrasound in Urology.* Baltimore: Williams & Wilkins, 1979.

21. UNEXPLAINED HEMATOCRIT DROP

Rule Out Perinephric Hematoma; Possible Perinephric Mass

ROGER C. SANDERS

SONOGRAM ABBREVIATIONS

Ao   Aorta

Du   Duodenum

IVC   Inferior vena cava

K   Kidney

L   Liver

P   Pancreas

Ps   Psoas muscle

QL   Quadratus lumborum muscle

KEY WORDS

Anticoagulant. Drug that increases the time needed for blood to clot; used in the treatment of pulmonary emboli and myocardial infarcts. Control of dosage is not always easy, and bleeding may ensue if there is overdosage.

Gerota's Fascia. Tissue plane around the kidney that includes the adrenals and much fat; important in the localization of hematomas and abscesses.

Hematocrit. A measurement of blood concentration; indicates the amount of blood in the body.

Hemophilia. Hereditary bleeding disorder seen in males. Those affected have a particular tendency to bleed into joints and the muscles in the retroperitoneum.

Retroperitoneum. Part of the body posterior to the peritoneum; includes the kidney and the pancreas, as well as many muscles in the paraspinous area.

Urinoma. Collection of urine outside the genitourinary tract.

THE CLINICAL PROBLEM

The retroperitoneum is a clinically silent area where fluid collections accumulate that cannot be diagnosed by conventional radiographic techniques. Such collections are commonly hematomas, abscesses, or urinomas.

Hematomas

An unexplained hematocrit drop indicates that a patient has bled internally. Often the site of the bleed is unclear to the clinician. Patients at risk for unexplained hematocrit drop are those who (1) have had recent surgery, (2) are taking anticoagulants, (3) have suffered a recent injury such as a road accident or stabbing, or (4) have bleeding or clotting problems such as hemophiliacs or leukemics. The most likely sites of such asymptomatic hematomas are (1) in the abdominal wall around an incision, (2) deep to an incision, (3) in a site where fluid collects adjacent to a surgical site (e.g., in the cul-de-sac, paracolic gutters, or subhepatic space), (4) around the spleen (perisplenic), liver (perihepatic), or kidney (perinephric), (5) in the retroperitoneum (this site is particularly likely in patients with no previous injury such as those on anticoagulants or suffering from bleeding problems), and (6) in the iliopsoas muscles, particularly in hemophiliacs.

Hematomas may develop into abscesses. They are a good culture medium for bacteria. Expansion of a hematoma on subsequent sonograms suggests that the lesion is infected. Normally hematomas slowly get smaller.

Urinomas (Urinipherous Pseudocysts)

Urinomas develop mainly in patients who have had trauma, who have passed a renal stone, or who have had operations such as a renal transplant. They may be asymptomatic and may be found years after the original process that caused them occurred. It is useful to follow the progress of urinomas that occur after surgery because they usually resolve spontaneously.

Abscesses

Abscesses occur in the retroperitoneum quite commonly. They may be relatively asymptomatic, particularly in the psoas muscle, presenting with fever rather than with localized symptoms.

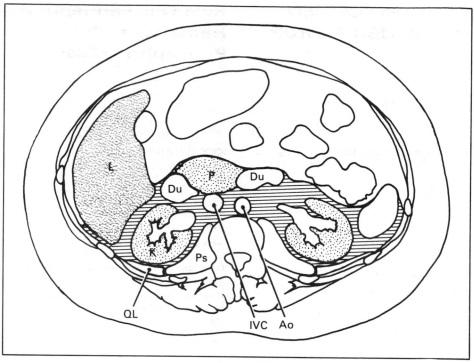

FIGURE 21-1. The cross-hatched area represents the retroperitoneum. Large structures in the retroperitoneum include the psoas muscles (Ps), quadratus lumborum muscles (QL), kidneys (K), and pancreas (P).

ANATOMY

Retroperitoneum

In practice, the retroperitoneum is a term used to describe the area that includes the kidney, the psoas, iliacus, and quadratus lumborum muscles, and the presacral area. Although the pancreas is technically within the retroperitoneum, this organ is not usually included in a retroperitoneal survey (Fig. 21-1).

Spaces Around the Kidney

The area around the kidney is traversed by several fibrous sheaths that form natural barriers to the passage of fluid and act as a guide for the site of origin of a collection. The retroperitoneum is divided into the following areas:

1. The *anterior pararenal space.* A space in front of the kidney that communicates with the opposite side around the pancreas.
2. The *perinephric space* within Gerota's fascia. This space may be open-ended inferiorly and encloses the kidneys, fat, and the adrenal glands.
3. The *posterior pararenal space.* This space extends behind the kidney into the lateral aspects of the abdominal wall.

   The fascial planes can be seen on a good quality sonogram in an obese patient when they are outlined by fat.

4. The *psoas muscles.* These muscles lie lateral to the spine and widen out as one progresses inferiorly (Figs. 21-2 and 21-3). They eventually join up with the iliacus muscles that arise on the anterior aspect of the iliac crest to form a joint muscle in the pelvis (Figs. 21-2 and 21-3).
5. The *quadratus lumborum muscles.* These muscles lie posterior to the kidney (Figs. 21-1 and 21-2) and are often surprisingly sonolucent, giving the impression that a collection is present. If one looks on the opposite side, a similar sonolucent area will be seen.

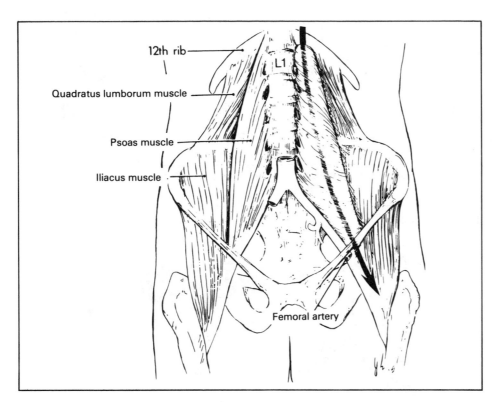

TECHNIQUE

Perinephric Area

As a rule, the prone or decubitus position gives the best view of the retroperitoneal areas around the kidneys down to the level of the iliac crest.

Psoas Muscles

The psoas and iliacus muscles may be visible on supine and supine oblique views, but gas may obscure the area (Fig. 21-3). It is usually best to perform a prone oblique decubitus view looking through the kidneys at the psoas muscles and at the area between the aorta and the inferior vena cava. This view is similar to the one used to look at the adrenal glands and the para-aortic nodes.

FIGURE 21-2. Diagram showing the normal location of the psoas, iliacus, and quadratus lumborum muscles.

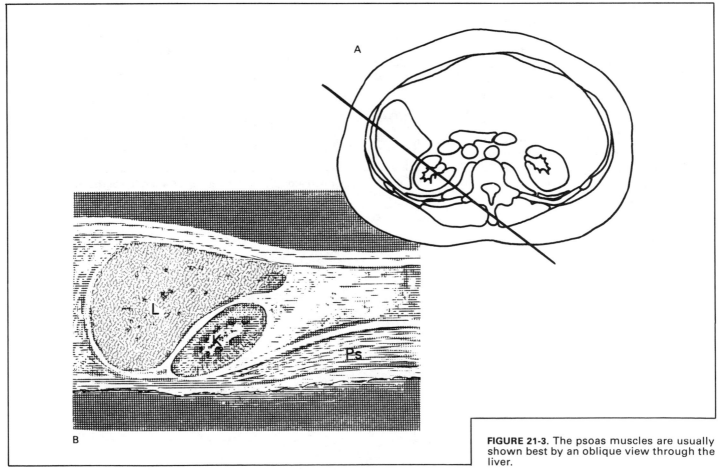

FIGURE 21-3. The psoas muscles are usually shown best by an oblique view through the liver.

Presacral Area

Visualizing the region anterior to the upper portion of the sacrum can be very difficult. A large bladder may be helpful in the supine position. Deep pressure using a linear array can displace the gut away from this area and allow views of the lower aorta and of the presacral area.

PATHOLOGY

Hematoma

SONOGRAPHIC APPEARANCES

Most hematomas in this area are sonolucent but alternatively may be evenly echogenic or clumpily echogenic (Fig. 21-4). Fluid-fluid levels may develop (Fig. 21-4). If the hematoma occurs following a penetrating injury, there may be visible distortion of an organ, for example, the kidney outline.

LOCATION

SUBCAPSULAR. If the hematoma is adjacent to the kidney in a subcapsular location, it will have a circular superior and inferior margin, and the shape of the kidney will be flattened (Fig. 21-5).

PERINEPHRIC. If the hematoma is in Gerota's fascia, it will usually be located postero-medially and will extend above and well below the level of the kidney.

POSTERIOR PARARENAL. A hematoma in the posterior pararenal space will extend up the lateral walls of the abdomen and displace the kidney anteriorly.

ANTERIOR PARARENAL. Hematomas in the anterior pararenal space lie anterior to the kidney and may extend medially into the region of the pancreas.

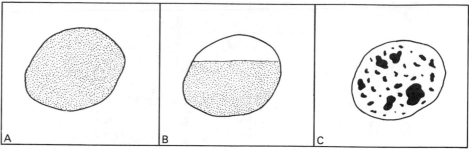

FIGURE 21-4. Sonographic patterns that suggest hematomas are, A, evenly echogenic; B, a fluid-fluid level; C, clumps of echoes.

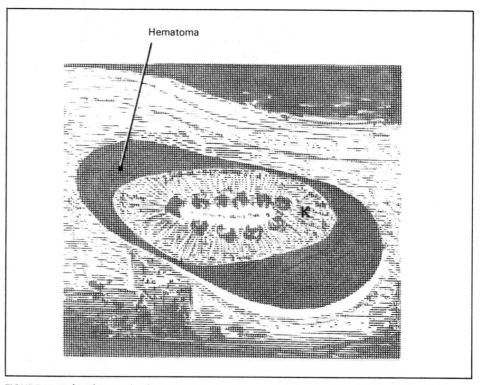

FIGURE 21-5. A subcapsular hematoma may be suggested when the border of the kidney is flattened and the capsular echogenic line is absent.

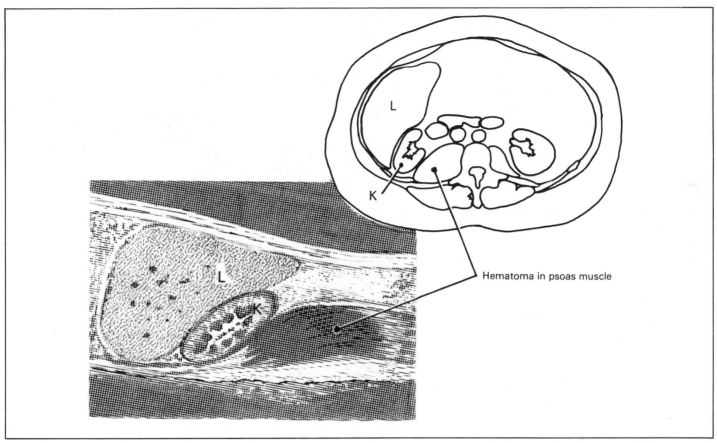

FIGURE 21-6. Sonolucent area that expands the psoas muscle due to a hematoma.

INTRAMUSCULAR. A hematoma in the psoas muscle will form an asymmetrical bulge within that muscle, displacing the kidney laterally. It will track down into the pelvis toward the iliacus muscle and the inguinal ligament (Fig. 21-6).

A hematoma secondary to deep cutting trauma (e.g., a stab wound) will not necessarily confine itself to the tissue planes already described.

Abscesses

Abscesses develop in the same area as hematomas and are difficult to distinguish from them sonographically. They may bulge more because they are not as well confined by the tissue planes, and evidence of a septum and loculation will be more apparent. The borders of abscesses are usually more irregular.

Other Fluid Collections

Urinomas may develop around the kidney, usually within Gerota's fascia. These are echo-free collections.

PITFALLS

1. *Collection versus shadowing.* Particularly in the prone position, it may be hard to distinguish between a true collection and rib shadowing. Attempts to view the suspect area in either the erect or the decubitus position are important. Alteration of the phase of respiration can help to clarify the issue.

2. *Echogenic hematoma.* At some stages in the course of its evolution a hematoma may be markedly echogenic. Do not miss it by scanning at too high a gain.

3. *Quadratus lumborum muscles.* The quadratus lumborum may be much less echogenic than other muscles and may mimic an abscess or hematoma. Comparison with the other side will show its true nature.

4. *Spleen versus collection.* It may be difficult to distinguish between the spleen and a mass at the upper pole of the left kidney. The interface between these two organs may be seen better with a decubitus view or with the patient in an erect postion. Angling up at a different phase of respiration is helpful.

5. *Gut versus collection.* It is important not to mistake the stomach or colon for a mass in the retroperitoneal pararenal area. Such masses will be fluid-filled. It is worth using real-time to check for peristalsis; if this is unsuccessful, one should consider performing a high-water enema to be sure that the mass is not gut.

6. *Duodenum.* The duodenum may lie anterior to the right kidney in the subhepatic space, mimicking a perinephric collection. Real-time will show peristalsis.

7. *Malrotated kidney versus collection.* The pelvis of a malrotated kidney lies anterior to the right kidney and may mimic a collection in the subhepatic space. Careful real-time analysis will show that the renal vein, renal artery, and ureter enter the supposed collection.

8. *Psoas versus masses.* In young patients the psoas muscles may be exceptionally prominent and may be mistaken for a mass; they will be symmetrically enlarged.

9. *Perinephric fat versus mass.* In obese patients considerable perinephric fat may be present, forming a relatively echogenic rim around the kidneys. Do not mistake this for a pathologic process. It will be bilateral.

WHERE ELSE TO LOOK

Psoas Abscess

These abscesses may track along the muscles into the hip (Fig. 21-2). A subtle collection in the hip may be seen near the femoral head.

SELECTED READING

Koenigsberg, M., Hoffman, J. C., and Schnur, M. J. Sonographic evaluation of the retroperitoneum. *Semin. Ultrasound* 3:79–96, 1982.

Kumari, S., Fulco, J. D., Karayalcin, G., et al. Gray scale ultrasound: Evaluation of iliopsoas hematomas in hemophiliacs. *A.J.R.* 133:103–106, 1979.

Spitz, H. B., and Wyatt, G. M. Rectus sheath hematoma. *J. Clin. Ultrasound.* 5:413–416, 1977.

22. RULE OUT PELVIC MASS

JOAN CAMPBELL

SONOGRAM ABBREVIATIONS

Bl   Bladder

C   Cervix
CE   Cervical endometrium
CdS Cul-de-sac
Co   Cornu

EC   Endometrial cavity

FNS Femoral nerve sheath

Ip   Iliopsoas muscle

OI   Obturator internus muscle
Ov   Ovary

PC   Pubococcygeal muscle
Pi   Piriformis muscle

Re   Rectum

Ut   Uterus

V   Vagina

KEY WORDS

Adenomyosis. Generalized enlargement of the uterus due to endometrial tissue within the myometrium; condition similar to endometriosis.

Chocolate Cyst. Blood-filled cyst associated with endometriosis.

Corpus Lutein Cyst. Cyst developing in the second half of the menstrual cycle and in pregnancy that regresses spontaneously.

Choriocarcinoma. The most severe form of trophoblastic disease; can metastasize throughout the body.

Cuff. After hysterectomy the blind end of the vagina is sutured and forms a fibrous mass, the cuff.

Dermoid. Form of teratoma that is benign and tends to occur in young women.

Endometriosis. Deposits of endometrial tissue on the ovaries, the exterior of the uterus, and the intestines, among other places. It bleeds at monthly intervals, causing development of hematomas and fibrosis.

Fibroid. A benign tumor of the smooth muscle of the uterus: (1) *submucosal,* a fibroid bordering on the endometrial cavity; (2) *subserosal,* a fibroid bordering on the peritoneal cavity.

Follicle. Developing ova within the ovary; can develop into a cyst.

Hematometrocolpos. Condition occurring at birth or at puberty due to an imperforate hymen. Blood or other fluid accumulates in the vagina and uterus.

Human Chorionic Gonadotropin (HCG). Hormone that increases in amount during pregnancy. Measurement of HCG levels in the blood is the most reliable way of detecting pregnancy.

Hydrosalpinx. Blocked fallopian tube that fills with sterile fluid as a consequence of previous infection.

Interstitial. Pregnancy located in the cornual segment of the fallopian tube. This form of ectopic pregnancy is particularly dangerous because it is likely to bleed copiously.

Nulliparous. A woman who has not been pregnant.

Parous. A woman with previous pregnancies.

Polycystic Ovary Syndrome (PCO, Stein-Leventhal syndrome). Multiple cysts developing in both ovaries. The condition is traditionally associated with obesity and male-like body hair.

Progesterone. Hormone secreted during pregnancy and the menstrual cycle.

Pseudomyxoma Peritonei. Condition that occurs when an ovarian cystic tumor bursts and its contents spread through the abdomen, forming additional lesions.

Pyometria. Pus within the uterine cavity.

Teratoma. Tumor composed of the various body tissues including skin, teeth, hair, and bone, among others. May be malignant but is usually benign in the pelvic area.

Theca Lutein Cysts. Multiple cysts that develop in association with trophoblastic disease due to increased human chorionic gonadotropin levels. May also occur with multiple pregnancy and induced ovulation.

Trophoblastic Disease. Neoplasms based on changes in the trophoblasts within the uterus; the term refers to hydatidiform mole, invasive mole, and choriocarcinoma.

THE CLINICAL PROBLEM

The sonographic characteristics of pelvic masses are usually nonspecific. Therefore, the efforts of the sonographer should be concentrated on fully evaluating the pelvis rather than on striving to make a specific diagnosis.

The questions that need to be answered for the clinician about a pelvic mass are

1. Is a pathologic pelvic mass present, or is the "mass" a normal anatomic variant?
2. Is the mass uterine or adnexal or neither?
3. Is the mass cystic, complex, or solid? If it is cystic, does it have septae?
4. Is the mass involving or invading any other pelvic structure?
5. Are other associated findings such as ascites, metastases, or hydronephrosis present?

Although the sonographic characteristics of many pelvic masses are similar, the clinical information may assist the sonologist in making a more focused diagnosis. Clinical management of pelvic masses is not always surgical. Pelvic mass assessment is helped by sonography in the following situations:

1. With ovarian cysts, if much solid material is found within a cyst or if a cyst is more than about 10 cm in size, surgery is more appropriate than expectant therapy.
2. When fibroids are not treated by surgery, they may be followed by serial sonograms.
3. Ovarian masses may be discovered in asymptomatic menopausal women.

ANATOMY

An overview of the effect of the normal menstrual cycle on the ovarian structures will make normal sonographic changes more readily understandable (Fig. 22-1).

Menstrual Cycle

Under the stimulation of the pituitary hormones follicle-stimulating hormone (FSH) and luteinizing hormone (LH), the ovary cyclically produces estrogen and progesterone. In the first half of the menstrual cycle, FSH stimulates a follicle, which contains an ovum, to grow and develop. This follicle grows to a size of about 22 to 25 mm at midcycle (large enough to be seen by ultrasound) and then bursts, releasing the ovum (i.e., ovulation). After ovulation the follicle transforms into the corpus luteum and produces progesterone, which prepares the endometrium to receive a fertilized egg. If the egg is not fertilized, the corpus luteum involutes and becomes a small white scar, the corpus albicans. The normal follicle and the corpus luteum can be recognized sonographically.

FIGURE 22-1. Diagram of the sequence of events during a normal menstrual cycle. The ovary contains several follicles, which slowly increase in size until one ovulates. At the site where ovulation takes place, the corpus luteum develops. The developing follicle (a sonographic cyst) ovulates when it reaches a size of about 22 mm. A degenerating corpus luteum has few internal echoes and a rather irregular border. The uterine endometrium thickens prior to menstruation.

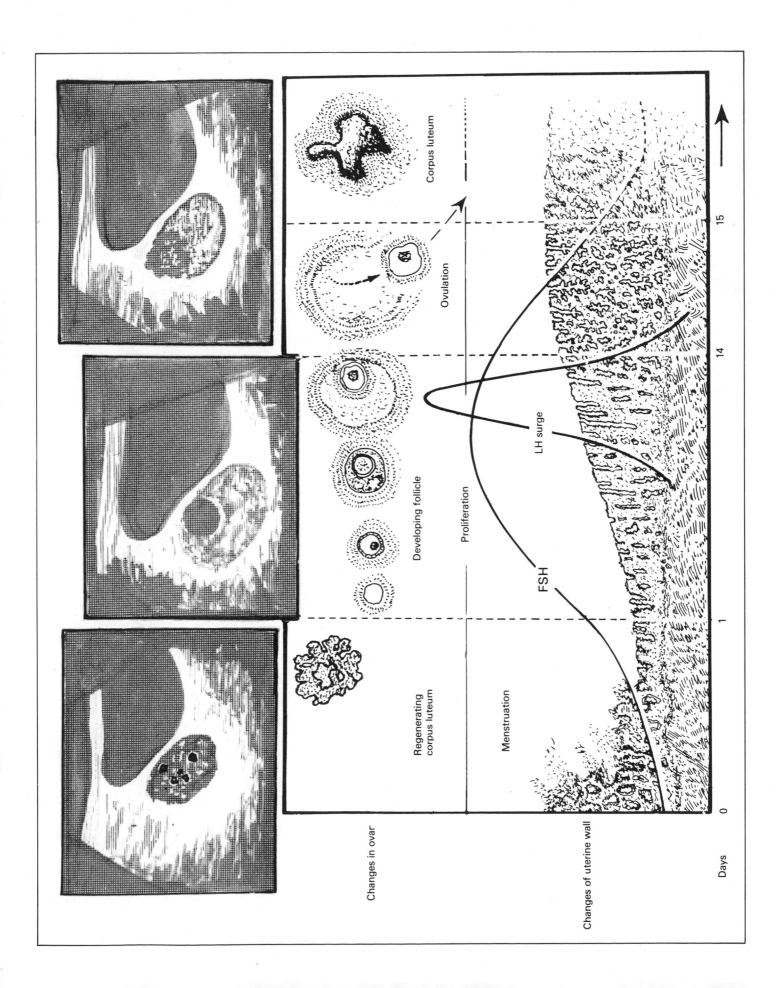

Changes in ovar

Regenerating corpus luteum

Developing follicle

Ovulation

Corpus luteum

Menstruation

Proliferation

FSH

LH surge

Changes of uterine wall

Days

0   1   14   15

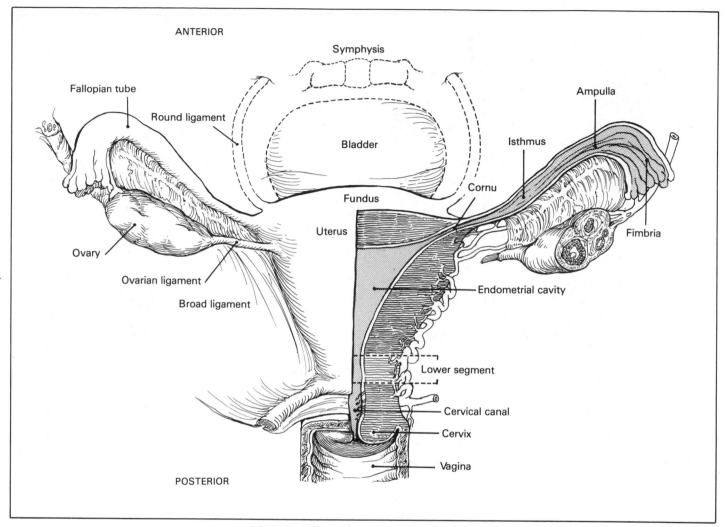

ANTERIOR

Symphysis

Fallopian tube

Round ligament

Ampulla

Bladder

Isthmus

Cornu

Fundus

Uterus

Ovary

Ovarian ligament

Broad ligament

Fimbria

Endometrial cavity

Lower segment

Cervical canal

Cervix

Vagina

POSTERIOR

FIGURE 22-2. Normal uterus and ovaries. The ovaries are suspended from the broad ligament and lie adjacent to the ampullary end of the fallopian tube. The fallopian tube arises from the cornu of the uterus. The lumen is rarely visible.

Uterus

The normal uterus in menstruating women ranges from 5 to 9 cm in length and up to about 5 cm in antero-posterior diameter and width (Figs. 22-2 and 22-3A). It is smaller in nulliparous women than in parous women. As a rule, the uterus lies behind the bladder (Fig. 22-2) and usually is slightly tilted anteriorly (Fig. 22-3A). However, the uterus may be retroverted, that is, pointing backward, as a normal variant (Fig. 22-3B). The sonographic appearance of the uterine endometrial cavity alters during the course of the menstrual cycle. In the later secretory phase the endometrial cavity becomes an echogenic line (Fig. 22-4). The uterus widens toward the fundus, and the cornual regions (Figs. 22-2 and 22-5), the lateral triangular areas extending bilaterally from the fundus, can be visualized. The cornu are the points of origin of the fallopian tubes (Figs. 22-2 and 22-5).

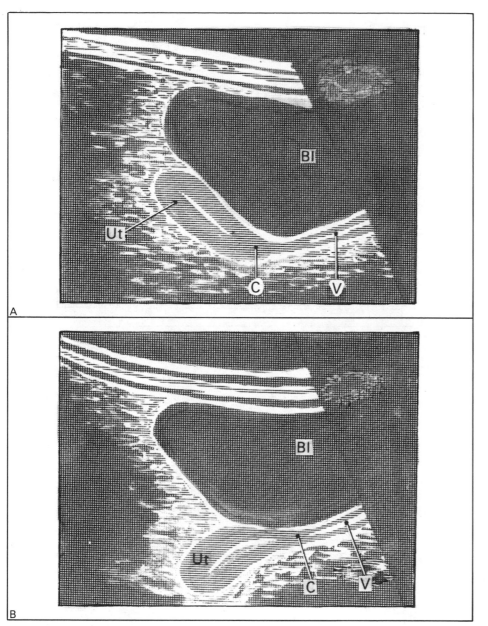

FIGURE 22-3. Uterus. A. Normal anteverted uterus with decidual reaction in the cavity. B. Normal retroverted uterus on longitudinal section.

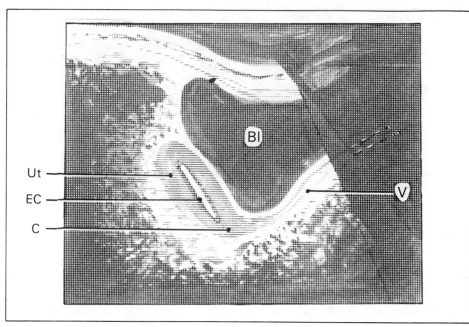

FIGURE 22-4. Anteverted uterus with a prominent decidual reaction surrounded by a sonolucent zone. This appearance is seen when menstruation is about to take place.

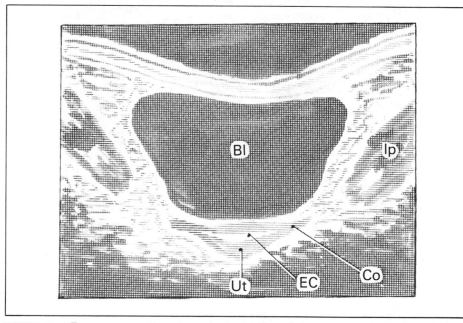

FIGURE 22-5. Transverse section through the fundus of the uterus and cornu; a decidual reaction is present.

A slight change in uterine size normally occurs during the course of the menstrual cycle. However, a dramatic increase in size takes place at menarche when the uterus grows rapidly from its small prepubertal size (Fig. 22-6). After the menopause, the uterus gradually decreases in size.

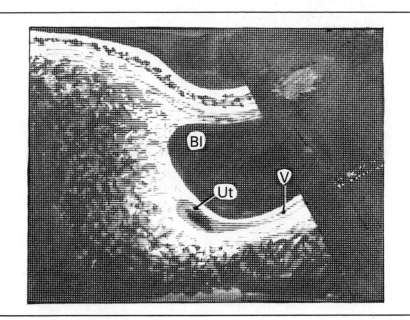

FIGURE 22-6. Prepubertal uterus. It will rapidly increase in size at puberty.

Ovaries

The ovaries are usually found at the level of the lateral fundus where the uterus becomes triangular (the cornu) (Figs. 22-2, 22-5, and 22-7B). The fallopian tube, seen as a linear sonolucent area, can sometimes be traced from the uterus to the region of the ovary. The ovary often lies adjacent to the iliopsoas muscle near an echogenic focus that is due to the femoral nerve sheath (Fig. 22-7B). The iliac vessels lie adjacent to the ovary. Ovaries in menstruating women measure up to 3 × 4 cm in size normally. Alteration in the size of the ovary takes place during the course of the menstrual cycle. Small cysts develop in the first half of the cycle that can reach a size of just over 2 cm (Fig. 22-1). Before menarche and after the menopause, the ovaries are smaller.

Pelvic Sidewalls

The pelvis is lined by muscle. In the inferior portion of the pelvis, the obturator internus muscles lie alongside the bony wall (Fig. 22-7A). At a higher level the iliopsoas muscle forms a more oblique muscular mass (Fig. 22-8B). The pubococcygeus and piriformis muscles can be seen posterior to the rectum, vagina, and uterus (Fig. 22-7A,B).

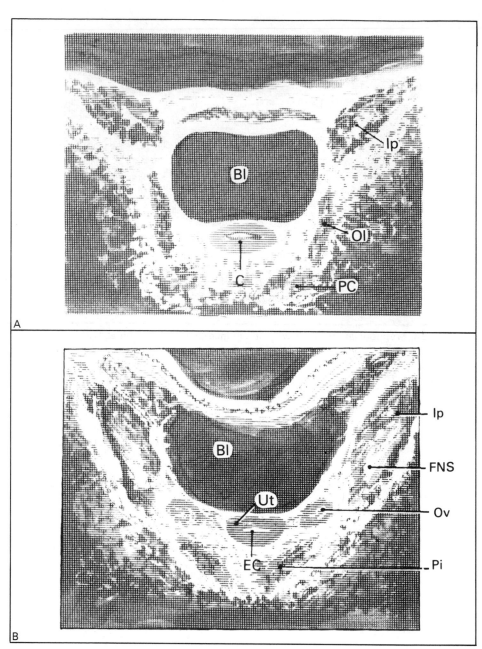

FIGURE 22-7. Transverse sections. A. Transverse section at the level of the cervix. Note the obturator muscles (OI). B. Transverse section at the fundus of the uterus through the ovaries. Note the iliopsoas muscles (Ip).

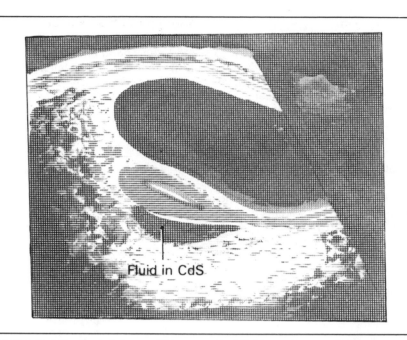

FIGURE 22-8. Fluid in the cul-de-sac. This amount of fluid may be seen in the course of the normal menstrual cycle.

Cul-de-sac

Small amounts of fluid may collect within the cul-de-sac behind the uterus during the course of the normal menstrual cycle, presumably due to rupture of follicular ovarian cysts (Fig. 22-8).

TECHNIQUE

Knowledge of the patient's clinical history and any specific questions to be answered is essential before beginning any pelvic scan.

Full Bladder

In all pelvic sonograms distention of the urinary bladder is imperative. The full bladder pushes the bowel superiorly and aligns the uterus in a more elongated fashion that is easier to scan (Fig. 22-9). The bladder also acts as an acoustic window for the pelvic structures.

A full bladder is essential, but beware of the "too full" bladder. Acoustic enhancement from a bladder that is too full is difficult to correct and will obscure some true information behind the bladder.

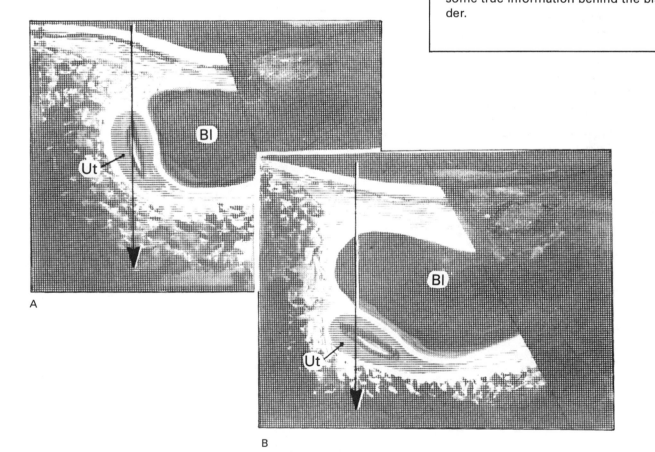

FIGURE 22-9A,B. Filling the bladder to alter the uterine axis. When this bladder was filled, B, the uterus became less anteflexed. Retroverted uteruses also usually adopt a more satisfactory position when the bladder is filled.

Uterus

The sonographic examination should begin in a longitudinal fashion by attempting to align the uterus with the vagina. The uterus can be recognized by the central line of the endometrial cavity and by the fact that it is contiguous with the vagina. The vagina is visualized as an echogenic center with relatively sonolucent walls.

The uterus is normally located in the midline, but it may be deviated to either side in an oblique axis. Make sure that the bladder is full when the uterus is examined. An anteflexed or retroverted uterus may become more normal in position and shape if the bladder is filled (Fig. 22-9).

Scanning at right angles to the axis of the uterus should demonstrate the location of the ovary. Triangular cornual regions near the uterine fundus indicate that the ovaries are somewhere nearby. Caudal angulation is helpful for visualizing the pelvic musculature and also a retroverted uterus.

Follow-up of ovarian follicles is carried out in patients who are infertile and are being treated with drugs such as Clomid (Fig. 22-1). Timing of ovulation is critical in conception. The follicles are followed with daily serial sonographic examinations until they reach a size of about 22 mm, when a chemical estimation of the time of ovulation is made.

Use of Real-Time

The axis of the uterus can be traced more easily with real-time. Real-time helps to distinguish between bowel and other periuterine structures because peristaltic motion will generally be seen.

A water enema can be helpful in the positive identification of bowel with or without the use of real-time. Only a small amount of fluid need be run into the rectum through a small enema tube during observation with real-time or performance of a static scan. A flickering motion is visible when the water is running through bowel. Do not mistake aortic pulsation or respiratory motion for peristalsis.

Angling the Transducer

When attempting to visualize the ovaries and other periuterine structures in a transverse scanning plane, an angulation of approximately 15° cephalad is helpful (Fig. 22-10).

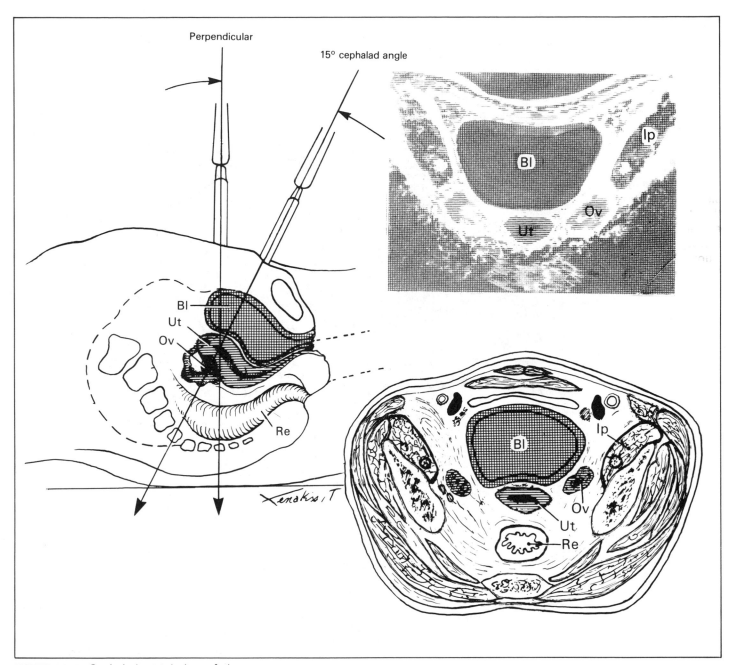

FIGURE 22-10. Cephalad angulation of the transducer helps in visualizing the ovaries because it increases the ability to use the bladder as an acoustic window.

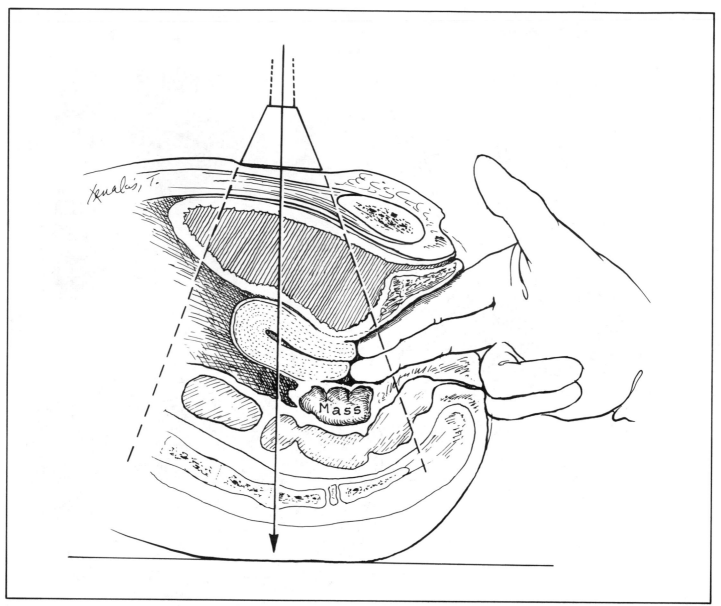

FIGURE 22-11. Vaginal examination by a gynecologist under real-time often allows one to distinguish a mass from the uterus, because the uterus will move separately from the mass.

Pelvic Examination

Pelvic examination by a physician during a real-time examination may help to clarify confusing masses (Fig. 22-11).

Trendelenburg Position

Placing a patient in the Trendelenburg position should shift free fluid in the cul-de-sac out of the pelvis.

PATHOLOGY

Pelvic masses can be divided into four basic groups: (1) single cystic masses, (2) multiple cystic masses, (3) complex masses, and (4) solid masses. Unfortunately, many of the following entities are not easy to distinguish from one another sonographically.

Cystic Masses

These masses have well-defined, smooth borders, show good through transmission, and are usually spherical.

SINGLE CYSTIC MASSES (REPRODUCTIVE AGE GROUP)

FOLLICULAR CYSTS. The cysts are caused by continued stimulation of a follicle that does not rupture. These cysts are usually small, although they may measure up to 10 cm in size, and usually disappear after one or two menstrual cycles (Fig. 22-12).

CORPUS LUTEUM CYSTS (REPRODUCTIVE AGE GROUP). These cysts are usually caused by HCG stimulation in pregnancy. Their size is variable, and occasionally they become quite large (up to 15 cm). They disappear before 20 weeks of gestation. Asymptomatic cysts are almost always simple. However, because bleeding into the cyst may occur, internal echoes may be noted.

PARAOVARIAN CYSTS (REPRODUCTIVE AGE GROUP). The cysts are indistinguishable from ovarian cysts. However, they may become very large, whereas single ovarian cysts are usually small. They represent embryonic remnants.

SEROUS CYSTADENOMA (REPRODUCTIVE AND POSTMENARCHE AGE GROUPS). The commonest benign tumor of the ovary, they are large, thin-walled cysts that may have septae within them (Fig. 22-13) and occur most commonly in women between the ages of 20 and 50. These cysts may be small but are usually large and may grow large enough to occupy most of the abdomen. About 30% are bilateral, but sonographically this may be difficult to document.

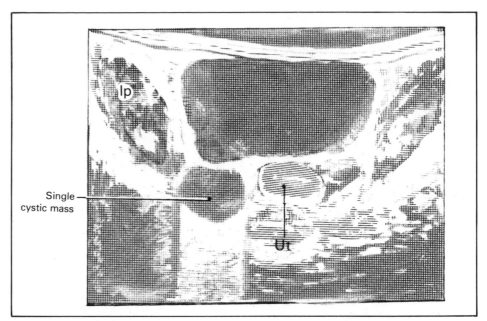

FIGURE 22-12. Cysts without internal structure in the adnexa are often follicular cysts that will disappear spontaneously.

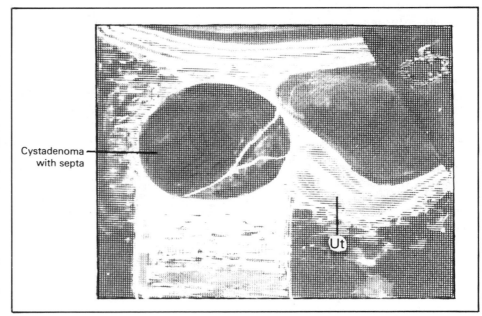

FIGURE 22-13. Serous cystadenoma and cystadenocarcinoma are cysts that contain septa. No sonographic features distinguish these two lesions.

HYDROSALPINX (REPRODUCTIVE AGE GROUP). Hydrosalpinx may be a sequela of pelvic inflammatory disease (PID) or any infection involving the fallopian tube. The pus in a pyosalpinx resorbs and is transformed into fluid. Hydrosalpinx may have a suggestive sonographic appearance because the tube folds over on itself and forms a funnel-shaped or kinked cystic structure (Fig. 22-14).

SINGLE CYSTIC MASSES SEEN WITHIN THE UTERUS

HYDROMETROCOLPOS (NEONATAL). This cyst comprises distention of the vagina and uterus with fluid, usually secondary to cervical or vaginal obstruction, for instance, imperforate hymen. Only the vagina may be distended while the uterus is still small or both uterus and vagina may be distended with fluid.

HEMATOMETROCOLPOS (PREMENARCHE). This condition occurs when the vagina and possibly the uterus are distended with blood rather than fluid. The findings are similar to those seen with hydrometrocolpos except that internal echoes may be present (Fig. 22-15). Hematometria, in which only the uterus is distended with blood, may be congenital or may follow radiation therapy for cancer of the cervix. It may occur with any cause of heavy uterine bleeding, for example, with an ectopic pregnancy or after uterine surgery.

PYOMETRIA (REPRODUCTIVE OR POST-MENARCHE). This condition, distention of the uterus with pus, usually occurs secondary to cervical obstruction of drainage of normal uterine secretions with subsequent superinfection.

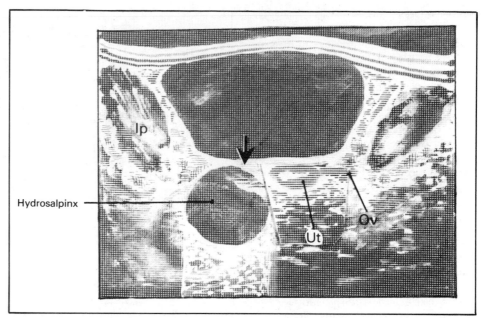

FIGURE 22-14. Hydrosalpinx sometimes has a rather characteristic appearance. The distal portion of the tube is dilated and circular; the proximal portion is much smaller and sometimes is not seen at all.

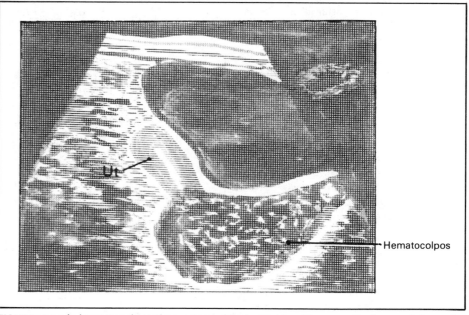

FIGURE 22-15. In hematocolpos the vagina is filled with blood because the hymen is imperforate. The uterus may or may not also be filled with blood. In this instance it is empty.

MULTIPLE CYSTIC MASSES

ENDOMETRIOSIS. A disease state that occurs during the reproductive years, endometriosis is caused by implantation of endometrial tissue in abnormal locations in the pelvis. This ectopic endometrial tissue responds to cyclic ovarian hormones and bleeds as if it were located within the uterus. Endometrial cysts may develop in these areas of bleeding. Small cysts are termed blebs, whereas larger ones, because of their contents (blood) and color, are called chocolate cysts. This type of cyst may occur singly, but more than one are generally seen. Because these cysts contain blood sonographically, they may contain internal echoes in the form of either many low-level echogenic structures or a dense echogenic "blob" (Fig. 22-16).

THECA LUTEIN CYSTS. These cysts are usually seen in conjuction with trophoblastic disease such as hydatidiform mole and choriocarcinoma. They form as a response to the abnormally high levels of HCG that are present in trophoblastic disease. They may become very large, have several septa, and are generally bilateral. Similar cysts are associated with drugs given for infertility (e.g., Pergonal), in which case they are known as hyperstimulation cysts (Fig. 22-17).

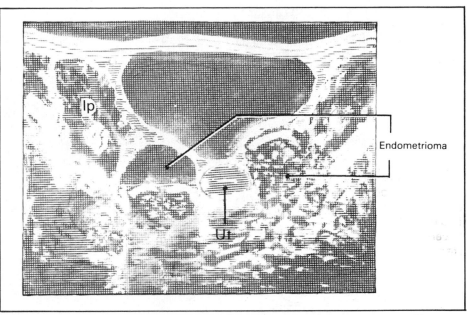

FIGURE 22-16. Endometrioma may have a variety of sonographic appearances. They may have fluid-fluid levels or may contain numerous internal echoes.

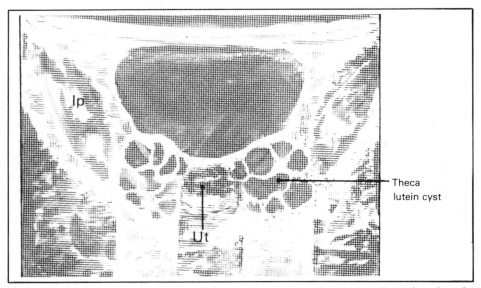

FIGURE 22-17. Theca lutein cysts contain numerous septa, are frequently bilateral, and can be very large. They are associated with hydatidiform mole and the hyperstimulation syndrome.

POLYCYSTIC OVARIES (PCO). PCO are generally found in the early reproductive years. Sonographically, multiple small cysts only 1 to 2 mm in diameter are noted in slightly enlarged ovaries (Fig. 22-18). Polycystic ovaries are often associated with hirsutism, oligomenorrhea, and infertility (Stein-Leventhal syndrome).

TUBO-OVARIAN ABSCESSES. These abscesses are irregularly shaped, thick-walled, fluid-filled structures in the adnexa that may develop a few internal echoes and even an internal fluid-fluid level (Fig. 22-19). Tubo-ovarian abscesses are usually bilateral, but occasionally a unilateral lesion is seen. These abscesses are usually not an isolated finding; multiple abscesses are often noted elsewhere.

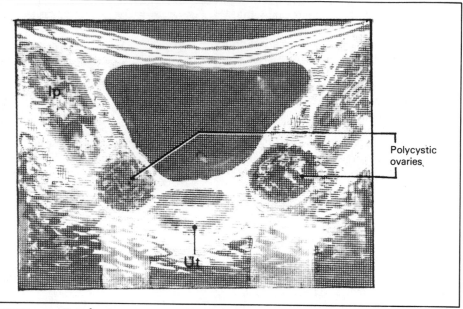

FIGURE 22-18. Polycystic ovaries are slightly enlarged and contain very small cysts. These cysts are small and are barely visible or seen only as echoes.

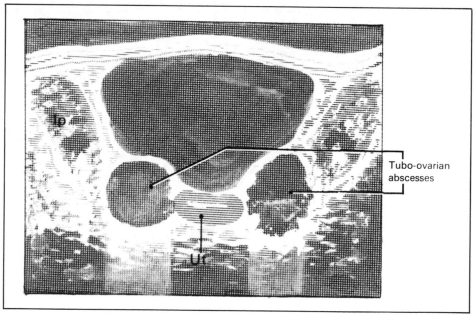

FIGURE 22-19. Tubo-ovarian abscesses may be circular, but more often they have a slightly irregular wall and contain low-level echoes.

Complex Masses

COMPLEX MASSES IN THE OVARY

These masses contain sonolucent and echogenic areas. The walls may be irregular or smooth; the shape is not necessarily spherical.

MUCINOUS CYSTADENOMA AND CYSTADE-NOCARCINOMA OF THE OVARY. These ovarian masses of the reproductive or postmenopausal age group are less common than the serous type and are more likely to be benign. They often have a characteristic sonographic appearance (Figs. 22-20 and 22-21). A cystic mass is present with many septa, and there is some solid material within the septa. When benign, the margins are usually well defined. Malignancy is suggested by large masses of solid tissue and ill-defined borders. Benign and malignant mucinous tumors may be associated with free peritoneal fluid and even with multiple cystic mesenteric masses (pseudomyxoma peritonei).

SEROUS CYSTADENOCARCINOMA. These cysts usually cannot be distinguished from the benign variety (Fig. 22-13). In fact, such cysts may be malignant when no internal material is present. However, features that suggest malignancy are poorly defined walls, considerable amounts of solid tissue, and ascites.

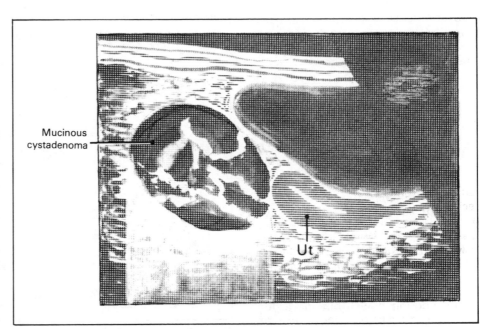

FIGURE 22-20. Mucinous cystadenomas have thick septa within.

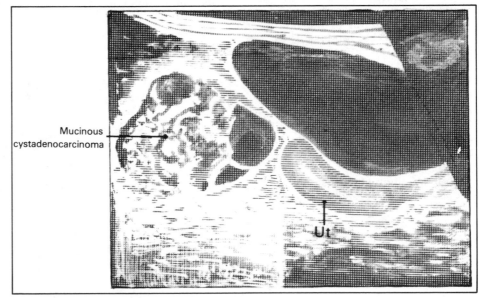

FIGURE 22-21. Mucinous cystadenocarcinomas often have echogenic material within as well as thick septa.

CYSTIC TERATOMAS (DERMOIDS). These cysts of the reproductive or premenarche age group have a wide variety of sonographic appearances:

1. *Mainly cystic.* These often have an echogenic area with acoustic shadowing due to calcium (Fig. 22-22). Teeth may be seen on a radiograph.
2. *Complex internal structure.* There are echogenic areas from fat, hair, or bone often with areas of shadowing. Fluid-fluid levels may be seen (Fig. 22-22).
3. *"Iceberg" appearance.* Often the echogenic material within the cysts shadows the main bulk of the lesion, rendering the mass invisible. A real-time study performed simultaneously with a pelvic examination will often reveal the true condition. In addition, the echogenic mass may blend in with neighboring bowel, but the lesion's presence will be revealed by an indentation of the bladder.
4. *Predominantly solid and homogenous.* Characteristically, dermoids lie in a position anterior to the uterus or adjacent to the fundus. They are common in teenagers.

OVARIAN CANCER. Ovarian cancer is one of the leading causes of death in women. An absolute diagnosis of malignancy cannot usually be made sonographically. However, several ultrasound features are strongly suggestive:

1. Poor definition of the lesion's borders due to tumor spread to adjacent organs
2. Bizarre, complex appearance
3. "Malignant" ascites—loculated fluid between fixed loops of bowel with peritoneal metastases (Fig. 22-23).

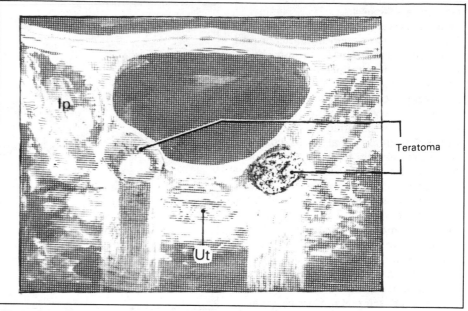

FIGURE 22-22. Teratomas have a number of sonographic patterns. In one of the most characteristic, echogenic material with acoustic shadowing (calcification) occurs within a cystic lesion (on the right). In another characteristic appearance, a mass containing high-level echoes develops (on the left).

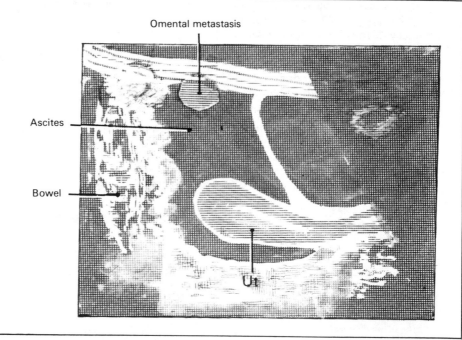

FIGURE 22-23. Malignant ascites. Loops of bowel are tethered to the anterior abdominal wall. Peritoneal metastatic lesions arise from the abdominal wall.

COMPLEX MASSES IN THE UTERUS

HYDATIDIFORM MOLE. This lesion is visualized as an enlarged uterus containing many echogenic cystic areas of varying sizes (Fig. 22-24). The echoes and small cysts represent the vesicles, and larger cystic areas represent areas of degeneration and hemorrhage. In about 40% of cases, theca lutein cysts, which may be quite large, are also seen. These cysts are multilocular.

MISSED ABORTION. A mass due to a missed abortion may appear as an enlarged uterus with an inhomogeneous collection of echoes in the center (as described in Chapter 24). A history of a positive pregnancy test will be obtained.

PYOMETRIA. A uterine cavity that usually contains a few internal echoes results from pyometria, but the appearances of this entity may be complex. Especially when significant debris or gas-forming organisms are present, highly echogenic areas with shadowing may occur.

Solid Masses

These masses contain only low-level echoes, show little or no through transmission, and have irregular or smooth walls.

OVARIAN MASSES

If a solid mass of the ovary is recognized sonographically, most often a specific diagnosis cannot be made. Nevertheless, the features of malignancy, as described previously, should be sought. Any solid ovarian mass in the postmenopausal age group, however, carries a high probability of malignancy. In the menstruating age group endometriosis should be considered.

UTERINE MASSES

FIBROIDS (LEIOMYOMAS). Fibroids represent an overgrowth of uterine smooth muscle that forms a tumor. Leiomyoma is the benign form and leiomyosarcoma the malignant form. Fibroids are the most common tumors in women. They may grow progressively during the menstrual years but usually shrink after menopause. Common symptoms are heavy, prolonged periods, infertility, and pelvic pain. They may be submucosal, interstitial, subserosal, or pedunculated. Sonographically, the features are as follows (Fig. 22-25):

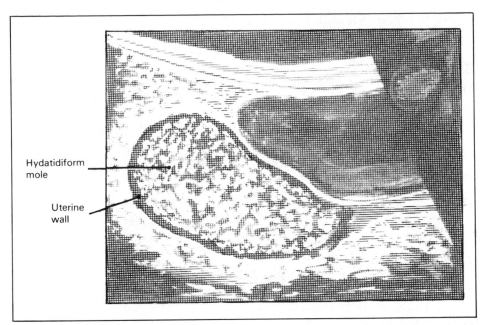

FIGURE 22-24. A hydatidiform mole fills the uterus with low-level echoes interspersed with anechoic spaces.

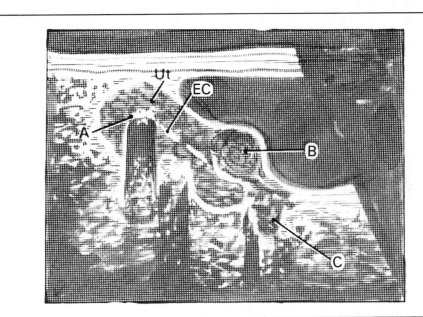

FIGURE 22-25. Fibroids can adopt a number of appearances. In type A there is calcification with acoustic shadowing. In type B, submucosal in location, a lobulated fibroid indents the bladder. Note the distortion of the endometrial cavity adjacent to this lesion. Type C, a subserosal paracervical fibroid, arises in the region of the cervix.

1. Enlarged uterus, often homogeneous unless fibroid degeneration has led to cystic or echogenic areas
2. Usually a lobulated uterine outline
3. Indentation of the bladder outline
4. Echogenic areas with shadowing that represents calcification

Patients with fibroids may need serial ultrasound scans for a period of months or years to rule out rapid growth; a change in size suggests malignancy.

ENDOMETRIAL CANCER. This cancer, a tumor of the uterine endometrial lining, is most common after menopause and is associated with abnormal bleeding. Sonography will show an enlarged uterus with solid tissue. The endometrial cavity often contains fluid. Endometrial cancer cannot always be distinguished from fibroids.

CERVICAL CANCER. The most common genital tract malignancy in women is cervical cancer. The peak age is in the fourth decade. Sonographically, the following may be seen:

1. Bulky cervix with an irregular outline, possibly extending into the vagina or peritoneum (Fig. 22-26)
2. A mass extending from the cervix to the pelvic sidewalls
3. Obstruction of the ureters, producing hydronephrosis
4. Invasion of the bladder, producing an irregular mass effect in the bladder wall

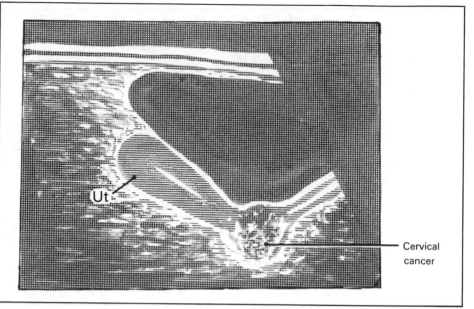

FIGURE 22-26. Cervical cancer causes a mass in the region of the cervix.

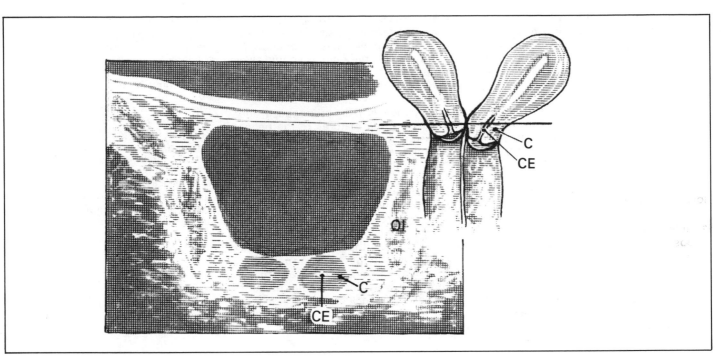

FIGURE 22-27. Diagram of one form of double uterus; there is complete separation of the uteruses with two adjacent cervices. In another form, the two uteruses are joined by a common midline septum.

DEVELOPMENTAL ANOMALY (DOUBLE UTERUS). The uterine shape is distorted; two completely separate uteruses, usually at an oblique axis to each other, may be seen (Fig. 22-27) or a bulky single "uterus," containing two endometrial cavities with a common central wall, may be present. With a bicornuate uterus two endometrial cavities can be seen at the fundus only.

PITFALLS

1. *An empty bladder* is the sonographer's worst enemy. Lesions may be missed if the bladder is empty. The bladder must always be adequately filled. In filling the bladder, three techniques may be used—oral hydration, intravenous hydration, or catheterization of the patient.

2. *Excessive rapid oral hydration* may result in fluid in the small bowel or the cul-de-sac that could be mistaken for a cystic lesion.

3. *Foreign bodies in the pelvis* (e.g., IUDs, metal clips in postoperative cancer patients, and tampons) may be mistaken for a pathologic lesion. Acoustic shadowing occurs with all these objects (see Chapter 25 for details about IUD appearance).

4. *Posthysterectomy changes* such as a large vaginal cuff may mimic a recurrent mass.

5. The fundus of the *retroverted uterus* may be difficult to delineate if the beam lies at the same angle as the uterus. When acutely retroverted, the fundus may lie adjacent to the cervix and simulate a mass. Because a retroverted uterus is globular in shape, enlargement is hard to assess. A fibroid may be mistakenly diagnosed.

6. With *uterine anomalies* such as bicornuate and double uterus, the second horn may be mistaken for an adjacent mass. Careful longitudinal scanning should demonstrate an endometrial cavity in each. With a double uterus two cervices and a vagina will be present.

7. By 1 week *postpartum* the *uterus* has decreased in size to about one half its size at delivery. During the next 4 to 7 weeks the uterus gradually returns to normal size. If the history is unknown, the enlarged uterus may be misdiagnosed as fibroids or other uterine mass.

8. *Pelvic musculature* can be confusing. The iliopsoas and piriform muscles may be misinterpreted as pelvic masses. A solid knowledge of pelvic anatomy is essential.

9. *Bowel,* especially if distended with fluid, may mimic a cystic mass. Observation with real-time should show peristalsis in bowel. Alternatively, a water enema may confirm that this "cystic mass" represents fluid-filled colon.

10. Ten to fifteen milliliters of *fluid* posterior to the *cul-de-sac* may be normal in women in the reproductive years. A portion of this fluid is derived from follicular rupture.

11. Make sure the supposed pelvic mass is not a *pelvic kidney*. A pelvic kidney will have a central group of sinus echoes and a reniform shape.

WHERE ELSE TO LOOK

1. When performing a scan of a patient with a large pelvic mass of ovarian or uterine origin, the *kidneys* should also be examined to rule out *hydronephrosis* caused by pressure on the ureters.

2. If the patient is in the menopausal age group and the features of the pelvic mass suggest *malignancy,* large size, complex echoes (e.g., internal structure), and ovarian origin, then a *search for metastatic lesions* should be carried out. The most common sites of metastatic lesions from pelvic masses are peritoneal, para-aortic nodes, and liver.

3. If you suspect that a *pelvic kidney* is present, examine the normal sites where the kidney should lie and make sure that two kidneys are not present in their usual location.

SELECTED READING

Gross, B. H., and Callen, P. W. Ultrasound of the Uterus. In P. W. Callen (Ed.), *Ultrasonography in Obstetrics and Gynecology.* Philadelphia: Saunders, 1983.

Morley, P., and Barnett, E. The Ovarian Mass. In R. C. Sanders and A. E. James (Eds.), *The Principles and Practice of Ultrasound in Obstetrics and Gynecology.* New York: Appleton-Century-Crofts, 1980.

Rosenberg, E. R., and Trought, W. S. The ultrasonographic evaluation of large cystic pelvic masses. *Am. J. Obstet. Gynecol.* 139:579–586, 1981.

Sample, W. F., Lippe, B. M., and Gyepes, M. T. Gray-scale ultrasonography of the normal female pelvis. *Radiology* 125:477, 1977.

23. ACUTE PELVIC PAIN

JOAN CAMPBELL

SONOGRAM ABBREVIATIONS

Ab   Abscess

Bl   Bladder

FP   Fetal pole

IUD   Intrauterine device

Ov   Ovary

Ut   Uterus

KEY WORDS

Abscess. Localized collection of pus.

Adnexa. The regions of the ovaries, fallopian tubes, and broad ligaments.

Adnexal Ring. A circular mass that has an echo-free center and an echogenic border, often seen with ectopic pregnancy. Usually it is formed from the remnants of a gestational sac, although there are many other causes.

Amenorrhea. Absence of menstrual periods in a woman of menstrual age.

Anteverted. The body of the uterus is tilted forward.

Corpus Luteum. Small structure that develops in the second half of the menstrual cycle within the ovary and secretes progesterone.

Cornu. Lateral horn of the uterus corresponding to the origin of the fallopian tube.

Cul-de-sac. An area posterior to the uterus and anterior to the rectum where fluid often collects.

Decidua. The modified mucous membrane of the uterus that has been transformed during the menstrual cycle in preparation for pregnancy. The decidua are expelled during menstruation if implantation of a fertilized ovum does not occur.

Dysmenorrhea. Difficult or painful menstruation.

Dyspareunia. Difficult or painful intercourse.

Ectopic Pregnancy. Pregnancy in any location other than the body of the uterus.

Endometritis. Infection of the endometrial cavity.

Endometrium. Mucous membrane lining of the uterus.

Endometrial Cavity, Canal. A potential space in the center of the uterus where blood or pus may collect.

Follicle (Graafian Follicle). An ovarian sac-like structure in which the ovum matures prior to rupture at ovulation. The follicle is visualized as an eccentric cavity with fluid.

Hematocrit. The percentage of red blood cells in a given volume of blood.

Hydrosalpinx. Accumulation of watery fluid in the fallopian tube. The tube is blocked at the peritoneal end by a prior infection with adhesions and fibrosis.

Interstitial Pregnancy. Pregnancy ectopically located in the proximal portion of the fallopian tube where it enters the wall of the uterus. This is a particularly dangerous type of ectopic pregnancy.

Laparoscopy. Surgically invasive technique for viewing the pelvic anatomy in situ through a small tube using fiberoptics. The tube is inserted into the perineum through a small incision near the umbilicus.

Leukocyte Count. The number of circulating white blood cells. This count increases when an inflammatory process is present as in PID but remains normal in ectopic pregnancy and endometriosis.

Myometrium. Smooth muscle of the uterus.

Pelvic Inflammatory Disease (PID). Infection that spreads from the uterine tubes and ovaries throughout the pelvis; commonly due to gonorrhea.

Peritonitis. Inflammation of the peritoneum, which is the serous membrane lining the abdominal cavity.

Purulent. Containing pus.

Pyosalpinx. Accumulation of pus in the fallopian tube.

Pregnancy Tests. (1) *Urine.* Urine pregnancy tests are not very reliable. Both false positive and false negative results occur. (2) *Blood (BHCG).* This test involves radioisotopic methods. It is not performed daily in most laboratories. The test is so sensitive that elevated HCG levels are detected even when the fetus has been dead for some time.

Retroverted Uterus. The long axis of the uterus points posteriorly toward the sacrum.

Tubo-Ovarian Abscess (TOA). An abscess involving the ovary and the fallopian tube.

Vulva. Region where the urethra and the vagina exit in the perineum.

Zygote. The fertilized ovum.

THE CLINICAL PROBLEM

A great number of gynecologic patients have acute pelvic pain. Obstetric disorders should be considered if the patient is of child-bearing age. The main differential diagnoses of acute pain are pelvic inflammatory disease (PID), ectopic pregnancy, and ruptured or twisted ovarian cyst. Endometriosis may have similar sonographic findings but does not usually have a similar clinical presentation.

Pelvic Inflammatory Disease

Patients with PID are usually febrile and often have a purulent vaginal discharge. On clinical examination an adnexal mass may be felt, and the patient may have pain associated with movement of the cervix. Often physical examination is so painful that a thorough search cannot be completed. In these cases a pelvic sonogram is needed as a supplemental examination, and at times it may replace the physical examination completely. To comprehend the sonographic appearances of PID, the pathophysiology must be thoroughly understood. Acute or chronic PID is most commonly caused by gonorrhea. Pyogenic (*Escherichia coli*) and tuberculous infections are the other primary causes. There is an association with the use of intrauterine contraceptive devices. PID due to gonorrhea spreads along the mucous membranes and travels from the vulva to the adnexa. However, the main site of localization is the fallopian tube. If left untreated, the course of tubal infection progresses as follows:

1. Endometritis (Fig. 23-1).
2. Acute salpingitis (Figs. 23-1 and 23-2).
3. Chronic salpingitis.
4. Pyosalpinx: A blockage of the peritoneal (fimbriated) end of the tube with an accumulation of pus (Fig. 23-4).
5. Tubo-ovarian abscess (TOA): Pus surrounded by tubal and ovarian tissue (Figs. 23-3 and 23-4).
6. Hydrosalpinx: The pus from a pyosalpinx resorbs and becomes sterile watery fluid (Fig. 23-4).
7. Pelvic abscess: Abscess outside of the tube in the region of the ovary or cul-de-sac (Figs. 23-1 and 23-3).

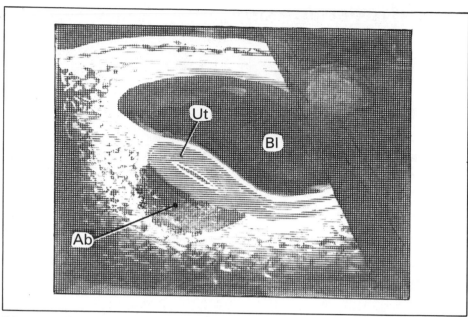

FIGURE 23-1. Pus in the cul-de-sac due to pelvic inflammatory disease. There is also a small amount of fluid in the endometrial cavity, a common finding with endometritis.

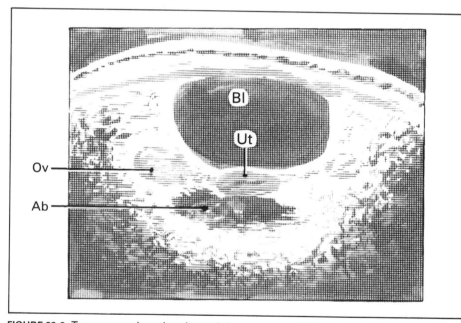

FIGURE 23-2. Transverse view showing cul-de-sac pus and inflammatory involvement of the right adnexal area.

The purulent contents of a TOA may escape the confines of the tube and ovary area and cause peritonitis or multiple pelvic abscesses. If an abscess is present, antibiotic treatment usually suffices, although surgical drainage may be contemplated. The pelvic sonogram will assist the clinician by determining the extent of the disease, including the presence and size of adnexal masses. If large echo-free areas compatible with pus are present, surgical drainage rather than antibiotic therapy may be appropriate. If antibiotic therapy is given, the response to therapy can be followed by means of serial sonograms.

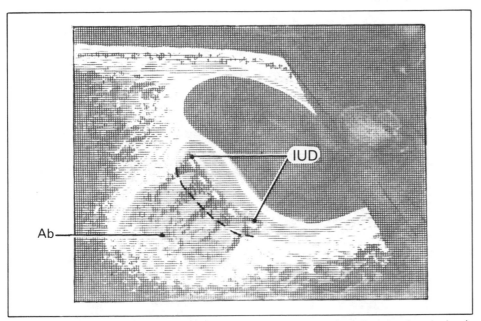

FIGURE 23-3. Tubo-ovarian abscess in the cul-de-sac resulting from intrauterine device (a Lippes loop). Note loss of the interface between the uterus and the abscess.

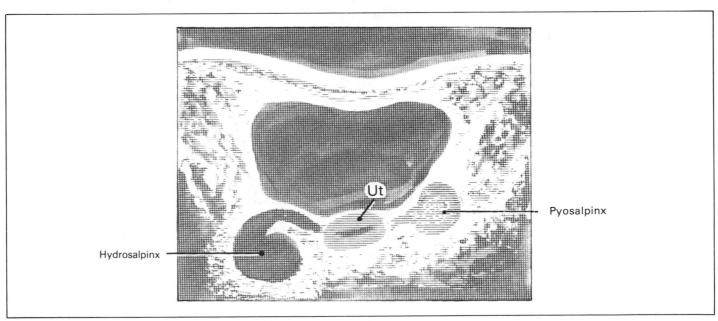

FIGURE 23-4. Fluid-filled lesion in the right adnexa with a shape suggestive of hydrosalpinx. In the left adnexa there is a collection with features that suggest a pyosalpinx.

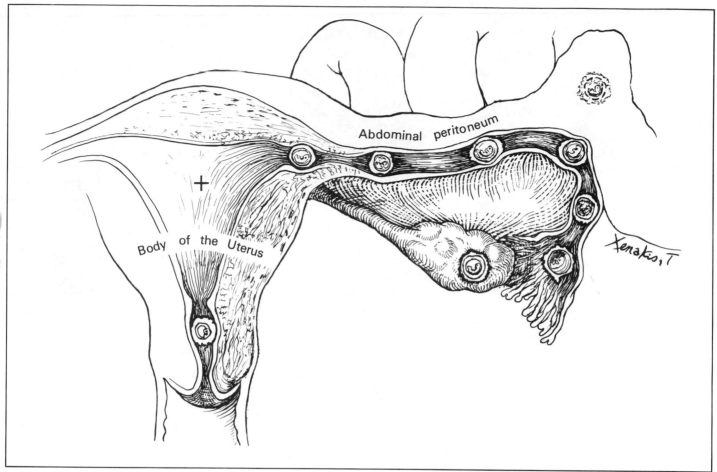

FIGURE 23-5. Possible sites of ectopic pregnancy.

Ectopic Pregnancy

After successful nonsurgical treatment of an infection, thickened and scarred fallopian tubes may still remain. Although these injured tubes may not prevent the passage of sperm for fertilization of ova, the scarring may retard the return of a fertilized zygote into the uterine cavity. The zygote may begin to develop and grow in the fallopian tube, and eventually pain will result due to distention and rupture of the fallopian tube. Ectopic pregnancy may also occur at other sites, because by definition such a pregnancy develops outside the body of the uterus. Possible sites include the abdominal cavity, the fallopian tubes as previously mentioned, the cornu of the uterus, and the cervix (Fig. 23-5). Pregnancies in the uterine cornu are the most difficult to diagnose because sonographically they appear at first to be partly in the uterine body. If misdiagnosed, they will progress to a more advanced stage before causing symptoms.

The clinical symptoms that suggest an ectopic pregnancy are:

1. Acute pelvic pain (before or after rupture)
2. Vaginal bleeding (before or after rupture)
3. Amenorrhea (consistent with pregnancy)
4. Adnexal mass (before or after rupture)
5. Positive pregnancy test (not always available or reliable in early gestation)
6. Cervical tenderness (usually after rupture)
7. A drop in hematocrit (usually after rupture)
8. Shock (after rupture)

Rupture usually occurs at or before the eighth week of gestation. An ectopic pregnancy is an urgent surgical emergency. The diagnosis usually cannot be made on clinical grounds alone so that pelvic sonography may be helpful in making a more specific diagnosis. Often sonography demonstrates an intrauterine pregnancy and thus precludes surgical intervention. Occasionally the sonographic picture of an ectopic pregnancy is so typical that the obstetrician can proceed straight to surgery (20% of cases). Further investigation of the remaining cases by means of laparoscopy is usually dictated by clinical signs, although some sonographic features may be supportive.

Abdominal pregnancy outside the tube and uterus is rare. Although abdominal pregnancies can be carried to term, they are most often removed when diagnosed. Clinically, in an advanced abdominal pregnancy the fetal parts are easily palpable.

Cystic Masses

Rupture or bleeding of any pelvic mass causes acute pelvic pain similar to that seen in rupture of an ectopic pregnancy. Torsion (a twisting of a cyst on a pedicle), hemorrhage, and rupture are the three complications that cause pain in cysts. Hemorrhage often results from torsion. The sonographic findings of ovarian cyst rupture are confusingly similar to those of ectopic pregnancy, but more specific changes are seen with hemorrhage and torsion, especially if there has been a previous sonogram showing a simple cyst.

Sonography helps (1) when clinical examination is not possible because of acute pain or obesity, (2) when accurate size estimation is necessary, (3) when it is unclear whether the mass is ovarian or uterine, and (4) in deciding whether a mass is cystic or solid.

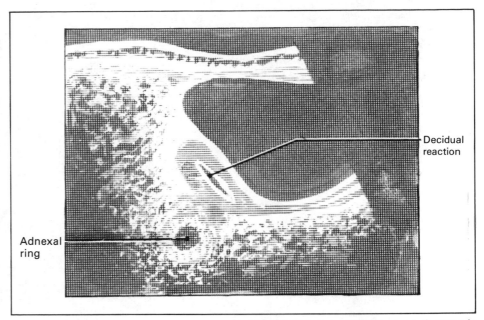

FIGURE 23-6. Ectopic pregnancy. A mass in the cul-de-sac has the configuration termed an adnexal ring. There is some fluid forming a decidual reaction within the endometrial cavity.

ANATOMY
See Chapter 22.

TECHNIQUE
See Chapter 22.

PATHOLOGY

Acute Pelvic Inflammatory Disease

There is an increase in echogenicity of the endometrial canal with separation due to fluid occasionally. Fluid may develop in a cul-de-sac. A loss of interfaces and blurring of the margins between the pelvic structures are usual. The ovaries may adhere to the sidewalls of the pelvis or the uterus and may not be easily seen (Figs. 23-1 to 23-4).

Fluid in an irregular, thick-walled cul-de-sac and cystic or complex masses located lateral, posterior, or superior to the uterus may represent pyosalpinx or TOAs. Fluid-fluid levels may develop.

Chronic Pelvic Inflammatory Disease

The uterus exhibits a normal echogenic pattern, but there is gross loss of the normal anatomic planes. Cystic or complex masses may represent pyosalpinx and tubo-ovarian abscesses, but in the chronic stage a hydrosalpinx is also possible. All structures may adhere in a central mass.

Ectopic Pregnancy

WITHOUT BLEED (BEFORE RUPTURE)

Features that suggest ectopic pregnancy include the following:

1. Uterine enlargement.
2. Decidual reaction in the endometrium without a gestational sac and an adnexal mass, which may be echo-filled or hypoechoic (Fig 23-6).
3. Gestational sac with thick rind in the adnexa with or without an identifiable fetal pole (Fig. 23-7). When this lesion is less well defined, the term *adnexal ring* is used (Fig. 23-6).
4. Cul-de-sac fluid.

WITH BLEED (AFTER RUPTURE)

If bleeding has occurred, there is a loss of uterine outline due to hematoma. Blood may surround the uterus, giving a "pseudo uterus" effect (Fig. 23-8); the presence of blood may not be obvious because it looks like the uterus.

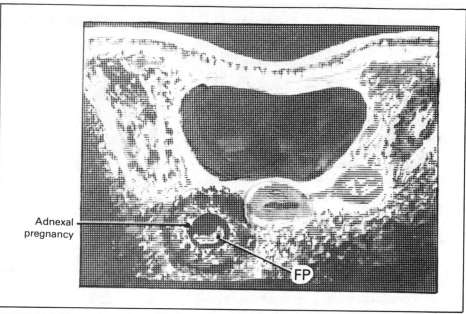

Adnexal pregnancy

FP

FIGURE 23-7. Transverse view showing typical appearances of ectopic gestational sac with viable fetal pole.

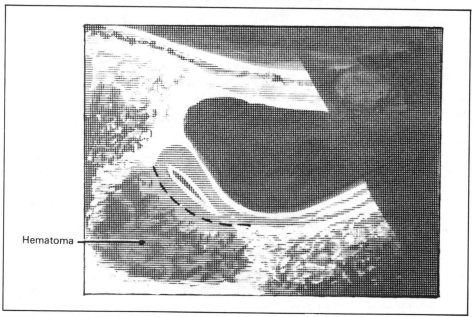

Hematoma

FIGURE 23-8. Ectopic pregnancy after rupture. A hematoma obscures the uterine outline.

Twisted Ovarian Cyst (Hemorrhagic Cyst)

These are fluid-filled cysts containing echoes that may form a fluid-fluid level (Fig. 23-9) or a clump-like pattern due to clot.

Ruptured Cyst

Common features of a ruptured cyst include the following:

1. An adnexal mass with an irregular shape
2. Cul-de-sac fluid
3. Evidence of bleeding with development of a relatively echogenic mass (hard to separate from the uterus), as in ruptured ectopic pregnancy.

PITFALLS

1. *Acoustic artifacts*
   a. *Enhancement.* Increased transmission through a cystic structure may obscure structures located posteriorly (the "too full" bladder).
   b. *Shadowing.* Decreased transmission through a solid structure may obscure structures located posteriorly.
2. *Nonspecificity of an adnexal ring.* A thick echogenic band around a predominantly cystic mass is known as an adnexal ring. Although this ring is sometimes a sign of ectopic pregnancy, it is not pathognomonic of this disorder. Other conditions such as dermoid, PID, and endometriosis not associated with pregnancy may also result in this appearance.
3. *Interstitial pregnancy.* Interstitial pregnancy may be misdiagnosed as intrauterine pregnancy. However, the gestational sac in an interstitial pregnancy is eccentrically located and surrounded by a thinner layer of myometrial tissue (Fig. 23-10) than usual. Unfortunately, similar findings are also seen with bicornuate pregnancy and some fibroids.

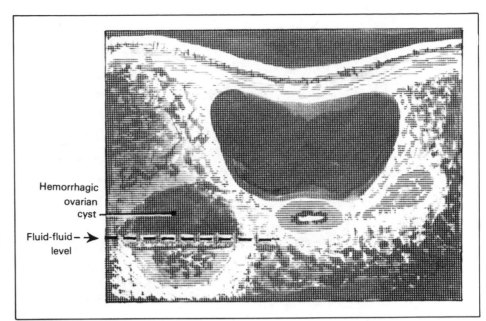

FIGURE 23-9. Hemorrhage into an ovarian cyst creates a fluid-fluid level, which changes position when the patient is shifted.

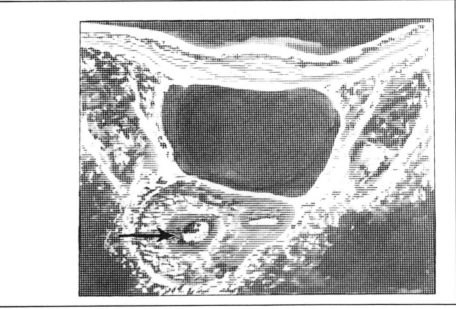

FIGURE 23-10. In an interstitial pregnancy the myometrium around the sac is barely visible.

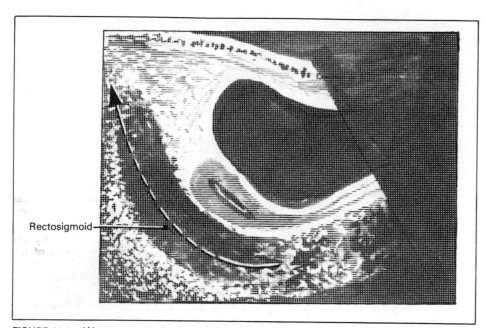

Rectosigmoid

FIGURE 23-11. Water enema. A small amount of fluid is introduced through a tube into the rectum and watched under real-time as it fills the rectosigmoid colon.

4. *Decidual casts.* A decidual cast is an echogenic line or circle within the endometrial cavity. It may resemble a gestational sac. An intrauterine pregnancy should be diagnosed only when a fetal pole is visible within the sac. If a fetal pole is not seen, continue searching the adnexal regions for abnormal masses or other signs of ectopic pregnancy. A double outline to a questionable sac favors an intrauterine pregnancy.

5. *Cul-de-sac fluid.* A small amount of fluid may appear in the region of the cul-de-sac during a normal menstrual period.

6. *Bowel.* Bowel may masquerade as an abnormal adnexal mass. This is such a common finding that any questionable complex mass must be proved to be truly pathologic. Real-time or a water enema allow the distinction to be made (Fig. 23-11).

SELECTED READING

Fleischer, A. C., Boehm, F. H., and James, A. E. Sonographic Evaluation of Ectopic Pregnancy. In R. C. Sanders and A. E. James (Eds.), *The Principles and Practice of Ultrasonography in Obstetrics and Gynecology.* New York: Appleton-Century-Crofts, 1980.

24. ABNORMAL VAGINAL BLEEDING

JOAN CAMPBELL

SONOGRAM ABBREVIATIONS

Bl   Bladder

C   Cervix

F   Fetus
FP   Fetal pole

GS   Gestational sac

Pl   Placenta

Ut   Uterus

KEY WORDS

Abortion. Termination of pregnancy prior to 20 weeks; various subdivisions of this term are discussed in the text.

Anembryonic. Gestation without development of a fetal pole (blighted ovum).

Dilatation and Curettage (D and C). Dilatation of the cervical canal and removal of the uterine contents.

Bleeding Dyscrasia. An abnormal and pathologic blood condition.

Endocrine. Pertains to organs that secrete hormones directly into the bloodstream.

Endometrium. Mucous lining of the uterus.

Estrogen. Hormone secreted by the ovary and in pregnancy by the placenta.

Fetal Pole. The early developing fetus. Consists of a small collection of echoes found within the gestational sac.

Gestational Sac. Sac-like structure that is normally within the uterus and represents the early developing pregnancy.

Human Chorionic Gonadotropin (HCG). Hormone that rises to very high levels in pregnancy. A radioimmunoassay test is used to assess it.

Hormone. A chemical substance produced by the body that has a specific effect on the activity of a certain organ or organs.

Macerated Fetus. The degenerative changes and eventual disintegration of a fetus retained in the uterus after fetal death.

Progesterone. Hormone produced by the corpus luteum in the second half of the menstrual cycle that modifies the endometrium in preparation for implantation of a fertilized ovum.

Septic. Pertaining to the presence of pathogenic bacteria and their products in blood or tissue.

Spontaneous Abortion. An unplanned abortion (miscarriage) of the fetus and gestational sac before 20 weeks' gestation. After 20 weeks the spontaneous loss of pregnancy is termed premature delivery.

Trophoblast. Tissue that supports the developing pregnancy, for example, the gestational sac.

THE CLINICAL PROBLEM

The uterus is the only organ in the body for which periodic loss of tissue with bleeding is a sign of health, not disease. A delicate balance of pituitary and ovarian hormones regulates this periodic loss of blood and tissue. Changes in progesterone and estrogen levels throughout the menstrual cycle first promote endometrial proliferation. Then, if implantation does not occur, the altered hormone levels withdraw support from the endometrium, resulting in menstrual flow. This flow of blood should be consistent in regularity, amount, and duration. Irregularity of any of these characteristics suggests pathology.

Conditions that may cause abnormal bleeding but do not distort the normal pelvic anatomy (e.g., bleeding dyscrasias) cannot be detected by sonography. However, many disorders that do distort the normal pelvic anatomy and result in abnormal bleeding can be diagnosed sonographically. Local uterine disorders include malignancies of the uterine body or cervix, benign submucosal fibroids, polyps, and adenomyosis. Local ovarian or adnexal disorders include malignancies, ovarian tumors (cystic or solid) that secrete steroid compounds, pelvic inflammatory disease, and endometriosis. Obstetric disorders that may also cause abnormal bleeding include abortion, ectopic pregnancy, premature separation of the placenta (abruption), placenta previa, and trophoblastic neoplastic conditions such as hydatidiform mole and choriocarcinoma.

Neoplasms (see Chapter 22) and second and third trimester bleeding problems such as placenta previa and abruptio placentae are discussed in Chapter 29. Therefore, this section will focus on spontaneous abortions.

The majority of spontaneous abortions occur between the fifth and twelfth weeks of pregnancy; a patient may therefore consult her physician for abnormal bleeding without suspecting that she is pregnant. A pregnancy test is usually performed. However, an early pregnancy of 5 to 6 weeks' gestation may give false negative results in a urine pregnancy test. The physician may then send the patient for a sonogram to determine the viability and location of the pregnancy. If the pregnancy is not viable, the subsequent management of the patient is usually the same regardless of the exact subcategory of abortion. Eventually, the patient will undergo dilatation and curettage (D and C) to clear the uterus of any remaining products of conception. The different types of spontaneous abortion that can be distinguished sonographically are (1) threatened abortion (a visible fetus with vaginal bleeding), (2) incomplete abortion (partial evacuation of the fetus and placenta), (3) complete abortion (no retained products), (4) missed abortion (retained fetus and placenta), (5) blighted ovum (anembryonic pregnancy), (6) inevitable abortion (abortion in progress), and (7) septic abortion (infected dead fetus or retained products).

Hydatidiform mole is a condition in which pregnancy develops abnormally into a form of neoplasm. The uterus is filled with grape-like structures (vesicles). This condition causes bleeding, vomiting, and an enlarged uterine size for date. The human chorionic gonadotropin titer (HCG) is very high. Dilatation and curettage is performed because the condition may develop into a neoplasm that spreads to other portions of the body.

ANATOMY

Uterus

The uterus enlarges in relation to the length of pregnancy. A gestational sac is visible as a well-defined circle of echoes in the fundus of the uterus. The sac can be seen as early as 4 weeks but only reliably by 6 weeks. At first, at 6 weeks, the sac should occupy less than one half of the total volume of the uterus and should appear echo-free because echoes from the fetal pole cannot yet be visualized. By 8 weeks the sac should occupy approximately one half of the uterine volume, and by 10 weeks the entire uterine cavity should be encompassed. The gestational sac is surrounded by a ring of echoes known as the gestational ring (Fig. 24-1). This ring should be well defined and of uniform thickness except at the site where the placenta will develop. A sonolucent extra gestational sac space ("implantation bleed") is not an uncommon feature of normal pregnancy between the sixth and tenth weeks (Fig. 24-2).

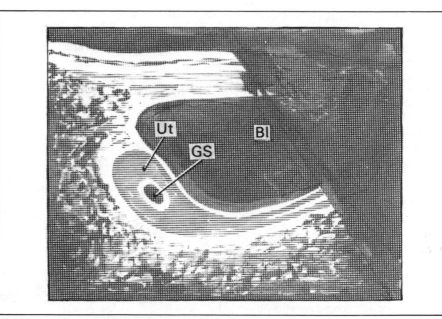

FIGURE 24-1. Normal gestational sac at 6 weeks.

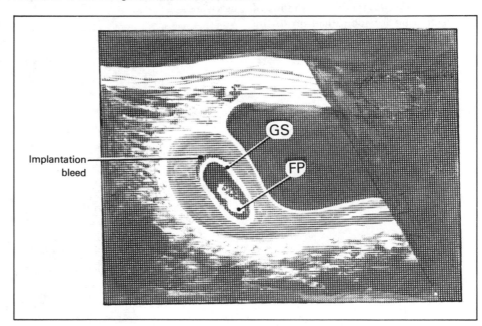

FIGURE 24-2. Normal gestational sac at 8 weeks; a fetal pole is visible.

Fetus

At 7 weeks, the fetus should be consistently seen within the uterus as a small collection of echoes known as a "fetal pole." Fetal heart and limb motion is visible at this early stage with high-quality ultrasound systems. This fetal pole may be seen as early as 6 weeks. At 8 to 9 weeks the fetal echo complex is much more well defined (Fig. 24-2). By 11 weeks some fetal structures can be identified (Fig 24-3).

TECHNIQUE

Real-Time

Real-time is essential in the positive identification of fetal limb motion or fetal heart motion.

Full Bladder Technique

The full bladder technique should always be used, especially when the cervix is the area of interest. For details of this technique for identification of the uterus and ovaries, see Chapter 22.

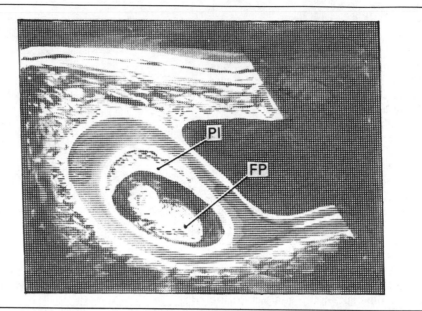

FIGURE 24-3. Normal fetal pole and gestational sac at 11 weeks. The placenta is beginning to be visible.

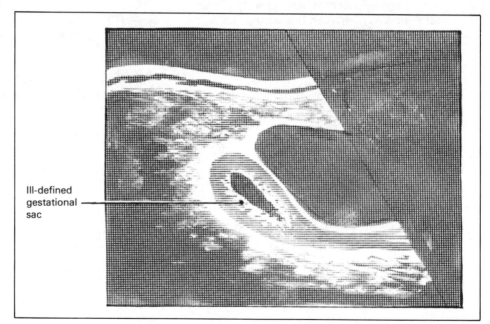

FIGURE 24-4. Incomplete abortion with empty ill-defined gestational sac.

PATHOLOGY

Threatened Abortion

Threatened abortion is not visible sonographically. This diagnosis is made whenever vaginal bleeding occurs within the first 20 weeks of pregnancy with a closed cervix. The sonogram should demonstrate a pregnancy corresponding to the patient's dates.

Most such pregnancies will proceed to term, but because of the threat of abortion and increased risk of bleeding later in pregnancy, serial sonograms during the pregnancy may be requested.

Incomplete Abortion

If a threatened abortion progresses and some of the products of conception are passed as tissue with bleeding, the clinical diagnosis is an incomplete abortion. However, portions of the placenta and some fetal parts may remain within the uterus, resulting in continued bleeding. Sonographically, the uterus appears enlarged. With incomplete abortion, the sonographer may note an empty, ill-defined gestational sac within the uterus or a sac with internal echoes that are not clearly fetal. Occasionally, no sac at all will be identified, but large clumps of echoes in the center of the uterus may be seen. This sonographic confirmation of diagnosis is useful because a dilatation and curettage may be necessary to complete the process of abortion (Figs. 24-4, 24-5, and 24-6).

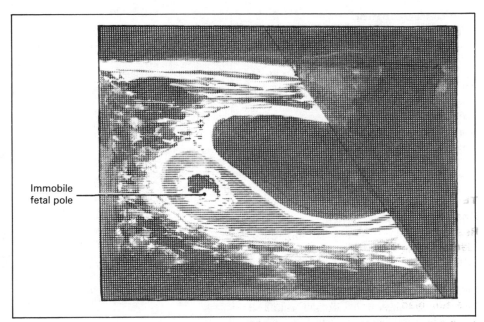

FIGURE 24-5. Incomplete abortion with immobile fetal pole within a relatively well defined gestational sac.

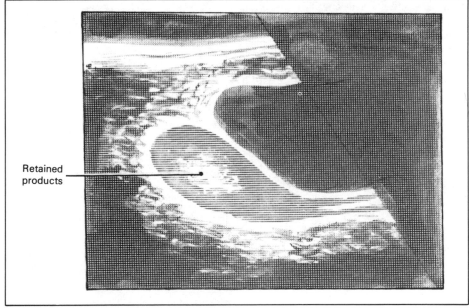

FIGURE 24-6. Incomplete abortion with retained products of conception. There is a featureless mass in the uterus.

Complete Abortion

With complete abortion, all products of conception pass. Sonographically, the uterus will appear enlarged, but a gestational sac or fetus will not be identified. However, a line of central echoes within the uterus may be present, which represent a decidual reaction. The uterus may remain enlarged up to 2 weeks after the abortion. After the initial passage of clots, bleeding is minimal, and the patient usually does not require any further treatment.

The sonographer's role is to confirm that the uterus is empty. Echoes within the cavity may represent blood rather than retained products of conception (Fig. 24-7).

Missed Abortion

When the fetus dies but is retained within the uterus, a missed abortion has occurred. Some bleeding may be noted with a missed abortion, but other clinical signs are usually present. The uterus is often too small for the expected dates. Most frequently, missed abortions occur between 10 and 14 weeks of gestation. This is a time when the fetus should be well defined sonographically, but with a missed abortion, the expected fetal and gestational sac characteristics are not present. Instead, a uterus containing a clump of shapeless echoes in its center may be visualized (Fig. 24-8). If the fetus is not macerated, the uterus will contain a gestational sac, but the fetal pole will show no evidence of movement or fetal heart motion (Fig. 24-5).

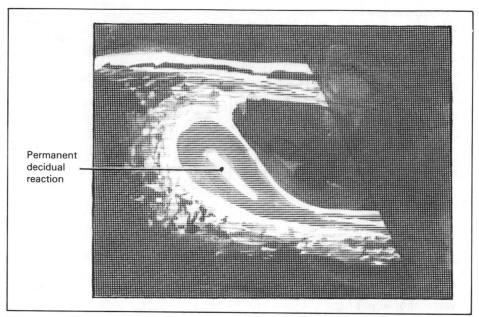

Permanent decidual reaction

FIGURE 24-7. Pronounced decidual reaction due to some retained products of conception.

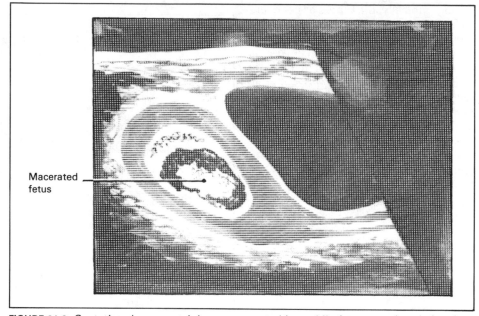

Macerated fetus

FIGURE 24-8. Gestational sac containing a macerated immobile fetus—a missed abortion.

Blighted Ovum

The definition of a blighted ovum is an anembryonic pregnancy. This means that the sac develops but the embryo does not. Clinically, the patient usually has slight vaginal bleeding. The pregnancy test may be positive even though no embryo is present because there is continued production of HCG by the trophoblasts in the sac. The growth of the sac will not increase as it would in a normal pregnancy. Although eventually a blighted ovum will abort, the physician may intervene with a D and C before that occurs.

The main sonographic finding is a trophoblastic ring within the uterus. This ring may have an appearance similar to that of a gestational sac, although the borders are usually less irregular and more ill defined (Fig. 24-9A,B). No fetal pole will be seen within the sac, and there may be a fluid-fluid level due to blood within the gestational sac; this is definitive evidence of fetal death. The absence of a fetal pole may be misleading because early normal gestational sacs also appear to be without a fetal pole. To solve this dilemma the patient may be asked to return in a week or two for a repeat sonogram. If on the second sonogram the sac has not grown and a fetal pole is still not present, the diagnosis of a blighted ovum can be made. There may be a discrepancy between the size of the sac and the uterine size, with the sac being too large or too small for the uterus (Fig. 24-9A,B).

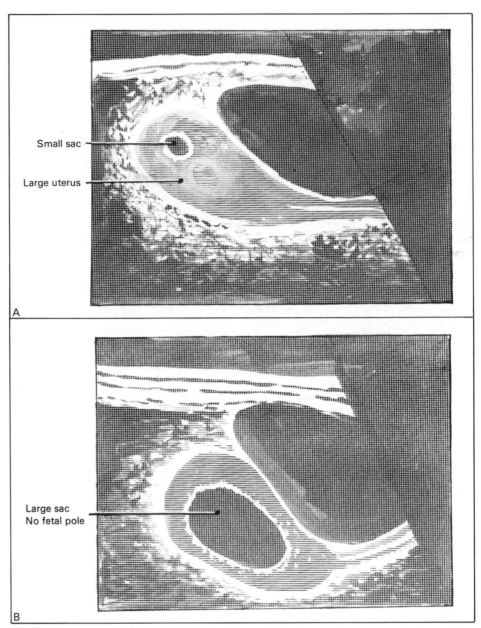

FIGURE 24-9. Blighted ovum. A. A small sac with a thin irregular trophoblastic ring in a large uterus. B. A large sac with a poorly defined border in a small uterus.

Inevitable Abortion

These pregnancies are usually clinically obvious. The patient consults her physician because she is experiencing some bleeding. The physican examines her and discovers that her cervix is dilating and the pregnancy is doomed to be aborted. Sonographically, the area of the cervix may appear to be widened and fluid-filled owing to blood and dilatation. A sonolucent space around the sac may be present where the sac has dissected away from the uterine wall. A fluid-fluid level may be present within the aborting sac. The gestational sac may lie at the level of the cervix and may be in the process of being aborted (Fig. 24-10).

Septic Abortion

In septic abortion there are infected products of conception in the uterus, perhaps as a result of surgical abortion with nonsterile devices. Alternatively, infection may occur in retained products after a spontaneous or induced abortion. Sonographically, the uterus will be enlarged, and there will be increased endometrial echoes. If the infection is caused by gas-forming organisms, areas of shadowing may be produced (Fig. 24-11).

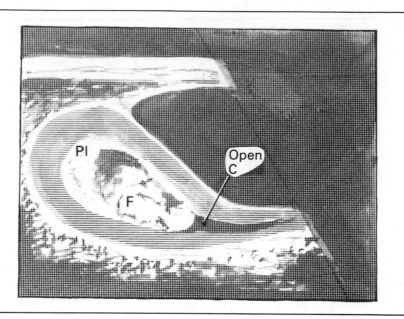

FIGURE 24-10. Incompetent cervix with inevitable abortion. One can see fluid in the cervix almost to the vagina. Note the irregular macerated fetus within the amniotic cavity. The fetus is in the process of being aborted.

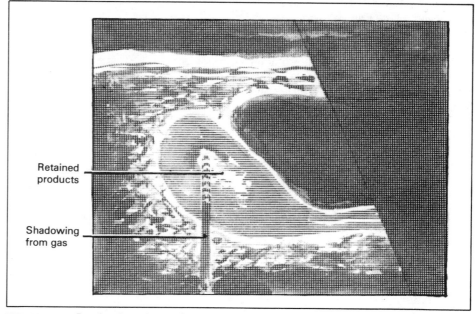

FIGURE 24-11. Retained products of conception with infection. Gas associated with retained products is responsible for some acoustic shadowing.

Hydatidiform Mole

Vaginal bleeding, vomiting (hyperemesis gravidarum), and high blood pressure suggest the presence of a mole. The uterus will be filled with echoes interspersed with echo-free spaces (Fig. 24-12). Occasionally, a fetus and a placenta are associated with a mole. Large echo-free spaces may occur with a mole, and the process may be confused with a missed abortion or a fibroid; however, the HCG titers will be markedly elevated.

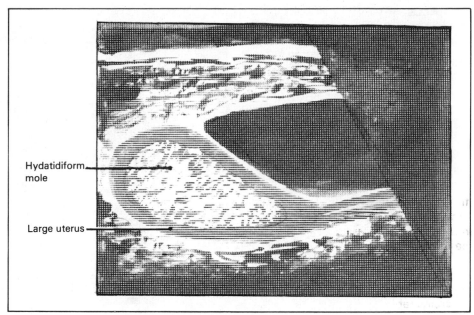

Hydatidiform mole

Large uterus

FIGURE 24-12. Hydatidiform mole. Irregular echoes and small sonolucent spaces fill the uterus.

PITFALLS

1. *Changes in sac shape* may be caused by external compression due to a distended bladder or bowel or to fibroids in the uterine wall (Fig 24-13).
2. *Placental sac thickening.* The placenta starts to develop at about 8 weeks' gestation. It is first seen as a thickened portion of the gestational ring. This thickening should not be misconstrued as an abnormality of the ring (Fig. 24-14).
3. *Mole mimics.* Other entities may mimic the complex echo pattern seen in a molar pregnancy. These include degenerating fibroid and missed abortion.
4. *Perisac sonolucent area.* Between the sixth and eighth weeks of pregnancy a sonolucent space may be seen around a portion of the gestational sac as a normal variant; this is thought to be due to an implantation bleed (Fig. 24-2).

SELECTED READING

Anderson, S. G. Management of threatened abortion with real-time sonography. *Obstet. Gynecol.* 55:2, 1980.

Bennett, M. J., and Kerr-Wilson, R. H. J. Evaluation of threatened abortion by ultrasound. *Obstet. Gynecol.* 17:382–384, 1980.

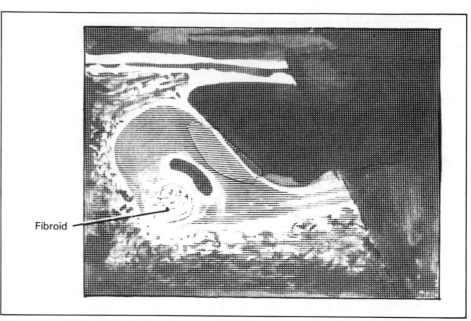

FIGURE 24-13. Fibroid distorting the uterus. This fibroid is more echogenic than the remainder of the uterus; other fibroids may be less echogenic.

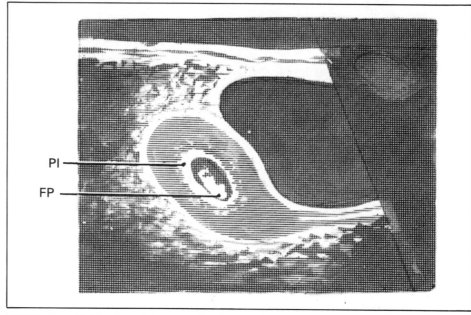

FIGURE 24-14. Thickening of the gestational sac at the site of the developing placenta may be mistaken for an abnormal finding.

25. INTRAUTERINE CONTRACEPTIVE DEVICES

"Lost IUD"

PATRICIA MAY KAPLAN

SONOGRAM ABBREVIATIONS

Bl Bladder

C   Cervix

E   Endometrium

Ip Iliopsoas muscle
IUD Intrauterine device

Ov Ovary

Ut Uterus

V   Vagina

KEY WORDS

Adnexa. Area of the broad ligament and ovaries.

Cul-de-sac. Area posterior to the uterus and anterior to the rectum, a common site for fluid collections.

Endometrial Cavity. Potential space in the center of the uterus where blood or pus may collect.

Myometrium. Uterine smooth muscle.

Os. (1) *External.* The mouth of the uterus at the level of the cervix as it joins the vagina. (2) *Internal.* Junction of the cervix and uterus proper.

Pelvic Inflammatory Disease (PID). Infection that spreads throughout the pelvis, often due to gonorrhea. If it is secondary to an IUD, other bacteria are usually found.

Retroverted. A uterus that points back toward the sacrum.

THE CLINICAL PROBLEM

Intrauterine contraceptive devices (IUD, IUCD) are the second most popular means of birth control after oral contraceptives. Although many varieties of IUDs are available, only the most commonly used devices will be discussed here.

The proper location of an IUD, regardless of type, is in the endometrial cavity at the uterine fundus. The remainder of the device should be above the cervix. A nylon thread, which extends from the uterus into the vagina, is attached to the proximal end of all IUDs. This string should be palpable or visible on pelvic examination. If this string can not be identified, the patient may be referred for evaluation of a "lost IUD."

Some patients have no complaint other than a lost string. Others, however, present with cramping, pain, or abnormal bleeding. In either case, the position of the IUD must be demonstrated. If the uterus is empty, the device has been expelled or has perforated the uterus. An IUD outside the uterus is usually not seen with ultrasound because it is surrounded by gut.

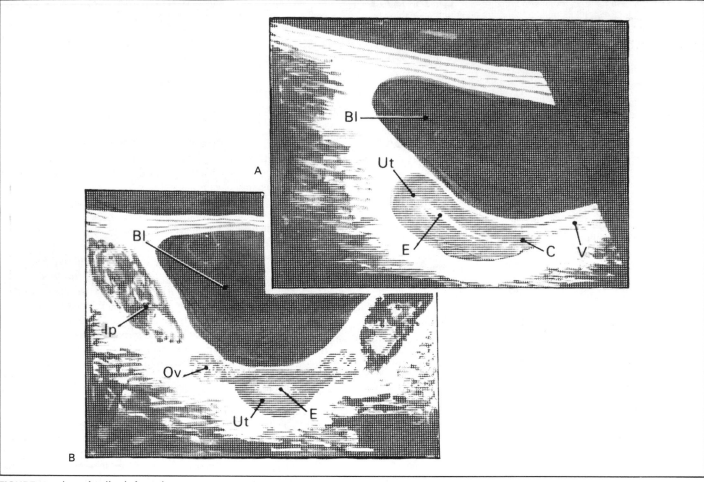

FIGURE 25-1. Longitudinal, A, and transverse, B, views of normal pelvic anatomy.

ANATOMY

Anatomy has been discussed already in Chapter 23. See also Figure 25-1.

TECHNIQUE

Longitudinal and transverse scans of the uterus are necessary to demonstrate the position of an IUD properly. A full bladder is essential to visualize the pelvic structures and adequately demonstrate the uterine fundus. IUDs may be difficult to see when the uterus is retroverted. A full bladder may push the uterus into an anteverted position.

Remember that not all patients have a midline uterus. It may be necessary to scan obliquely in order to obtain a long axis view of the uterus. Transverse scans are useful in demonstrating that the entire device is within the endometrial cavity and has not penetrated or perforated the myometrium.

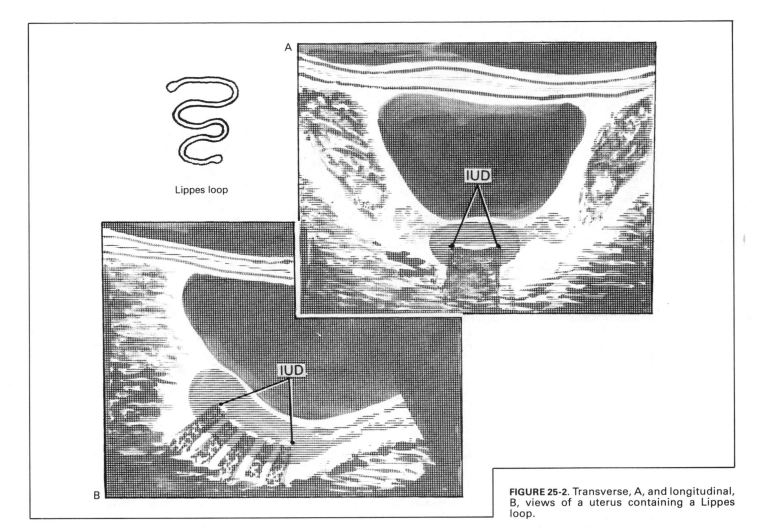

Lippes loop

FIGURE 25-2. Transverse, A, and longitudinal, B, views of a uterus containing a Lippes loop.

PATHOLOGY

Types of Device

LIPPES LOOP

The Lippes loop is the most widely used IUD. In a long-axis view, the loop appears as two to five dashes depending on whether or not a true long-axis IUD view has been obtained (Fig. 25-2B). Transversely, the device is visualized as a single line (Fig. 25-2A).

SAF-T-COIL

If the Saf-T-Coil is scanned along its central portion, the device is visualized as a solid line. However, if the Saf-T-Coil is scanned along the coil portion, an appearance similar to that of a Lippes loop is obtained with an interrupted line (Fig. 25-3).

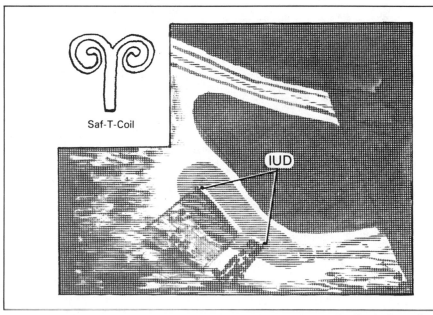

Saf-T-Coil

FIGURE 25-3. Longitudinal view of a uterus containing a Saf-T-Coil. Note shadowing behind the IUD.

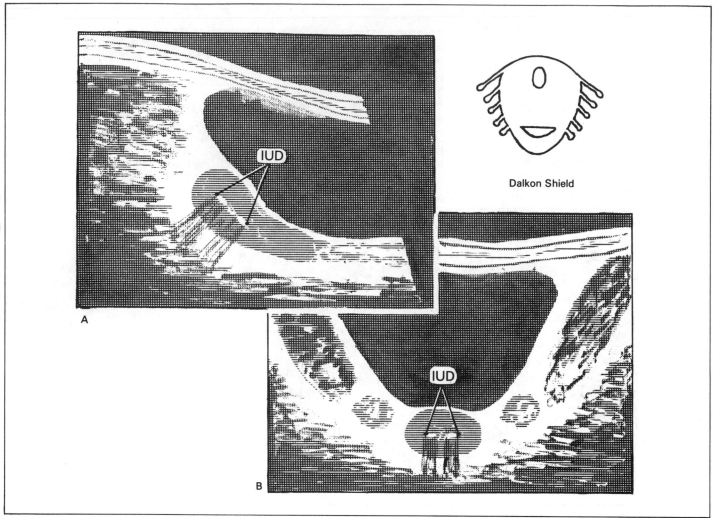

Dalkon Shield

FIGURE 25-4. Longitudinal, A, and transverse, B, views of a uterus containing a Dalkon shield.

DALKON SHIELD

Insertion of the Dalkon shield has been suspended because of a large number of associated infections. However, there are still a number of women using the device. The Dalkon shield is the smallest of the IUDs. On both longitudinal and transverse scans, it appears as two echogenic foci (Fig. 25-4A,B).

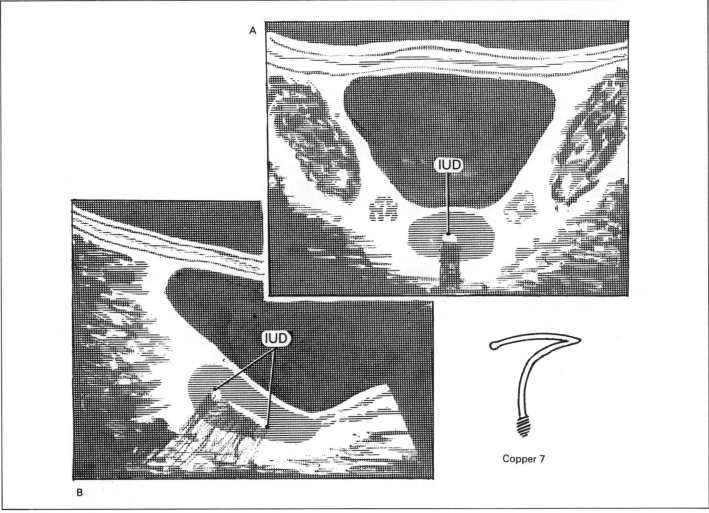

Copper 7

FIGURE 25-5. Transverse view of a uterus containing a Copper 7 (Cu 7) IUD. Note shadowing behind the IUD.

COPPER 7 AND COPPER T

These devices differ from the others in that a band of copper is wound around one end. On long-axis views both usually appear as a line with thickening at the upper end of the bend that forms the 7 or the T and at the lower end due to the band of copper. Transversely, the devices will appear as a dot except at the upper end, where a short line can be seen owing to the 7 or T configuration (Fig. 25-5).

Perforation

If an IUD is not in the endometrial cavity, a perforated uterus must be considered. This perforation may be complete or incomplete. If incomplete, a portion of the IUD may be demonstrated within the uterine wall. If a complete perforation has occurred, the IUD may be invisible because of overlying bowel gas.

A radiographic procedure (hysterogram) may determine if the IUD has perforated the uterus when the device is not centrally located within the uterus.

Pregnancy

Pregnancy can occasionally occur with IUDs. When an IUD with a coexisting pregnancy is discovered, one should determine the relationship of the device to the gestational sac (i.e., superior or inferior). This is important in deciding whether an IUD can be safely removed. If it is left in place, a severe infection may occur. In the later stages of pregnancy the location of the IUD (if it can be located at all) is difficult to determine because of the large volume of the uterus occupied by the fetus.

Pelvic Inflammatory Disease

IUDs are associated with an increased incidence of PID. If a patient presents with pain or bleeding and the IUD is properly positioned, check the adnexal areas and the cul-de-sac for evidence of PID (as discussed in Chapter 23).

IUD Position

The position and relationship of the IUD to the uterus should be clearly shown. An IUD located in the lower uterine segment and extending into the vagina, or one that is too large for the uterine cavity will probably be expelled. An IUD may lie outside the cavity within the wall of the uterus in an unsatisfactory position.

PITFALLS

The decidual reaction in the endometrial cavity may be mistaken for an IUD. IUD echoes are more readily reproducible, are associated with shadowing, and are generally stronger than decidual echoes. If the gain is decreased, IUD echoes will still be visible.

WHERE ELSE TO LOOK

If the sonographer is unable to find the IUD despite a thorough search, and pregnancy has been ruled out, an abdominal radiograph may reveal the location of a migrated IUD or prove that the IUD has been expelled.

SELECTED READING

Callen, P. W. Ultrasonography in the Detection of Intrauterine Contraceptive Devices. In P. W. Callen (Ed.), *Ultrasonography in Obstetrics and Gynecology.* Philadelphia: Saunders, 1983.

Sanders, R. C., and James, A. E. (Eds.). *The Principles and Practice of Ultrasonography in Obstetrics and Gynecology.* New York: Appleton-Century-Crofts, 1980.

26. UNCERTAIN DATES

Elective Cesarean Section, Late Registration, or Unknown Fetal Lie

ROGER C. SANDERS

SONOGRAM ABBREVIATIONS

Ao   Aorta

Bl   Bladder

D   Diaphragm
DV   Ductus venosus

FH   Fetal head
FS   Fetal spine

H   Heart

L   Liver

SP   Symphysis pubis
St   Stomach

U   Umbilicus

KEY WORDS

Amniocentesis. Procedure involving the insertion of a small needle into the amniotic cavity to obtain fluid for cytogenic or biochemical analysis.

Brachycephaly. Short, wide fetal head—a third-trimester normal variant.

Breech Presentation. The fetal head is situated at the fundus of the uterus.

Cephalic Presentation. The fetal head is the presenting part in the cervical area; also known as a vertex presentation.

DeLee's Test. The first time the fetal heart can be heard with the fetal stethoscope, usually at about 16 weeks' gestation.

Dolichocephaly. Long, flattened fetal head—a third trimester normal variant.

Ductus Venosus. Fetal vein that connects the umbilical vein to the inferior vena cava and runs in an oblique axis through the liver.

Gravid. Pregnant.

High-Risk Pregnancy (HRP). Pregnancy at high risk for an abnormal outcome. Typical examples of high-risk pregnancies are (1) maternal disease (e.g., kidney or heart disease), (2) maternal drug ingestion (e.g., alcohol or cigarettes), (3) previous pregnancy with a small fetus, and (4) family history of congenital malformations.

Hydrocephalus. Enlargement of the cerebral ventricles. Associated with spina bifida.

Late Registration. A pregnant woman who first attends the obstetric clinic when she is about 20 weeks pregnant or more is termed a late registrant. At this stage of pregnancy, clinical dating is difficult because several important dating landmarks have passed (e.g., quickening and the DeLee's test).

Microcephaly. Unduly small skull and brain. Associated with mental deficiency.

Para. Term used to describe how many pregnancies a woman has undergone. The first number represents the total number of full-term pregnancies. The second number represents the number of premature births. The third number indicates the total number of abortions, and the fourth number shows the total number of living children. For example, para 2113 represents two full-term pregnancies, one premature birth, one abortion, and three live children.

Quickening. The time when the mother first feels the baby move—about 16 to 18 weeks.

Shoulder Presentation. The fetal shoulder is the presenting part.

Transverse Lie. A fetus that is lying transversely so that head and trunk are at approximately the same level.

Umbilical Vein and Arteries. Vessels within the cord. There are two arteries and one vein.

Vertex Presentation. The fetal head is the presenting part. This is the usual presentation; it can be face first or brow first.

THE CLINICAL PROBLEM

One of the common reasons for referral for an ultrasonic examination is uncertainty about when the mother became pregnant. The mother (1) may be uncertain whether the last menstrual period was a genuine period, (2) may have a history of infrequent periods, or (3) may first attend the clinic after dating landmarks such as the DeLees test, quickening, and the first trimester physical examination have already passed. Such a patient is termed a *late registrant.* When a woman has had a previous cesarean section, another cesarean section is often performed with any subsequent pregnancy. In such patients the gestational age must be accurately determined so that a cesarean section will not be performed too early, which can result in a child with immature fetal lungs. A sonogram is usually recommended for such mothers to confirm the maternal dates.

Dating by ultrasound should take place before 28 weeks because at a later stage in pregnancy, the biparietal diameter may vary within a 4-week range of possible dates. Ideally, a dating sonogram should be performed between 17 and 20 weeks so that the timely diagnosis of twins, fetal anomalies, or placenta previa can be made.

It can be difficult for the clinician to decide which part of the baby is going to be delivered first. Most babies are delivered head first (cephalic or vertex presentation). Others are delivered foot or bottom first (breech presentation). The latter is a much more dangerous mode of delivery and may require cesarean section. Other dangerous fetal positions are shoulder presentation and transverse lie. The sonographer should therefore make a point of mentioning the fetal position in the preliminary report.

An obstetric sonogram (even one for the simple problem of uncertain dates) should never be a routine series of sonographic sections performed at set intervals from the midline. Once the fetal lie has been determined, views along the long axis of the fetus and transverse views at key levels such as the umbilical vein and the bladder should be obtained. A number of organs should be specifically identified and shown to be normal. These include the fetal stomach, bladder, heart, lungs, liver, spine, cerebral ventricles, limbs, and kidneys. The amount of amniotic fluid should be roughly quantified, and the location of the placenta should be demonstrated so that the physician interpreting the examination knows that the placenta is clear of the cervix. The cord position should be established if amniocentesis is being considered.

The sonographer's preliminary report on obstetric sonograms should include (1) fetal position, (2) number of pregnancies, (3) placental position, (4) biparietal diameter, and (5) whether evidence of fetal movement or fetal heart movement was observed.

ANATOMY

Fetal Head

Cross-sectional anatomy of the fetal head should be defined at varying levels, starting at the level of the lateral ventricles (Fig. 26-1) and moving inferiorly (Figs. 26-2 and 26-3). Structures that should be routinely identified are the thalamus (Fig. 26-2), the lateral ventricles (Fig. 26-1), the cavum septum pellucidum (Fig. 26-2), the sylvian fissures (Fig. 26-2), the hippocampus (Fig. 26-3), and the vermis of the cerebellum (see Chapter 27, Fig. 27-1).

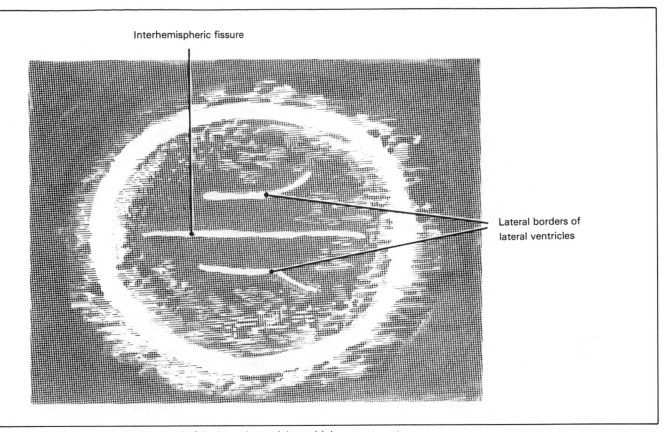

Interhemispheric fissure

Lateral borders of
lateral ventricles

FIGURE 26-1. View through the skull at the level of the lateral ventricles, which are seen as two
slightly curved lines.

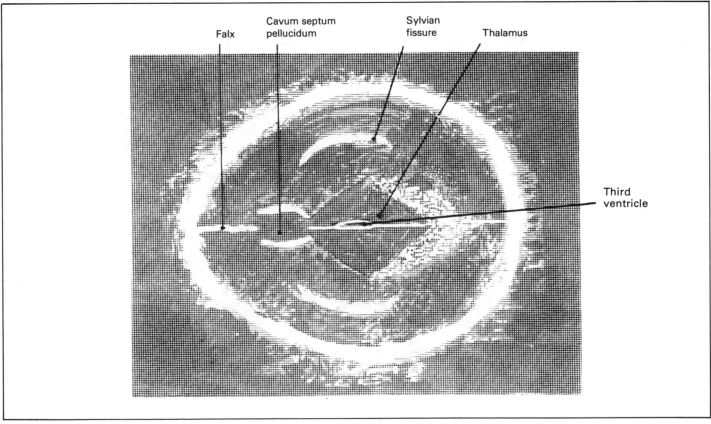

Falx

Cavum septum
pellucidum

Sylvian
fissure

Thalamus

Third
ventricle

FIGURE 26-2. View at the level of the thalamus showing the sylvian fissure, cavum septum
pellucidum, and third ventricle.

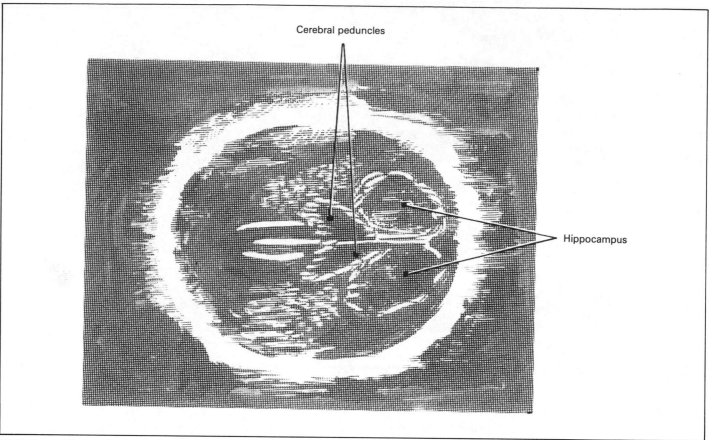

Cerebral peduncles

Hippocampus

FIGURE 26-3. View at the level of the cerebral peduncles showing the hippocampus.

Fetal Chest

On either side of the heart one can see the fetal lungs, which are evenly echogenic but have a slightly different texture from the liver. The diaphragm can be seen with real-time between the liver and the lung in spite of this similarity (Fig. 26-4). Fetal breathing with movement of the diaphragm is commonly present. The ribs cast acoustic shadows across the chest (Fig. 26-4).

Fetal Heart

The four chambers of the fetal heart (Fig. 26-4) can be identified, and an attempt should be made to obtain longitudinal and transverse axis views if congenital heart disease is a clinical concern. The pulmonary artery and the aortic arch with its branches into the neck can be traced on other sections.

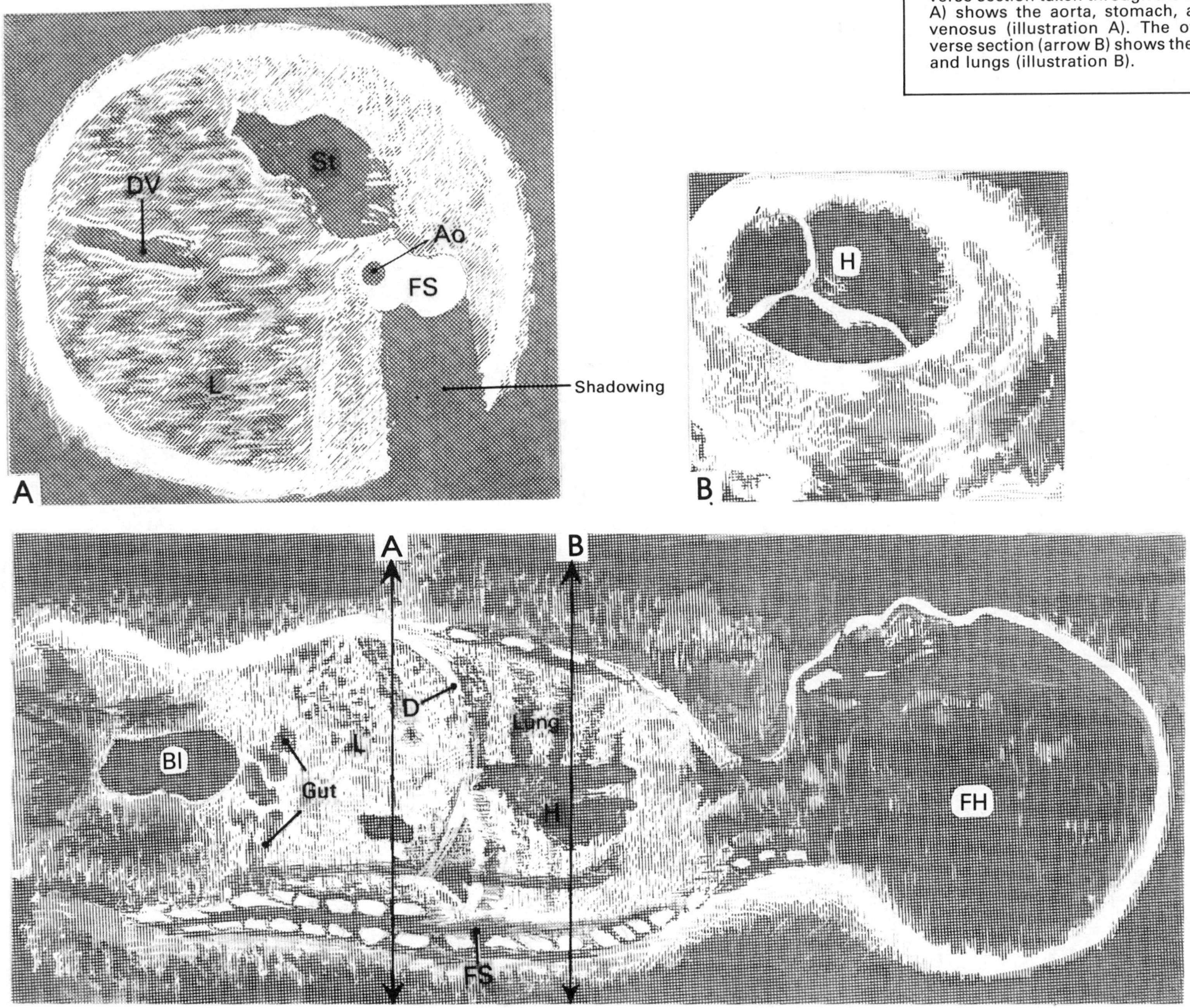

FIGURE 26-4. Longitudinal section of the fetus through the chest and abdomen. A transverse section taken through the liver (arrow A) shows the aorta, stomach, and ductus venosus (illustration A). The other transverse section (arrow B) shows the fetal heart and lungs (illustration B).

Limbs

The forearm and thigh, which are single-boned limbs, generate only a single echo, whereas the distal limbs generate two parallel linear echoes. Bones are seen as echogenic lines with acoustic shadowing. Individual digits can be counted from about 16 weeks' gestational age.

Fetal Abdomen

On a high transverse section the liver, ductus venosus, stomach, aorta, and spine should be visible (Fig. 26-4A). On lower sections the fetal kidneys can be seen (Fig. 26-5A,B). They are paraspinous and have a configuration similar to that of adult kidneys. A small degree of dilatation of the central sinus echoes is permissible as a normal variant.

At a still lower section the fetal bladder should be recognizable (Fig. 26-6).

Fetal Spine

On a long-axis view the spinal cord, which has a central linear echo from the spinal canal, can be seen (Fig. 26-4A). Vertebral bodies can be identified. The normal fetal spine widens slightly in the cervical and lumbar areas (see Fig. 31-2A). To rule out spina bifida, serial transverse sections must be made throughout the spine, making sure that a complete spinal canal is present at every level (Figs. 26-5B and 31-2A). The canal will be seen as a ring. The posterior borders are formed by the lamina of the spine. The spine gives rise to an area of acoustic shadowing (Fig. 26-5B).

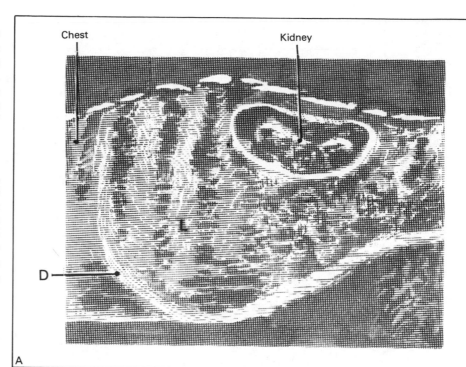

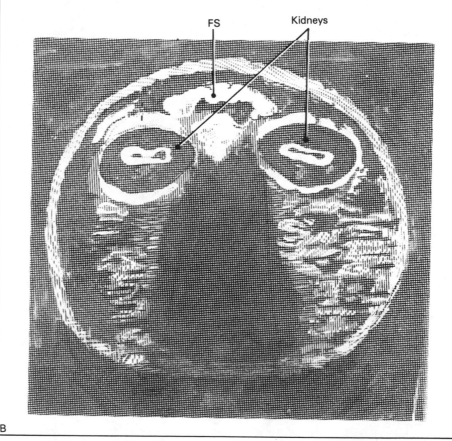

FIGURE 26-5. Fetal kidneys. A. Long section of the fetus showing the fetal kidneys. The diaphragm can also be seen. B. Transverse section through the kidneys showing the fetal spine.

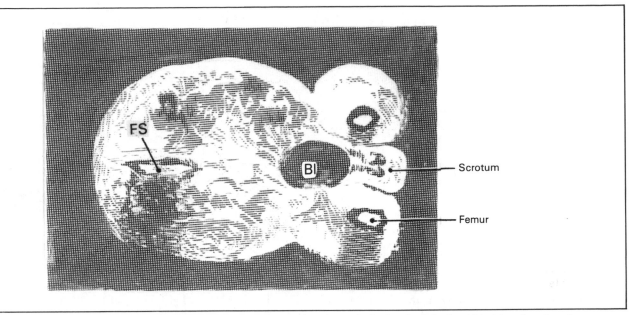

FIGURE 26-6. Transverse section through the level of the fetal bladder showing the scrotum and hips.

TECHNIQUE

Routine Views

The following routine is desirable when examining a woman with an apparently normal pregnancy.

REAL-TIME VIEWS

LONG AXIS VIEWS OF FETUS. Obtain a view that shows the relative appearance of the lung and liver and long axis views of the spine, kidney, stomach, and bladder (Fig. 26-4). The lung-liver view may also show the fetal heart.

TRANSVERSE SECTIONS. Obtain views of the biparietal diameter and of the ventricles to exclude a diagnosis of hydrocephalus. In the abdomen show (1) the normal kidneys (Fig. 26-5B), (2) the level of the liver, the umbilical vein and stomach (Fig. 26-4A), and (3) the fetal bladder (Fig. 26-6).

OBLIQUE AXIS VIEWS. Be sure to obtain long axis views of the femur (Fig. 26-7), and if necessary document the appearances of the lower limbs and digits.

MOVEMENT. Note whether the fetal heart and limbs are moving and whether there is fetal breathing.

STATIC SCANS. Obtain a view that shows the relationship of the fetal axis to the uterus and maternal bladder so that the interpreter of the scan will know whether it is a cephalic or a breech presentation. Document the amount of amniotic fluid and the placental position with static scans.

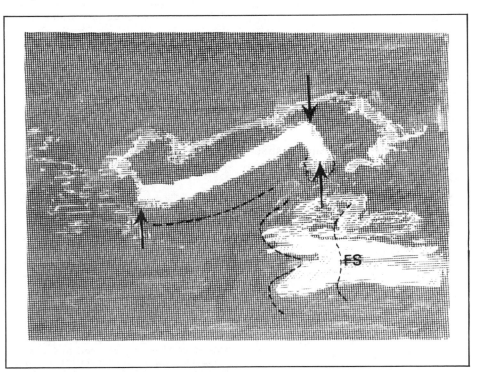

FIGURE 26-7. View of the femur showing the angulation at the level of the greater trochanter (single arrow). The femoral length is measured along the shaft (arrows).

MEASUREMENTS TO PERFORM

CROWN-RUMP LENGTH. In a dating examination performed in the first trimester, the crown-rump length (CRL) is the optimal method of establishing fetal age. This measurement is performed using a real-time system by finding the longest axis of the rapidly mobile fetus. This value can be obtained between approximately 7 and 12 weeks quite easily if real-time is available. If only a static scanner is available, discover the axis of the fetus by multiple longitudinal scans and then perform an oblique scan along the fetal axis (Fig. 26-8; see also Appendices 3 and 4).

BIPARIETAL DIAMETER. For dating after 12 weeks, the biparietal diameter (BPD) is used. This examination is also simple with a real-time system. Find the widest axis of the fetal skull, normally at the level of the thalami (Fig. 26-2), which are recognizable as diamond-shaped structures in the center of brain. Structures visible at the desirable level include the thalamus, the third ventricle, and the cavum septum pellucidum. Do not take a biparietal measurement at the level of the lateral ventricles, which are too high on the skull and are visible as two lines parallel to the midline (Fig. 26-1). To obtain this measurement with a static scanner, the degree of flexion of the fetal head (the angle of asynclitism) should be determined and the transducer angled this amount (Fig. 26-9). Transverse views at different angulations are then performed to obtain the ovoid shape that is desirable. Measurements are made from the near side of the skull echoes to the near side of the distal skull echoes (Fig. 26-10). Accuracy with this technique is ± 1 week prior to 20 weeks and ± 10 days until about 28 weeks. Beyond this point accuracy diminishes to ± 2 to 4 weeks; therefore, dating by biparietal diameter measurement is undesirable after about 28 weeks (see Appendix 8).

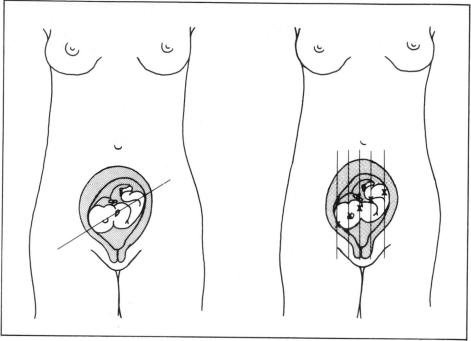

FIGURE 26-8. Technique used with a static B-scanner to find the crown-rump length.

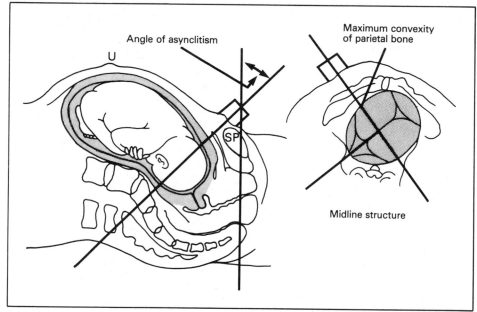

FIGURE 26-9. Technique used to find the biparietal diameter with a static scanner. First discover the angle of asynclitism on a longitudinal section and then, moving the transducer transversely, set it to a similar angle to get transverse views.

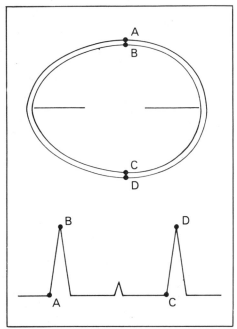

FIGURE 26-10. Diagram of the usual site of biparietal diameter measurements. A and C are the usual measurement sites used.

FEMORAL LENGTH. If a technical problem arises with the biparietal diameter because the fetal head is too deep in the pelvis or if the fetal head appears abnormal (either hydrocephalic or microcephalic), the femoral length (FL) can be employed as an alternative method of estimating gestational age. The longest axis of the fetal femoral shaft is obtained at a point where its angulation with respect to the greater trochanter can be observed (Fig. 26-7). Tables of normal values are available (see Appendix 9). This measurement can be obtained only with a real-time system. The ratio of biparietal diameter to femoral length should be 0.79 ± 0.03.

OCCIPITOFRONTAL DIAMETER. A ratio of the biparietal diameter to the longest distance from the front of the head to the back of the head (occipito-frontal diameter, OFD) is useful in the diagnosis of dolichocephaly. This normal variant—a long, flattened fetal head in the third trimester—produces erroneous biparietal diameters. The normal ratio is 0.74 ± 0.08.

ABDOMINAL AND HEAD CIRCUMFERENCES. These measurements are usually used for detecting IUGR (see Chapter 27). They can also be used for dating the fetus (Appendixes 5,6,7).

PITFALLS

1. An *inadequate biparietal diameter* is obtained if
   a. The biparietal diameter is not taken at the level of the thalamus and cavum septum pellucidum.
   b. The head is round or flattened rather than ovoid.
   c. The head measurement is taken at a point where the distance between one side of the skull and the midline is not the same and is asymmetrical.
   d. There is no well-defined line around the fetal head to measure.
   e. The measurement is obtained in the third trimester when there is a wide variation of normal for any given measurement.
2. The *crown-rump length* is inaccurate if it is obtained after 12 weeks or when no strong effort is made to obtain the longest axis of the fetus.
3. The *femoral length* may be underestimated if a real-time system is not used in a fashion that shows the true length rather than an oblique axis.
4. The *biparietal diameter* in the third trimester is less than caliper measurements at birth because of the measurement site used.

WHERE ELSE TO LOOK

1. If the biparietal diameter and femoral length do not indicate the same fetal age, perform the measurements suggested for intrauterine growth retardation (see Chapter 27).

2. If the biparietal diameter is less than expected, consider the possibility of microcephalus and compare the measurement with the femoral length (see Chapter 31).

3. If the biparietal diameter is more than expected, make sure that hydrocephalus is not present (see Chapter 31).

4. If the femoral length is too small, consider the possibility of dwarfism and perform a head-trunk ratio. Note how many digits or distal bones there are because some limb anomalies are associated with absence or an excessive number of these bones.

SELECTED READING

Athey, P. A., and Hadlock, F. P. (Eds.). *Ultrasound in Obstetrics and Gynecology.* St. Louis: Mosby, 1981.

Callen, P. W. (Ed.). *Ultrasonography in Obstetrics and Gynecology.* Philadelphia: Saunders, 1983.

Sanders, R. C., and James, A. E. (Eds.). *The Principles and Practice of Ultrasonography in Obstetrics and Gynecology.* New York: Appleton-Century-Crofts, 1980.

27. SMALL FOR DATES

ROGER C. SANDERS

KEY WORDS

Amenorrhea. Absence of menstruation.

Eclampsia. High blood pressure occurring in pregnancy. In its most severe form it is associated with epileptic seizure. It is a very serious condition that causes IUGR and often leads to fetal death.

Hyaline Membrane Disease (Respiratory Distress Syndrome). Respiratory condition occurring in the neonate as a consequence of delivery when the fetal lungs are still immature.

Intrauterine Growth Retardation (IUGR). A fetus is suffering from IUGR when it is below the tenth percentile for weight at a given gestational age or weighs less than 2500 g at 36 weeks' gestational age.

Oligohydramnios. Too little amniotic fluid. No fluid, or only small pockets of fluid are present.

Preeclamptic Toxemia. High blood pressure and proteinuria that precedes eclampsia.

Trimester. Pregnancy is divided into three periods of 13 weeks each, known as trimesters. Obstetric problems are conveniently related to a given trimester.

THE CLINICAL PROBLEM

Three possibilities should be considered when a fetus is *small for dates.*

1. The *mother's dates are wrong* and the fetus is actually younger than indicated by her dates.
2. *Palpation is misleading* because of obesity or unusual uterine lie.
3. A small uterus with *oligohydramnios* is present owing to (a) premature rupture of membranes, (b) intrauterine growth retardation (IUGR) with a small fetus, placenta, and diminished amniotic fluid, or (c) fetal renal anomaly (see Chapter 31).

Premature Rupture of Membranes

The rupture of membranes (a "show") early in pregnancy is an obstetric management problem. If the fetus is too small to survive outside the womb, no efforts are made to salvage it. If the fetus is large enough to survive, the mother is put on bedrest and treated with antibiotics to stop infection of the uterine contents. Ultrasound is valuable in showing how large the fetus is and in giving an idea of the mother's true dates. This is an obstetric emergency study.

Intrauterine Growth Retardation

In IUGR, insufficient food is supplied to the fetus. Fetuses are at risk if (1) the mother is chronically ill (e.g., chronic heart disease), (2) the mother is taking drugs (e.g., alcohol or cigarettes), (3) the mother does not eat enough, or (4) the mother is very young (under 17) or elderly (over 35).

In *symmetrical* IUGR the entire fetus is smaller than normal. In *asymmetrical* IUGR, on the other hand, the fetal trunk is small but the skull is more or less normal in size. The latter type of IUGR is thought to be associated with placental problems that result in defective transfer of food from the mother to the fetus. When the onset of fetal nutritional insufficiency is abrupt, the fetal brain is relatively spared, but the liver is severely affected, leading to an asymmetrical growth pattern.

Diagnosis of symmetrical IUGR requires accurate dating at an early stage. Some sonologists feel that a routine biparietal diameter measurement at 17 to 20 weeks' gestation is desirable in mothers who are at risk for IUGR so that accurate dates are known. IUGR is usually diagnosed by ultrasound when growth is less than expected in the third trimester. Establishing the diagnosis is crucial because of increased risk of difficult delivery and of stunted stature and intellect at a later age if the condition is not detected in utero. The fetal condition can be improved by maternal bedrest and other maneuvers such as eliminating cigarette smoking. The ultrasonic diagnosis depends on comparing the sizes of different structures in the fetal body, such as the overall size of the abdomen including the liver, with the head size and correlating these measurements with those expected according to standard experience for a given obstetric date.

ANATOMY

For the standard approach to the fetal anatomy, see Chapter 26.

TECHNIQUE

See the techniques described in Chapter 26.

Renal Anomalies

Eliminate the possibility of a *renal anomaly* by finding the kidneys and looking for the fetal bladder (see Chapter 26). If the bladder is present, the possibility of agenesis (absence) of the kidneys can be discarded. The bladder normally fills and partially empties over the course of about an hour. Slower rates of filling are associated with IUGR.

Measurements

Intrauterine growth retardation is diagnosed by obtaining the following measurements.

BIPARIETAL DIAMETER

Standard normal growth charts of the biparietal diameter according to week of pregnancy are available. If the mother has accurate dates or has been dated by an earlier biparietal diameter measurement before 26 weeks, a diagnosis of IUGR can be made if a subsequent sonogram shows unduly small growth for the stage of pregnancy (see Appendix 8, and Chapter 26).

TRUNK CIRCUMFERENCE

This measurement is taken at the level of the ductus venosus and the liver (Fig. 27-1). Adequate abdominal circumference measurements can be made using real-time if the fetal trunk is not too large for the field of view. If a static scanner is used, make sure that the transverse axis is angled as the fetus is flexed and is truly transverse (Fig. 27-2).

Make sure that the trunk is more or less round at the point of measurement and that the ductus venosus, aorta, stomach, and spine are visible. If the kidneys are present, the section is too low. To obtain a trunk circumference, run a map measurer around the trunk or use a digital computer tracer. The latter is more accurate. Calculations of fetal weight can also be made from the trunk diameter. Two trunk diameters at right angles are measured and their averages calculated to yield an average trunk diameter (ATD). The circumference can be derived from the diameter by using the formula πD. A weight estimation can then be made by taking the biparietal and the trunk circumference or diameter and using Appendix 10 to make the calculation.

The abdominal circumference also represents another method of dating the fetus (Appendix 5).

HEAD CIRCUMFERENCE

This measurement is valuable because the head-to-trunk ratio will allow the diagnosis of asymmetrical IUGR. The head circumerence should be obtained at a level that shows the thalami, the cavum septum pellucidum, the falx cerebri, and the third ventricle as for calculating a biparietal diameter. Dating tables based on the head circumference are available (Appendix 7).

HEAD-TRUNK CIRCUMFERENCE RATIO

Finding the head-abdomen ratio and comparing it with normal tables (see Appendix 11) allows the recognition of asymmetrical intrauterine growth retardation when the liver is unusually small. If there is an abnormal head-abdomen ratio, consider the possibility that the fetus has hydrocephalus, which will give similar findings. A low head-abdomen ratio suggests the possibility of microcephalus or a large fetus with macrosomia.

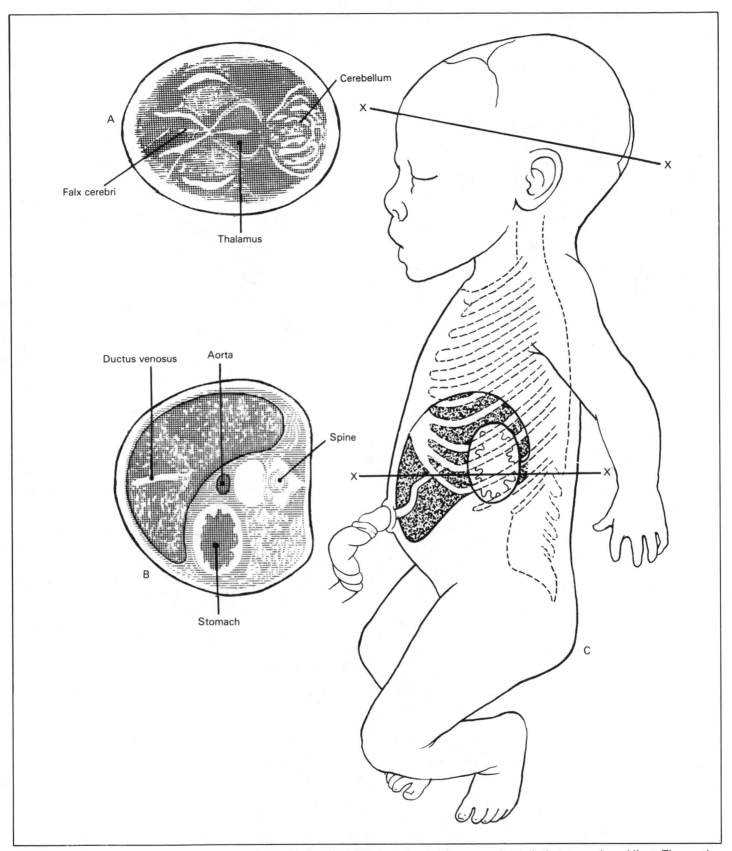

FIGURE 27-1A–C. The trunk circumference or trunk diameter is obtained at a level that passes through the stomach and liver. The section should show the ductus venosus, aorta, stomach, and spine, B. The appropriate head circumference for comparison is made through the thalamus and falx cerebri, A.

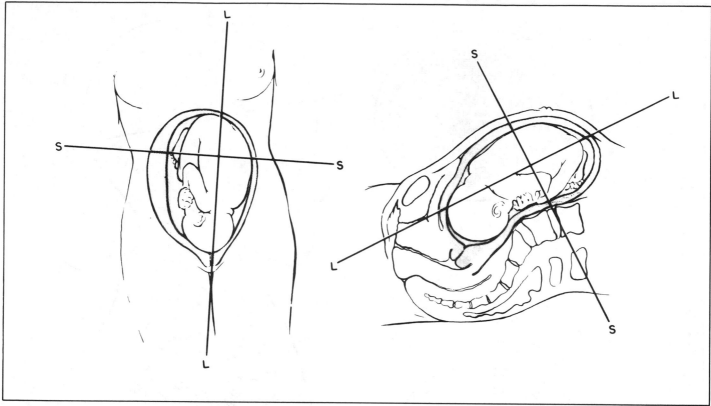

FIGURE 27-2. Technique for obtaining the trunk circumference with a B-scanner. First, find the axis of the fetus (L) and set the arm of the scanner (S) at right angles to it; then find the longitudinal section and set the degree of flexion so that right-angle sections of the fetus are obtained.

TOTAL INTRAUTERINE VOLUME (TIUV)

This overall measurement of intrauterine size is obtained by taking the longest width, length, and height of the uterus and multiplying by 0.5233 (Appendix 12, Fig. 27-3). The TIUV is a crude method of ascertaining whether or not IUGR is likely to be present and whether more complex measurements should be obtained. Exclude the myometrium when obtaining this measurement.

FEMORAL LENGTH

This measurement has already been described in Chapter 26 and is valuable in diagnosing IUGR because it represents another method of determining whether adequate fetal growth has occurred (Appendix 9).

FEMORAL LENGTH—BIPARIETAL DIAMETER RATIO

This ratio is a useful method of detecting growth problems. The femoral length–biparietal diameter ratio should be 0.79 ± 0.03. If it is not, either the biparietal diameter or the femoral length is suboptimal, the fetus is a dwarf or hydrocephalic, or growth is retarded.

Fetal Anatomy

The fetal anatomy should be examined in considerable detail because about 10% of IUGR cases are due to a congenital fetal anomaly.

Placental Maturation

The placenta is likely to be small with IUGR. Signs of premature placental aging prior to 36 weeks suggest IUGR (Fig. 27-4). Grade III placental changes almost always indicate that the fetal lungs are mature and that amniocentesis can be avoided.

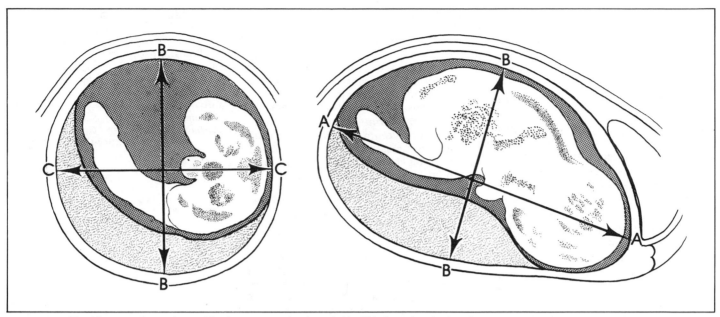

FIGURE 27-3. Total intrauterine volume. The longest uterine length (A–A) is found at the level of the cervix. Measurements are made from the inner aspect of the myometrium. The greatest antero-posterior (AP) diameter (B–B) is also measured. A width measurement (C–C) is made at the site of the AP measurement.

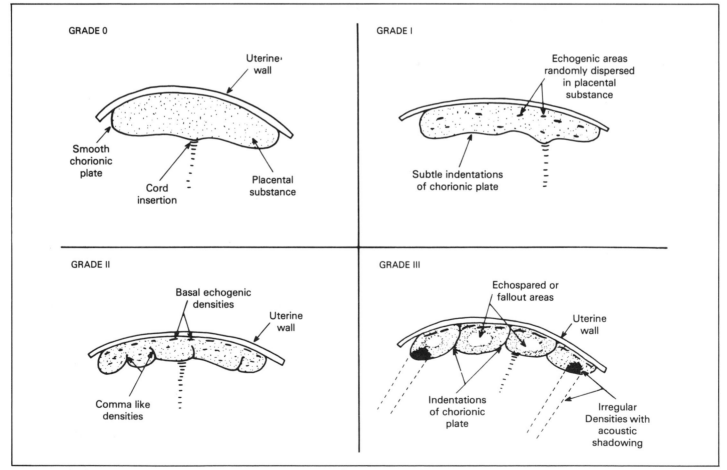

FIGURE 27-4. Diagram showing placental grading appearances. (Reproduced with permission from Grannum P, Berkowitz R, and Hobbins J. The ultrasonic changes in the maturing placenta and their relation to fetal pulmonic maturity. *Am J Obstet Gynecol* 133; 915–922, 1979.)

Amount of Amniotic Fluid

The amount of amniotic fluid is low in most cases of IUGR (oligohydramnios). Reduced amounts of amniotic fluid are normally seen in the third trimester.

Biophysical Profile (Fetal Planning Score)

Fetuses with IUGR are at risk for problems at delivery such as difficulty in breathing. The biophysical profile attempts to gauge fetal well-being by examining muscle tone, limb movement, fetal breathing, and amount of amniotic fluid. The results of these tests, together with the nonstress test (a test in which the obstetrician observes with Doppler how the fetal heart rate responds to fetal movement and uterine contraction), are used to compute a score of fetal well-being. During the course of a half-hour observation period a score of 8 is given if (1) fetal breathing is observed for 30 seconds (2 points), (2) fetal movements are seen (2 points), (3) the fetus is able to extend and flex a limb vigorously (2 points), and (4) a space of over 1 cm of amniotic fluid is observed (2 points). If the score is 4 or less, problems at delivery can be expected; they are not invariable.

PITFALLS

1. *IUGR versus hydrocephalus.* Remember that an abnormal head-to-trunk ratio may occur not only with intrauterine growth retardation but also with hydrocephalus. Examine the ventricles carefully if you find an abnormally high head-to-trunk ratio.
2. *Total intrauterine volume.* The total intrauterine volume (TIUV) is rather difficult to measure. Make sure that you do not include the walls of the uterus in addition to the uterine cavity. This error makes a considerable difference in the accuracy of the measurements.
3. *Trunk circumference.* The trunk circumference is often quite difficult to obtain. Try to obtain a more or less round appearance because if the trunk is ovoid, it suggests that the fetus was not at a direct right angle to the spine. Do not press too vigorously with the transducer or you will distort the shape of the fetal trunk.

SELECTED READING

Athey, P. A., and Hadlock, F. P. (Eds.). *Ultrasound in Obstetrics and Gynecology.* St. Louis: Mosby, 1981.

Callen, P. W. (Ed.). *Ultrasonography in Obstetrics and Gynecology.* Philadelphia: Saunders, 1983.

Sanders, R. C., and James, A. E. (Eds.). *The Principles and Practice of Ultrasonography in Obstetrics and Gynecology.* New York: Appleton-Century-Crofts, 1980.

28. LARGE FOR DATES

ROGER C. SANDERS

SONOGRAM ABBREVIATIONS

Bl   Bladder

FH   Fetal heart
FT   Fetal trunk

Pl   Placenta

KEY WORDS

Corpus Lutein Cyst. A cyst developing as a response to human chorionic gonadotropin (HCG) in the first few weeks of pregnancy. Such cysts usually disappear by 14 to 16 weeks after the last menstrual period.

Dizygotic, Dichorionic. Twin pregnancies in which there are two nonidentical fetuses.

Erythroblastosis Fetalis (Rh Incompatibility). A form of fetal anemia in which the fetal red cells are destroyed by contact with a maternal antibody produced in response to a previous fetus. Severe fetal heart failure results.

Hydrops Fetalis. The fetal abdomen contains ascites and the skin is thickened by excess fluid. This condition has a variety of causes, of which the most well known is Rh (rhesus) incompatibility. Other causes are grouped as "nonimmune hydrops" (see Chapter 31).

Locking Twins. Because no amniotic sac membrane is present, the twins interlock and are consequently difficult to deliver.

Macrosomia. Exceptionally large infant with fat deposition in the subcutaneous tissues; seen in fetuses of diabetic mothers.

Monozygotic, Monochorionic. Twin pregnancies in which the fetuses are identical; usually an amniotic sac membrane is present between the two amniotic cavities, but this may be absent.

Multiple Pregnancy. More than a singleton fetus (e.g., twins, triplets, or quadruplets).

Polyhydramnios. Excessive amniotic fluid. Defined as more than 2 liters at term.

Rubella. Viral disease occurring in utero with a number of associated fetal anomalies including congenital heart disease.

Siamese Twins (Conjoined). Twins that are joined at some point in their bodies.

Toxoplasmosis. Viral disease affecting the fetus in utero, often resulting in intracranial calcification.

Twin Transfusion Syndrome. When monozygotic twins share a placenta, most of the blood from the placenta may be appropriated by one fetus at the expense of the other. One twin becomes excessively large and the other unduly small.

THE CLINICAL PROBLEM

If the pregnancy appears clinically more advanced than predicted by dates, several detectable causes should be considered by the sonographer. Most commonly the mother is wrong about her dates. Other possible causes of a uterus that is too large for dates include (1) polyhydramnios, (2) multiple pregnancy, (3) a large fetus, (4) a mass in addition to the uterus, and (5) a large placenta.

Hydramnios (Polyhydramnios)

In polyhydramnios there is excess amniotic fluid; consequently, the limbs stand out separated by large echo-free areas devoid of any fetal structures. Detailed sonographic visualization of the fetal gastrointestinal (GI) tract and the skeletal and central nervous systems (CNS) is required because anomalies in these areas are associated with polyhydramnios (see Chapter 31 for more detail). Other causes of polyhydramnios include diabetic pregnancy, multiple pregnancy, hydrops, and viral infections such as toxoplasmosis and rubella. Most often, especially between 20 and 30 weeks, polyhydramnios is a normal variant.

Twins

Multiple pregnancy is a very important cause of a fetus that is large for dates. Twins are at risk for a number of problems during pregnancy and have to be followed with serial sonograms to see that growth is adequate, that death has not occurred, and that one twin is not growing at the expense of the other. Careful sonographic examination of multiple pregnancy is necessary because the fetuses often adopt an unusual fetal lie. Triplets can easily be missed if careful scanning is not performed.

Macrosomia

Unduly large fetuses (over 3000 g) are a problem for the obstetrician because they are difficult to deliver. They are often the fetuses of diabetic mothers. Weight estimation is important here because the obstetrician must decide whether to perform a cesarean section and must be alert to the delivery problems that occur with the fetuses of diabetic mothers.

Mass and Fetus

Additional masses may give the impression that the uterus is larger than it really is, as with fibroids or ovarian cysts. Such problems are particularly important if an abortion is being considered because the clinician may incorrectly estimate the dates as being beyond the legal limits for abortion. Fibroids cause a number of problems during pregnancy, such as spontaneous abortion and difficulty in delivery, so that size estimation and location of fibroids are important.

ANATOMY

See Chapter 26 for a discussion of the relevant anatomy.

TECHNIQUE

Appropriate technique is described in Chapter 26.

PATHOLOGY

Unduly Large Baby

Exceptionally large fetuses cause discrepancies between estimation of dates and examination findings. Sometimes these fetuses are normally large infants. Often the mother has diabetes mellitus and the fetus is *macrosomic*.

When a large fetus is found the following procedures are in order:

1. Measure the biparietal diameter.
2. Measure the trunk circumference (the normal head-to-trunk ratios are inappropriate in such babies, but the fetal weight can still be estimated).
3. Search for evidence of scalp or trunk edema, which will be apparent as a second line running around the skull or trunk. This is a common finding in infants of diabetic mothers due to subcutaneous deposition of fat.
4. Examine the placenta. The placenta is often increased in size in diabetic mothers.
5. Fetal anomalies related to the genitourinary tract, CNS, and the cardiovascular system are more common in diabetic pregnancies than in others. Make sure that these areas are examined in detail.

Multiple Pregnancy

A comprehensive real-time survey of the whole uterus should be performed in all pregnancies but particularly when the uterus is large for dates. When a multiple pregnancy is found, make an attempt to show all fetuses on the same view (Fig. 28-1). Static scans showing all fetuses are desirable. Polyhydramnios, which may occur with multiple pregnancy, raises the question of a monochorionic pregnancy or a fetal anomaly. There are specific features to look for in a multiple pregnancy.

DEATH

Make sure all fetuses are alive—there is an increased incidence of fetal death in multiple pregnancy.

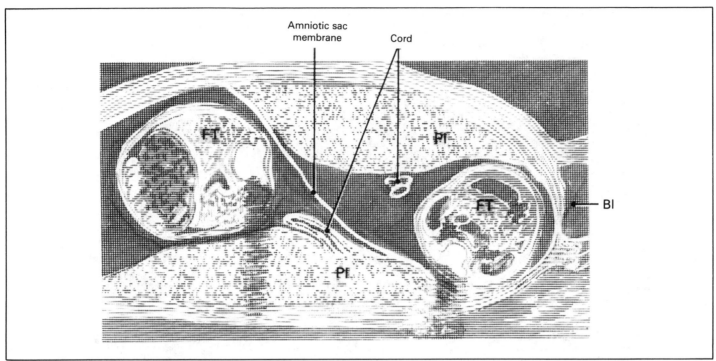

Amniotic sac
membrane

Cord

FT

PT

FT

BI

PT

PT

FIGURE 28-1. Twin pregnancy. Note the amniotic sac membranes separating the two fetal trunks and the presence of two placentas.

AMNIOTIC SAC MEMBRANE

Make an attempt to show the membrane that separates the amniotic sacs (Fig. 28-1). This membrane is almost always present whether the twins are identical (monochorionic) or nonidentical (dichorionic). However, the membrane is absent in about 10% of monochorionic pregnancies. Absence of the membrane suggests the possibility of many associated anomalies (e.g., Siamese twins, locking twins, polyhydramnios, asymmetrical growth). Such a membrane may rarely be seen in a singleton pregnancy but is generally incomplete.

ANOMALIES

Siamese and locking twins should be ruled out in any twin pregnancy by noting position changes. Make sure that there are two heads and trunks and adequate limbs when a twin pregnancy is present.

AMNIOCENTESIS

When amniocentesis is to be performed in a twin pregnancy, identify the amniotic sac membrane and show the obstetrician where to place the needle to obtain fluid from two separate sacs.

PLACENTA

Try to determine whether one or two placentas are present. The presence of two placentas almost always indicates nonidentical twins, whereas a single placenta is of little diagnostic significance.

GROWTH PROBLEMS

Look for IUGR or asymmetrical growth. One twin may grow at the expense of the other (twin transfusion syndrome). On follow-up examinations, measure the biparietal diameter, trunk circumference, and head-abdomen ratio on both twins every time. These measurements may be difficult because multiple pregnancies often result in an unusual fetal lie. If one twin is bigger than the other and the twin transfusion syndrome seems possible, look for ascites in the larger twin—an early indication of heart failure.

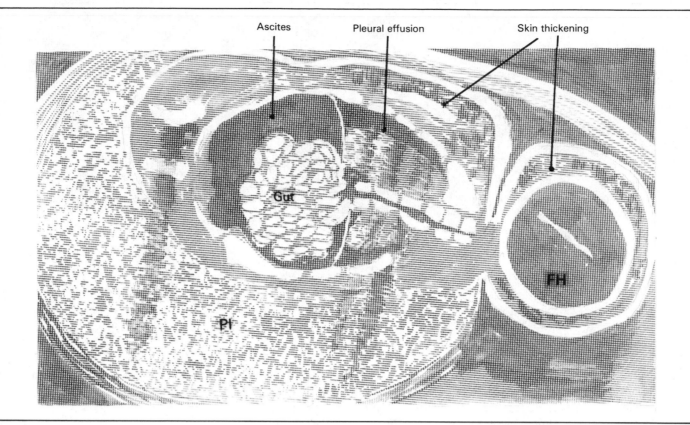

Ascites   Pleural effusion   Skin thickening

Gut

FH

Pl

FIGURE 28-2. In fetal hydrops fluid accumulates in a number of body sites. There is skin thickening around the trunk and skull. Pleural effusions, a pericardial effusion, and fetal ascites develop. The placenta enlarges and has a more echogenic texture.

Fetal Hydrops

A large-for-dates fetus may be the first indication of fetal hydrops with polyhydramnios. Until a few years ago this condition was almost always due to Rh incompatibility (erythroblastosis fetalis), but now hydrops is more commonly due to a group of congenital fetal anomalies or infections known collectively as nonimmune hydrops, which have particular sonographic findings.

FETAL EDEMA

The fetus may show evidence of scalp and skin edema as a second line around the fetal parts. In more severe cases, fetal ascites, pleural and pericardial effusions will be present (Fig. 28-2).

PLACENTAL ENLARGEMENT

The placenta is often markedly enlarged and has an abnormal echogenic texture. A large placenta is most likely to occur with Rh incompatibility, placental tumors, and fetal cardiac problems.

UMBILICAL CORD DILATATION

The umbilical cord will appear enlarged. Cross sections through the cord, both within the amniotic fluid and through the umbilical vein as it enters the fetal liver, should be obtained. Dilatation of the umbilical vein is an early indication of fetal heart failure (Fig. 28-3).

UNDERLYING CAUSES

Nonimmune hydrops is a consequence of a number of different conditions, some of which can be detected ultrasonically.

PLACENTAL TUMORS. These tumors syphon off the blood destined for the fetus, and the fetus becomes anemic. Make sure that a mass is not adjacent to or within the placenta (Fig. 28-4).

CARDIAC AND CHEST ANOMALIES AND FETAL TUMORS. Such anomalies may be the cause of hydrops (see Chapter 31).

VIRAL DISEASES. Diseases such as toxoplasmosis, cytomegalic inclusion disease, and rubella are causes of fetal hydrops. Cytomegalic inclusion disease and toxoplasmosis may be associated with intracranial calcification and acoustic shadowing within the brain. Large placentas may be seen with these conditions. Rubella is known to be associated with cardiac anomalies.

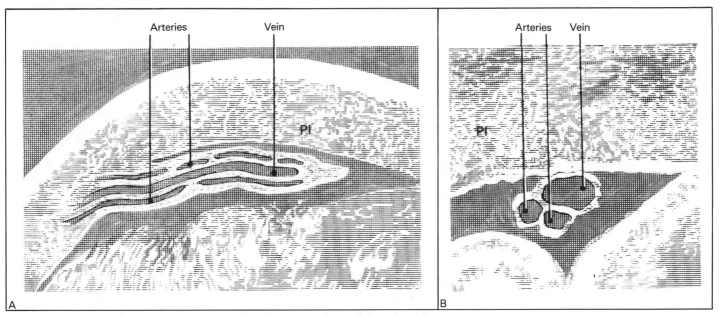

FIGURE 28-3A,B. View of the umbilical cord showing the two arteries and the vein as they enter the placenta.

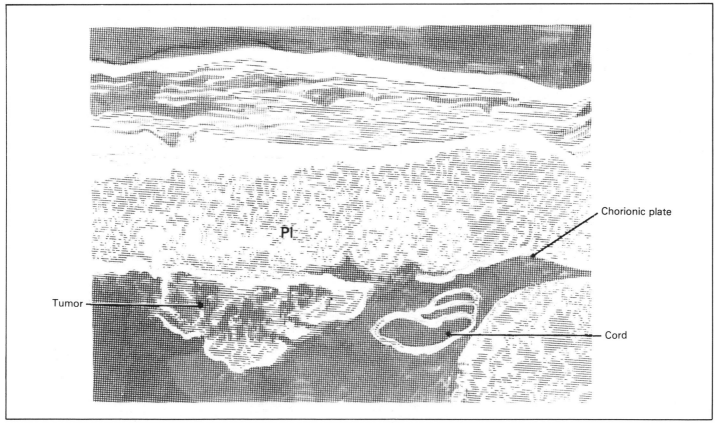

FIGURE 28-4. A placental tumor is arising from the placenta. It has a slightly different texture and usually shows pulsation on real-time.

Additional Masses

The uterus may appear large for dates because of a mass. Either a cyst or a uterine mass may be present in addition to pregnancy.

FIBROIDS

Fibroids (leiomyomas) are a common cause of apparent uterine enlargement. Fibroids may be confused with the placenta because they have a somewhat similar acoustic texture, but the texture of a fibroid is more disorganized and tends to bulge in a more localized fashion than the placenta. Fibroids located in the lower uterine segment near the cervix are clinically important because they can interfere with delivery. As fibroids are followed through pregnancy, they may change in texture, becoming less echogenic due to cystic degeneration.

OVARIAN CYSTS

Physiological ovarian cysts, known as corpus lutein cysts, are common in pregnancy. In the first few weeks of pregnancy, the increased amount of human chorionic gonadotropin (HCG) stimulates the development of such cysts. They may achieve a large size (up to 10 cm) but involute spontaneously as pregnancy continues and usually disappear by 16 weeks. They are echo-free apart from an occasional septum unless bleeding has occurred within them.

Other types of cysts may occur in the ovaries, notably dermoids and serous cystadenomas. These cysts often contain internal structures such as calcification or septa and do not decrease in size on follow-up sonograms. Cysts arising from the kidney or liver may appear on palpation to be associated with the uterus.

ABSCESS FORMATION

Abscess formation due to a ruptured appendix or pelvic inflammatory disease may occur at the same time as pregnancy. An abscess has a complicated internal texture, as described elsewhere in this book, and is usually tender locally.

PITFALLS

1. *Fibroids versus myometrial contraction.* Uterine contractions occur throughout pregnancy and are known as Braxton-Hicks' contractions (see Fig. 29-10). They last for up to a half hour and may simulate a fibroid or placenta while present, although the internal texture is much more even than a fibroid and different from placenta. To differentiate a Braxton-Hicks contraction from a fibroid, re-examine the patient after approximately half an hour.

2. *Cysts versus bladder.* Cysts located anterior to the uterus have been mistaken for the bladder. The normal bladder should have a typical shape. Ovarian cysts are generally spherical. Asking the patient to void or fill the bladder will solve the problem.

3. *Overlooking a triplet or twin.* A thorough search of the entire uterine cavity is the only way to avoid this disaster.

WHERE ELSE TO LOOK

Cystic masses should have a follow-up examination because most, but not all, will go away. Those that do not disappear or even grow may be surgically removed.

SELECTED READING

Athey, P. A., and Hadlock, F. P. (Eds.). *Ultrasound in Obstetrics and Gynecology.* St. Louis: Mosby, 1981.

Callen, P. W. (Ed.). *Ultrasonography in Obstetrics and Gynecology.* Philadelphia: Saunders, 1983.

Sanders, R. C., and James, A. E. (Eds.). *The Principles and Practice of Ultrasonography in Obstetrics and Gynecology.* New York: Appleton-Century-Crofts, 1980.

29. SECOND AND THIRD TRIMESTER BLEEDING

ROGER C. SANDERS

SONOGRAM ABBREVIATIONS

Bl   Bladder

FH   Fetal head
FT   Fetal trunk

M   Myometrium

Pl   Placenta

KEY WORDS

Abruptio Placentae (Accidental Hemorrhage). A placental bleed. A serious condition that threatens the life of the fetus and the mother. It is seen by the sonographer only when it is relatively mild; other cases go straight to the operating room.

Amnion. The membrane that lines the fluid cavity (amniotic cavity) within the uterus in pregnancy.

Amniotic Sac Membrane. This membrane surrounds the amniotic fluid. It is not normally seen sonographically except when the separation between two amniotic sacs is visualized in a multiple pregnancy.

Braxton Hicks' Contraction (Myometrial Contraction). Slow contraction of the uterine muscles (not felt by the mother) occurring in the second and third trimesters. Such local myometrial thickening may mimic a placenta or fibroid sonographically.

Cervix. Most inferior segment of the uterus, which is more than 5 cm long during a normal pregnancy but decreases (effaces) in length during labor.

Cesarean Section (C-Section). Operation performed to deliver a fetus. An incision is made in the lower anterior wall of the uterus. In a "classic" cesarean section, the incision is made at the fundus of the uterus.

Chorionic Plate. A membrane that lines the amniotic aspects of the placenta.

"Double Set-Up." Examination performed by an obstetrician on a patient with a suspected placenta previa. Due to the risks of placental rupture, the examination is performed in the operating room so that a cesarean section can be done immediately if necessary.

Infarct of the Placenta. Loss of tissue blood supply due to arterial occlusion.

Low-Lying Placenta. The inferior edge of the placenta is close to but does not cover the inner aspect of the cervical os.

Marginal Placenta Previa. The edge of the placenta is at the margin of the internal os.

Migration. Term used to describe the shift in position of the placenta from the cervical to the fundal area that often occurs during the course of pregnancy.

Myometrium. The muscle that forms the wall of the uterus.

Os. Term used to describe the upper (internal) and lower (external) entrances to the cervical canal (see Fig. 29-1).

Partial Placenta Previa. Part of the internal os is covered by the placenta.

Placenta Previa (Total). The placenta completely covers the internal os.

Succenturiate Lobe. Anomaly in which the placenta is divided into two segments that are connected by blood vessels. The second lobe may be so small that it is overlooked sonographically. This anomaly occurs in less than 1% of cases.

THE CLINICAL PROBLEM
Vaginal bleeding in the second or third trimester is an ominous clinical sign. Although such bleeding may be due to unimportant conditions such as cervical erosions or vaginal piles, it may signify placenta previa or abruptio placentae.

Placenta Previa
In placenta previa the placenta covers the internal os of the cervix and bleeds because the placenta has separated from the myometrium. When the placenta covers the cervix (total placenta previa), cesarean section is necessary because vaginal delivery would endanger the fetus. Unless a double set-up has been prepared, a pelvic examination is avoided because it may provoke bleeding. With lesser degrees of placenta previa vaginal delivery can be attempted. Ultrasound is the best noninvasive method of establishing a diagnosis of placenta previa.

Abruptio Placentae
Although abruptio placentae is more common in clinical practice than placenta previa, ultrasonic examinations are not often performed because most patients with abruptio are taken straight to the operating room as a clinical emergency. The primary event is a bleed between the placenta and the uterine wall, but blood also frequently enters the amniotic cavity, where it can be visualized sonographically. Abruptio may be present yet not visualized sonographically.

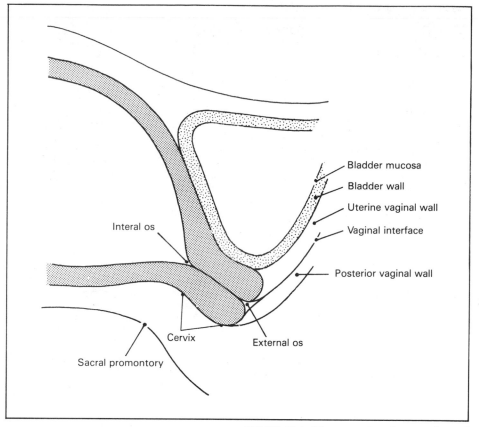

FIGURE 29-1. Diagram showing cervix and surrounding structures.

ANATOMY
In the second trimester the placenta is evenly echogenic with a smooth, well-defined border marginated by the chorionic plate. An irregular border and textural changes often occur in the third trimester (see Placental maturation in Chapter 27). Holes in the placenta in a subchorionic location are a normal finding. Other sonolucent areas of uncertain significance may be seen in the placenta. With the bladder full, the vagina can be seen as an echogenic line with echo-free walls. It ends at the cervix. With luck, the internal os, external os, and cervical canal can be seen within the cervix (Fig. 29-1).

TECHNIQUE

Filled Bladder and Uterus
With the patient's bladder moderately filled, the placental position should be determined. If the placenta extends into the lower uterine segment, demonstrate the vagina and cervix (Fig. 29-1) because it may represent a placenta previa. The axis of the vagina and cervix may not be longitudinal, and oblique sections may be required to show this critical relationship. If the placenta appears to lie adjacent to the cervix, scan transversely at right angles to see whether the placenta is centrally located or whether it lies to one side of the cervix and lower uterine segment (Fig. 29-2). This relationship is easy to determine if the fetus is breech but more difficult with a cephalic (vertex) presentation.

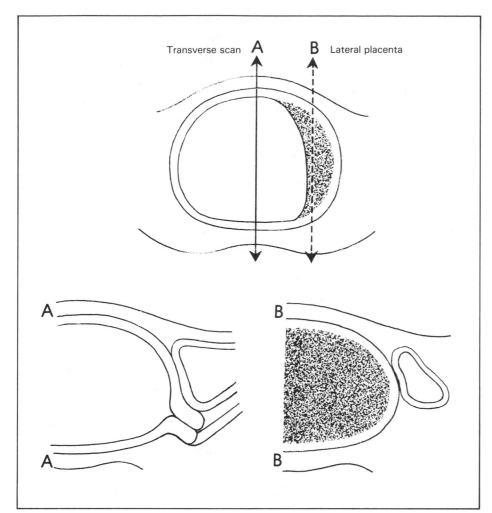

Maneuvers Used to Show Possible Placenta Previa

If the fetal head lies more than 2 cm distant from the sacrum, the possibility of placenta previa exists, and particular maneuvers should be performed to show the area behind the fetal head.

1. Push the transducer into the maternal abdomen just superior to the pubic symphysis and arch it longitudinally toward the patient's head.
2. Perform longitudinal sections with similar pressure above the pubic symphysis with the transducer in a more lateral position, angling medially.
3. By placing the patient head down in the Trendelenburg position, the fetal head may float out of the pelvis.
4. Have a physician move and hold the fetal head out of the pelvis with an abdominal rather than a vaginal approach and scan the lower uterine segment as described above (Fig. 29-3A,B).

FIGURE 29-2. Longitudinal section at level B gives the impression of a placenta previa, but the placenta is off to the left. A longitudinal section at level A in the midline through the vagina shows no placenta covering the cervix.

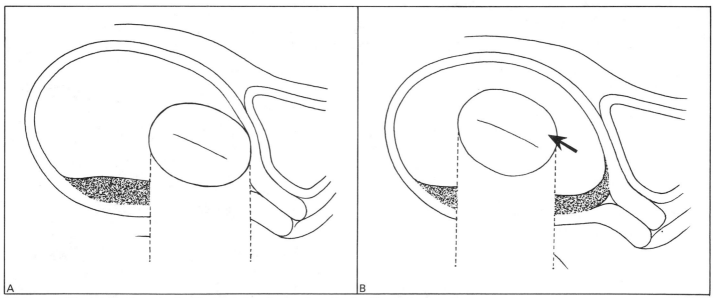

FIGURE 29-3. Shadowing from the fetal head. A. Shadowing from the fetal head obscures the region of the internal os. B. With the fetal head elevated superiorly, the placenta previa is revealed.

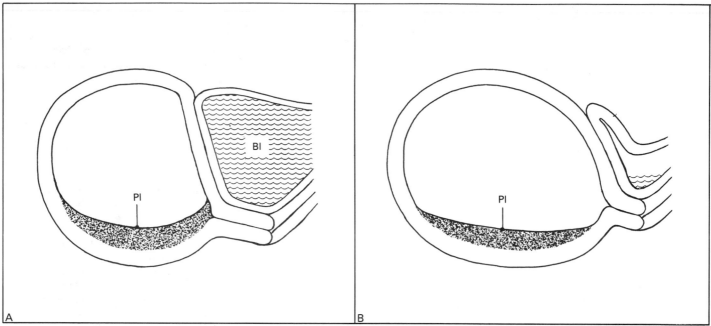

FIGURE 29-4. Overdistended bladder and placenta previa. A. An overdistended bladder may compress the anterior wall of the uterus against the posterior wall, causing an appearance resembling a placenta previa. B. With the bladder empty, the true length of the cervix is seen; the placenta ends above the cervix.

Postvoiding View

If, after performing these maneuvers, you are convinced that the placenta lies adjacent to the cervix, repeat the examination after voiding. The anterior wall of the uterus may be compressed against the placenta, giving a false impression of placenta previa when the bladder is filled (Fig. 29-4A,B).

PATHOLOGY

Placenta Previa

This condition is present whenever the placenta can be shown to lie adjacent to the internal cervical os. It is divided into three types:

1. *Low-lying* when the placenta is close to the os but not overlying it (Fig. 29-5A)
2. *Marginal or partial* when it incompletely covers the internal os (Fig. 29-5B).
3. *Complete or total* when it completely overlies the internal os (Fig. 29-5C).

From a practical point of view, the first two conditions cannot be separated ultrasonically. The maneuvers described under Technique must be followed to prove ultrasonically that there is a placenta previa.

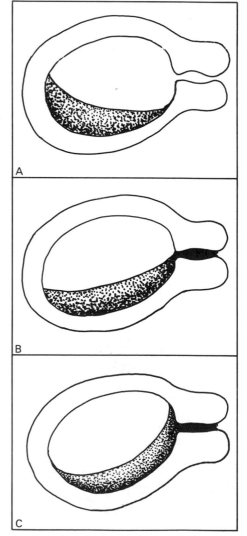

FIGURE 29-5. The types of placenta previa. A. Low-lying, abutting on the internal os but not covering it. B. Partial, partly covering the internal os. C. Total, completely covering the internal os.

Serial ultrasonic examinations are necessary when placenta previa is discovered because the placenta changes its position during the course of pregnancy (migration). At term, it frequently lies at the fundus, while previously it was close to the cervix (Fig. 29-6). In asymptomatic patients, the placenta often lies near the cervical os. A sonolucent gap with internal echoes between the placenta and the cervix may represent blood. It can be supporting evidence that a placenta previa is the cause of symptoms in a patient who is bleeding from the vagina (Fig. 29-7).

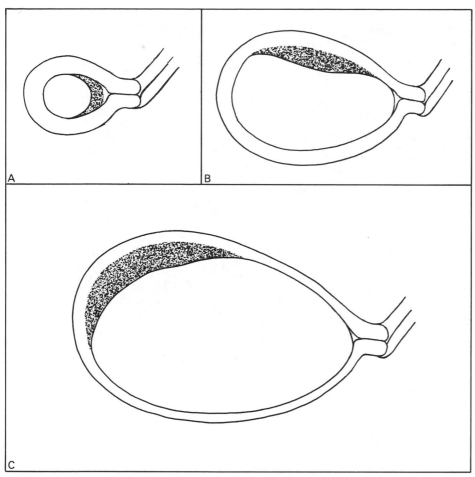

FIGURE 29-6. Placental migration. A. Early in pregnancy the placenta overlies the internal os. B. With selective growth of the lower uterine segment the placenta moves to an anterior site. C. Late in pregnancy the placenta lies at the fundus of the uterus.

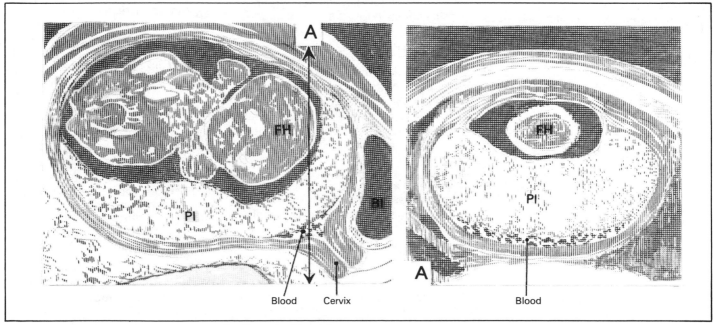

FIGURE 29-7. Total posterior placenta previa. Note the blood between the cervix and the placenta.

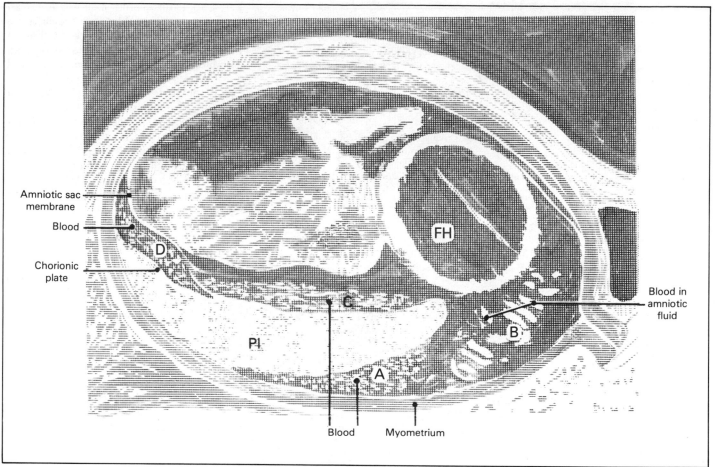

Amniotic sac membrane

Blood

Chorionic plate

PI

Blood

Myometrium

FH

Blood in amniotic fluid

FIGURE 29-8. Appearences of abruptio placentae. A. Blood may lie between the placenta and the myometrium. B. There may be blood mixed with the amniotic fluid. C. A fluid-fluid level may be formed by the blood and amniotic fluid. D. There may be blood between the amniotic sac membrane and the chorionic plate.

Abruptio Placentae (Accidental Hemorrhage)

This condition has several sonographic manifestations (Fig. 29-8).

A GAP BETWEEN THE MYOMETRIUM AND THE PLACENTA

This collection may be completely sonolucent, or it may contain low-level internal echoes due to blood. The border of the placenta will be displaced away from the myometrium with an obvious separation.

ECHOES WITHIN THE AMNIOTIC FLUID DUE TO BLOOD

These echoes may be focal and present in small clumps, or they may be evenly echogenic and extensive and even form a fluid-fluid level.

BLEEDING BETWEEN THE CHORIONIC PLATE AND THE AMNIOTIC SAC MEMBRANE

The blood within this space may be relatively similar in texture to that of the placenta, but it will eventually become sonolucent. The amniotic sac membrane may be displaced away from the chorionic plate at sites other than the placenta.

PITFALLS

1. *Placental and uterine vessels.* Sometimes the blood vessels that supply the placenta are large and form spaces in the myometrium adjacent to the placenta (Fig. 29-9A,B) which may be mistaken for abruptio placentae. Real-time visualization will document pulsation in this area.

2. *Septa.* Septa within the amniotic fluid of little pathologic significance may occur and may be mistaken for displacement of the amniotic sac membrane away from the wall of the uterus by blood. Septa may also be seen normally in twins.

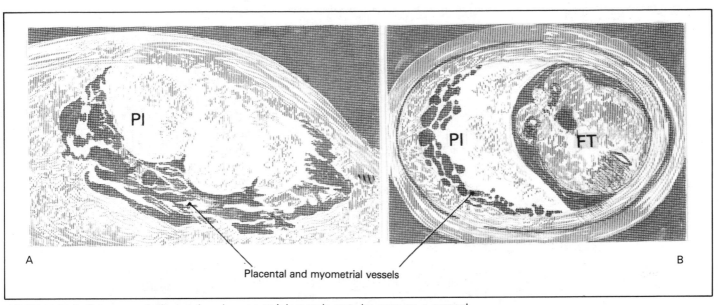

Placental and myometrial vessels

FIGURE 29-9A,B. Pronounced placental and myometrial vessels may be seen as a normal variant. These vessels may be confused with abruptio placentae.

Braxton-Hicks' contraction

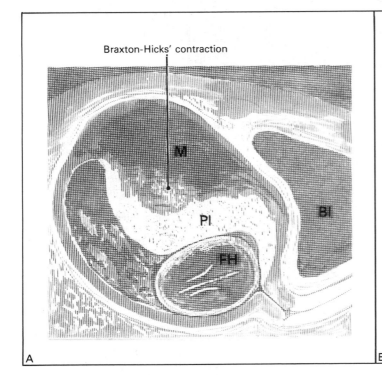

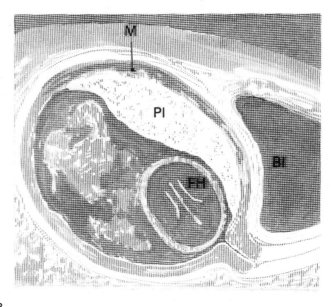

FIGURE 29-10. Braxton Hicks' contractions. A. The placenta bulges into the amniotic cavity. A Braxton Hicks' contraction of the myometrium is responsible. B. After a wait of approximately 30 minutes, such contractions disappear. Fibroids do not have the regular texture of thickened myometrium.

3. *Overdistended bladder.* An overdistended bladder may cause an appearance that suggests a placenta previa because the anterior wall of the uterus is compressed against the posterior wall (Fig. 29-4). Postvoiding films resolve this false positive finding.

4. *Myometrium.* Mistaking the myometrium (uterine wall) for abruptio is possible. The normal sonolucent space around the placenta should be symmetrical at all sites, although this space is particularly obvious at the fundus of the uterus.

5. *Braxton-Hicks' contraction.* A myometrial contraction (Braxton-Hicks' contraction) can be mistaken for a placenta previa when the contraction occurs in the lower uterine segment (Fig. 29-10). If the placenta appears to be visible at two separate sites, rescan after 30 minutes. One of the possible placentas will usually turn out to be a myometrial contraction. These are painless contractions of the uterus wall of no pathologic significance.

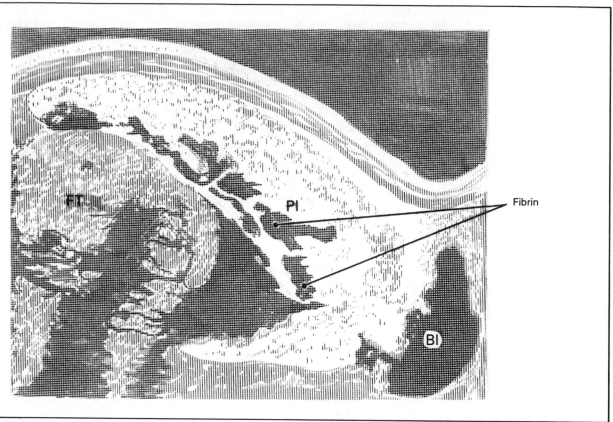

Fibrin

FIGURE 29-11. Sonolucent areas within the chorionic aspect of the placenta due to fibrin deposition or prominent vessels. These are a normal variant.

6. *Succenturiate lobe.* Succenturiate lobe, a rare variant of placenta (occurring in approximately 1% of cases), occurs when the placenta is split into two parts. If the second part is small and located adjacent to the cervix, sonographic detection may be impossible.

7. *Low-lying placenta.* Placentas lying in the lower uterine segment in a lateral position may mimic a placenta previa unless a thorough effort to define the relationship between the cervix and the placenta is made.

8. *Fibrin deposition.* Sonolucent areas may be seen adjacent to the chorionic plate within the placenta. These represent either fibrin deposition or large placental vessels and are of no pathologic significance (Fig. 29-11).

9. *Low lateral placenta mimicking a placenta previa.* If the placenta lies lateral to the cervix but in the region of the lower segment, casual scanning may give the impression of a placenta previa (see Fig. 29-2). Make sure that a section is taken through the cervix and lower uterine segment simultaneously to be confident that a placenta previa is present.

SELECTED READING

Athey, P. A., and Hadlock, F. P. (Eds.). *Ultrasound in Obstetrics and Gynecology.* St. Louis: Mosby, 1981.

Callen, P. W. (Ed.). *Ultrasonography in Obstetrics and Gynecology.* Philadelphia: Saunders, 1983.

Sanders, R. C., and James, A. E. (Eds.). *The Principles and Practice of Ultrasonography in Obstetrics and Gynecology.* New York: Appleton-Century-Crofts, 1980.

30. FETAL DEATH

ROGER C. SANDERS
MARY B. SILBERSTEIN

SONOGRAM ABBREVIATIONS
Pl   Placenta

KEY WORDS

FDIU. Fetal death in utero.

FH. Fetal heart or fundal height.

Maceration. Disintegration of the fetus after intrauterine death occurs. The amniotic fluid is filled with partially digested segments of the fetus.

Spalding's Sign. Overlapping of the fetal skull bones.

THE CLINICAL PROBLEM

Fetal death can occur at any stage in pregnancy but is most common in the first few weeks, that is, in spontaneous abortion (see Chapter 24). This chapter will center on fetal death occurring in the second and third trimesters. Usually fetal death occurs in association with known predisposing causes such as intrauterine growth retardation, abruptio placentae, and congenital malformations, but it may occur unexpectedly. As a rule, the diagnosis is suspected because of the absence of fetal movement. The patient is usually sent for an ultrasonic examination after failure to detect fetal heart motion by Doppler examination in the obstetrics clinic. However, in our experience, a false positive diagnosis of fetal death by Doppler examination is not unusual. Because fetal death is often treated by evacuation of the uterus, confirmation of death by real-time ultrasound is essential. The sonographer, in cooperation with the physician, therefore, carries a heavy responsibility in establishing this diagnosis.

ANATOMY

Fetal heart and limb motion can be detected by real-time ultrasound beginning from 6 to 7 weeks after the last menstrual period. Fetal activity is considerable between approximately 8 and 20 weeks but decreases in the third trimester because less space is available for fetal movement. The normal fetal pulse beats approximately 140 times per minute. Slowing of the fetal pulse suggests impending fetal death.

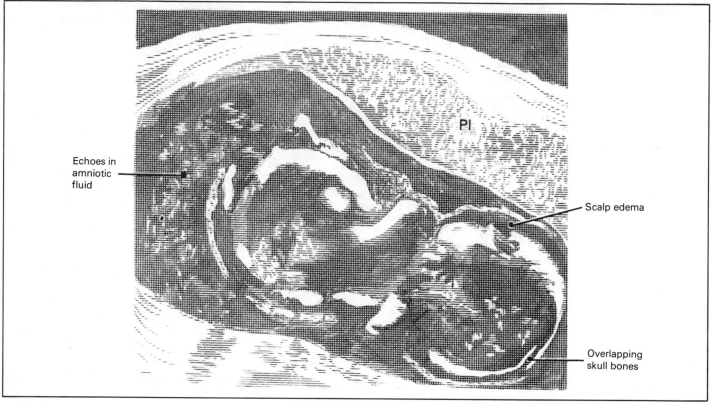

Echoes in amniotic fluid

Pl

Scalp edema

Overlapping skull bones

FIGURE 30-1. Signs of fetal death on a B-scan include scalp edema, overlapping of skull bones, unusual fetal position, and extra echoes in the amniotic fluid due to maceration of the tissues.

TECHNIQUE
Real-Time

A real-time examination is by far the best technique for detecting fetal death. Identify the anatomy of the chest and make sure that a sonolucent area within the segment surrounded by the ribs is visible. Count the pulsations of the apparent fetal heart. Evidence of fetal limb movement makes visualization of fetal heart motion redundant. If no fetal heart motion has occurred after 3 minutes of observation, a videotape may be desirable as a permanent legal record, especially with obese patients.

Slow B-Scan

If real-time is not available, a slow B-scan over the fetal heart should show evidence of fetal heart motion. With very slow scanning, a wiggle will be seen from the septum that divides the two ventricles.

Combined Use of B-Scan with A-Mode and Fetal Echocardiography

These techniques have been used in the past but are no longer needed now that real-time equipment is available.

B-Scan Signs of Fetal Death

About 3 days after death, the fetus shows changes in shape and position that indicate fetal death (Fig. 30-1).

1. With subcutaneous edema a *double outline* develops that extends around to the skull and trunk. Skin thickening may also be seen with a variety of other conditions such as infants of diabetic mothers and hydrops.
2. Adoption of an *unusual fetal position* occurs, with the fetus curled into a ball. This position will be unchanged on serial sonographic examinations.
3. *Overlapping of the skull bones* (Spalding's sign) is seen in labor as a normal phenomenon but at other times indicates fetal death.
4. *Loss of definition of structures in the fetal trunk* occurs over a period of time. Echoes start to appear in the fetal brain.
5. *Gross echoes in the amniotic fluid* develop due to maceration.

PITFALLS

1. Some motion of the gestational sac and fetal pole may be derived from the maternal aorta. Make sure that apparent pulsations are not due to maternal pulsations by counting the maternal pulse.
2. The umbilical cord may pulsate even when the fetus is dead.

SELECTED READING

Athey, P. A., and Hadlock, F. P. (Eds.). *Ultrasound in Obstetrics and Gynecology.* St. Louis: Mosby, 1981.

Callen, P. W. (Ed.). *Ultrasonography in Obstetrics and Gynecology.* Philadelphia: Saunders, 1983.

Sanders, R. C., and James, A. E. (Eds.). *The Principles and Practice of Ultrasonography in Obstetrics and Gynecology.* New York: Appleton-Century-Crofts, 1980.

31. FETAL ANOMALIES

ROGER C. SANDERS

SONOGRAM ABBREVIATIONS

Bl Bladder

D Diaphragm

FH Fetal head
FS Fetal spine

K Kidney

L Liver

Pl Placenta

KEY WORDS

Achondrogenesis. A type of dwarfism.

Achondroplasia. A type of dwarfism—the usual circus dwarf with bulging forehead and short limbs.

Alpha-Fetoprotein. An enzyme found in maternal blood and amniotic fluid that is elevated in the presence of neural crest anomalies, most gastrointestinal anomalies, fetal death, twins, wrong estimation of dates, and maternal liver problems.

Anal Atresia. Intestinal obstruction at the anal level due to failure to form the rectum; the large and small bowel are fluid filled. May occur without polyhydramnios.

Anencephalus. Most common fetal intracranial anomaly. Only the base of the brain and face are present, resulting in a very small "head."

Closed Neural Defects. Neural defects in which the spinal cord and brain are not in contact with the amniotic fluid and thus are not associated with an elevated alpha-fetoprotein level.

Cystic Adenomatoid Malformation. Anomaly in which a part of the lung is replaced by cysts.

Cystic Hygroma. Large fluid-containing sac usually filled with lymph and usually located in the region of the neck. Not fatal but very disfiguring and difficult to treat surgically.

Cytomegalic Inclusion Disease. Fetal viral disease with consequent intracranial calcification, microcephaly, and mental deficiency.

Diaphragmatic Hernia. A portion of one diaphragm is missing, and the bowel or liver lies in the chest.

Down's Syndrome (Mongolism). Syndrome seen predominantly in the fetuses of women who are over 35 years old; recognizable on amniotic fluid analysis by the presence of abnormal chromosomes. It is associated with congenital heart disease and duodenal atresia.

Double Bubble Sign. Sign of duodenal atresia in which two circular, fluid-filled structures, representing the stomach and duodenum, are seen in the upper abdomen.

Duodenal Atresia. Intestinal obstruction at a duodenal level with subsequent distention of the duodenum and stomach by fluid. Associated with polyhydramnios and Down's syndrome.

Ellis-van Creveld Syndrome (Six-Fingered Dwarfism). Type of dwarfism in which there are extra digits.

Encephalocele. Herniation of the coverings of the brain through an anterior or posterior midline defect in the skull. Brain tissue is contained within the herniation, although usually most of the contents of the sac are fluid.

Gastroschisis. Condition similar to omphalocele except that no membrane covers the herniated material. Gut floats freely in the amniotic fluid. The herniation is paraumbilical.

Holt-Oram Syndrome. Congenital syndrome consisting of a combination of heart disease and absence of a digit or the radius in the arm.

Hydrocephalus. Marked enlargement of the cerebral ventricles.

Hydranencephaly. Replacement of most of the brain except the brain stem with cerebrospinal fluid.

Hydronephrosis. An obstructed kidney with a dilated collecting system.

Hypoplastic Left Heart Syndrome. Congenital abnormality in which the aorta is too small. This condition is not compatible with life.

Hydrops Fetalis. The fetal abdomen contains ascites and the skin is thickened by excess fluid. This condition has a variety of causes, of which the most well known is rhesus incompatibility (Rh disease). Other causes are grouped as "nonimmune hydrops."

Ileal Atresia. Intestinal obstruction at a midgut level. Filling of small bowel loops with fluid is associated with polyhydramnios.

Infantile Polycystic Kidney. A congenital condition in which large kidneys are filled with tiny cysts.

Iniencephaly. Defect consisting of an encephalocele that involves the posterior aspects of the skull and the cervical vertebrae; some vertebrae may be missing.

Lamina. Lateral bridge of bone covering the posterior spinal canal.

Lymphangioma. See *Cystic hygroma* (above).

Meckel's Syndrome. A syndrome consisting of infantile polycystic kidney, encephalocele, and extra digits (polydactyl).

Meconium. Contents of the fetal bowel.

Meconium Peritonitis. Bowel rupture in utero leads to meconium spillage with consequent calcification. There is usually bowel obstruction.

Meningocele. Spinal bone defect with cerebrospinal fluid pouch.

Meningomyelocele. Bone defect associated with expansion of the spinal cord and a fluid-containing cavity at the level of the abnormality.

Microcephaly. Unduly small skull and brain associated with mental deficiency.

Multicystic (Dysplastic) Kidney. Developmental abnormality of the kidney in which the normal renal parenchyma is totally replaced by cysts of varying sizes. If bilateral, it is not compatible with survival.

Myelocele. Spinal bone defect with spinal cord protrusion, but no cerebrospinal fluid pouch.

Neural Crest Anomaly. Spinal defect in which there is no skin covering on the spine, and therefore contact between some portion of the central nervous system and the amniotic fluid occurs. This combination gives rise to a raised alpha-fetoprotein level.

Omphalocele. Herniation of much of the gut, often including the liver, out of the abdomen through an umbilical opening (see *Gastroschisis,* above). A membrane covers the herniated contents. Associated with other congenital anomalies.

Osteogenesis Imperfecta. Congenital anomaly in which bone fractures occur.

Posterior Urethral Valves. Valves situated in the posterior urethra that cause obstruction of the bladder, ureters, and kidneys. Complete blockage of the urethra may be present.

Potter's Syndrome. Fetus with bilateral renal abnormalities, which may consist of absent kidneys, bilateral hydronephrosis, bilateral multicystic dysplastic kidneys, or infantile polycystic kidney. Oligohydramnios accompanies this syndrome. The consequences of too little amniotic fluid—unusual face, deformed limbs, and hypoplastic lungs—will be seen at birth. Most such fetuses are stillborn.

Prune-Belly (Eagle-Barrett) Syndrome (Agenesis of the Abdominal Muscles). Congenital condition in which there are weakened or absent abdominal wall muscles, markedly distended ureters with tiny or hydronephrotic kidneys, and a large bladder.

Rhesus (Rh) Incompatibility (Erythroblastosis Fetalis). The fetal blood possesses a different Rh blood group from the maternal blood. When maternal blood cells leak into the fetal circulation, they interact, forming antibodies. In the next pregnancy there is hemolysis, and the fetus is left anemic with hydrops.

Rubella. Viral disease occurring in utero associated with a number of fetal anomalies including congenital heart disease.

Spina Bifida. Bony spinal defect over the spinal canal. The spinal cord at the affected level is abnormal.

Teratoma. Tumor composed of multiple different tissues arising anywhere in the body but usually in the region of the sacrum.

Thanatophoric Dwarf. Form of dwarfism that affects not only the limbs but also the chest, which is too small. Invariably fatal.

Toxoplasmosis. Viral disease affecting the fetus in utero and causing intracranial calcification.

Tracheoesophageal Fistula. Obstruction of the esophagus composed of a fistula to the trachea and sometimes a connection to the stomach through the trachea. In the most severe form no fluid reaches the stomach.

THE CLINICAL PROBLEM

Many congenital disorders are detectable at less than 24 weeks' pregnancy (early enough for an elective termination) by abnormal biochemical findings in the amniotic fluid or are associated with structural sonographic changes of more than 2 cm in size. Some patients with a familial history of a defect such as dwarfism are sent directly for an ultrasound examination. Other patients are referred because of an abnormality found on maternal serum or amniotic fluid analysis. Mothers who are over 35 years old have an increased chance of carrying a fetus with Down's syndrome (mongolism) and are therefore screened by amniocentesis to detect chromosomal abnormalities in the amniotic fluid. At the same time as amniocentesis, various biochemical tests are conducted on the amniotic fluid, notably, an alpha-fetoprotein determination.

Amniotic alpha-fetoprotein elevation occurs in association with open neural crest anomalies such as anencephaly or spina bifida and encephalocele and is also associated with gastrointestinal problems such as omphalocele and duodenal atresia. All these structural problems can be identified with ultrasound. Because alpha-fetoprotein elevation can also be detected in the mother's blood, biochemical tests for this substance are now performed as a screening procedure. Fetal anomalies of course can be detected in other women being screened for ultrasound for various clinical reasons, such as a discrepancy between expected dates and examination results or placenta previa.

Fetal anomalies of more than 2 cm in size can be readily discovered by an accomplished sonographer. Thus, all sonographers should have a detailed knowledge of normal fetal anatomy. It is desirable that anomalies be discovered before the fetus is 23 to 24 weeks old, because therapeutic abortions currently cannot be legally performed after 6 months' gestational age. Nevertheless, discovery of an anomaly at a later stage of pregnancy is of practical importance because the optimal fashion and time of delivery can be arranged, and the presence of the fetal anomaly will prompt early transfer to a hospital that has neonatal care and pediatric surgical facilities. Fetuses with anomalies that may rupture at the time of delivery (such as an omphalocele) are best delivered by cesarean section. If the fetal prognosis is very poor, those with a fluid-distended abdomen or head may be decompressed under ultrasound control prior to delivery in order to avoid a needless cesarean section. Some anomalies such as hydronephrosis or hydrocephalus may be treated with in utero decompression.

ANATOMY

The relevant anatomy is described in Chapter 26.

TECHNIQUE

See Chapter 26 for appropriate technique.

PATHOLOGY

Renal Anomalies

CYSTS AND HYDRONEPHROSIS

Renal anomalies may involve a single kidney or may be bilateral, as in multicystic kidney or hydronephrosis. If renal involvement is bilateral, oligohydramnios is usual, although polyhydramnios may occur with hydronephrosis even when the condition is bilateral. Cystic spaces in the location of the normal kidneys are found if hydronephrosis or multicystic kidney is present. Multicystic kidney is likely if the cysts are variable in size and do not appear to connect (Fig. 31-1). In hydronephrosis there is usually a central dilated pelvis with dilated calyces arising from it (Fig. 31-2). If both kidneys are involved, hydronephrosis may be due to obstruction of the urethra, in which case the bladder will be greatly distended. Bilateral multicystic kidney may be associated with ureteric and urethral atresia although the bladder may still be visible. Prune-belly syndrome, a variant of hydronephrosis, can be confusing because tortuous distended ureters appear as cystic spaces. Fetal ascites may be present with this condition, and the fetal abdomen bulges.

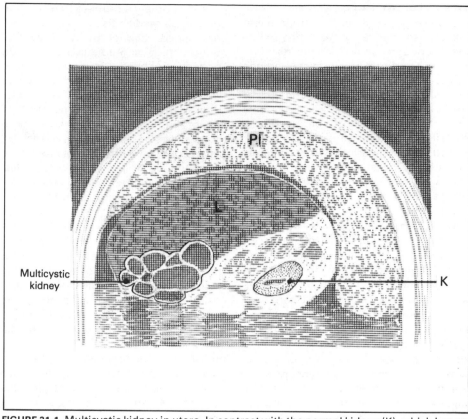

FIGURE 31-1. Multicystic kidney in utero. In contrast with the normal kidney (K), which has an echogenic center and an even renal parenchyma, a multicystic kidney contains cysts that vary in size and shape.

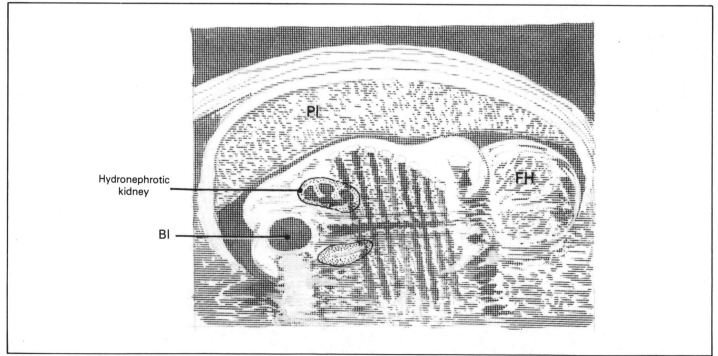

FIGURE 31-2. A hydronephrotic kidney contains fluid-filled areas that communicate and form a glove-like pattern.

INFANTILE POLYCYSTIC KIDNEY

Infantile polycystic kidney is another cause of oligohydramnios. The kidneys are much enlarged and are densely echogenic without visible cysts (Fig. 31-3). The trunk circumference will be wider than usual. Meckel's syndrome is a variant of infantile polycystic kidney in which there is an encephalocele and extra digits in addition to the kidney anomaly.

Gastrointestinal Tract Anomalies

Most gastrointestinal anomalies are associated with polyhydramnios. One should look for the following problems.

OMPHALOCELE

Some portion of the intestines and abdominal organs, usually the liver, are contained in a sac that lies outside the normal confines of the trunk (Fig. 31-4).

GASTROSCHISIS

Gastroschisis is a condition similar to omphalocele, but because the gut contents are not confined within a membrane, the intestines spread out through the amniotic fluid.

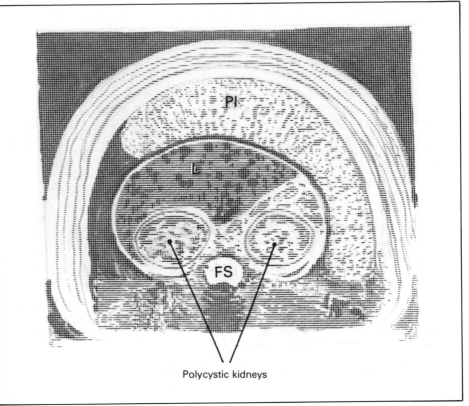

Polycystic kidneys

FIGURE 31-3. In infantile polycystic kidney the kidneys are large and echogenic. Both kidneys are involved.

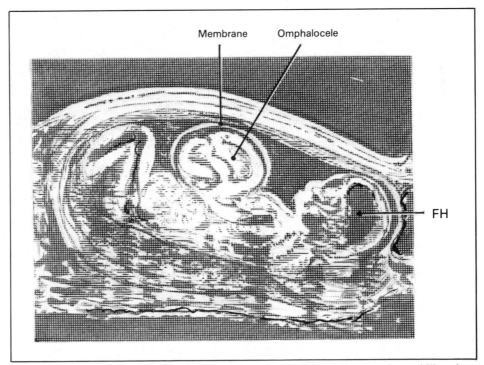

Membrane   Omphalocele

FH

FIGURE 31-4. With omphalocele the abdominal contents prolapse through the umbilicus into a sac in front of the abdomen.

DUODENAL ATRESIA

Two large sonolucent spaces (the double bubble sign) are visible within the upper abdomen. These can be shown to connect if a real-time system is used and represent the distended fluid-filled stomach and duodenum (Fig. 31-5).

INTESTINAL OBSTRUCTION

Long tubular structures within the fetal abdomen are seen (Fig. 31-6). Lower gastrointestinal tract obstruction may not be associated with polyhydramnios (e.g., anal atresia).

TRACHEOESOPHAGEAL FISTULA

The stomach bubble is not seen in one rare type; the more common types have not yet been diagnosed by ultrasound.

MECONIUM PERITONITIS

Spillage of fetal intestinal contents (the meconium) results in calcification, usually in a ring-like form in the fetal abdomen. This condition is usually associated with bowel obstruction.

Limb Anomalies

Many forms of dwarfism are familial. Dwarfism may not be seen in utero or may develop only after 24 weeks—too late for a therapeutic abortion. Some types of dwarfism (e.g., thanatophoric and achondrogenic) can be recognized in time for a therapeutic abortion. The following features suggest dwarfism.

SHORTENING OF LIMBS

The femur and humerus should be measured. Normal femoral length tables are available (Appendix 9).

There may be disproportionate shortening of the distal limb bones (i.e., the tibia and fibula and the radius and ulna). See Appendix 2 for normal lengths of fetal long bones. The distal or proximal portion of the extremity can be identified once it has been determined whether one or two bones are present.

DIGIT COUNTING

After 15 to 16 weeks, the number of fetal digits (fingers or toes) can be counted. This is crucial in certain syndromes in which extra digits are present (e.g., Ellis-van Creveld syndrome) or in which a digit is missing (e.g., Holt-Oram syndrome).

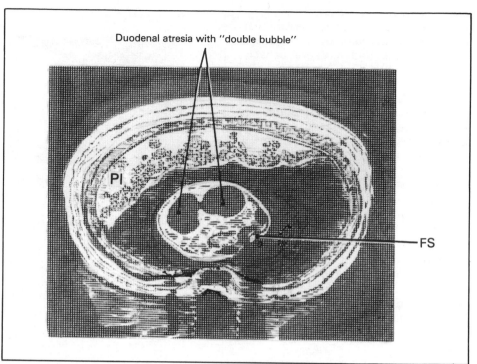

FIGURE 31-5. In duodenal atresia there are two large upper abdominal, round, fluid-filled cavities that can be shown with real-time to communicate.

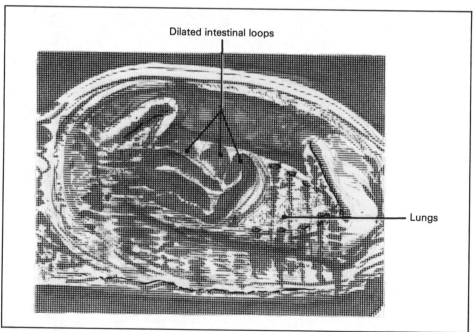

FIGURE 31-6. With intestinal obstruction, fluid-filled tubes will be seen within the fetal abdomen.

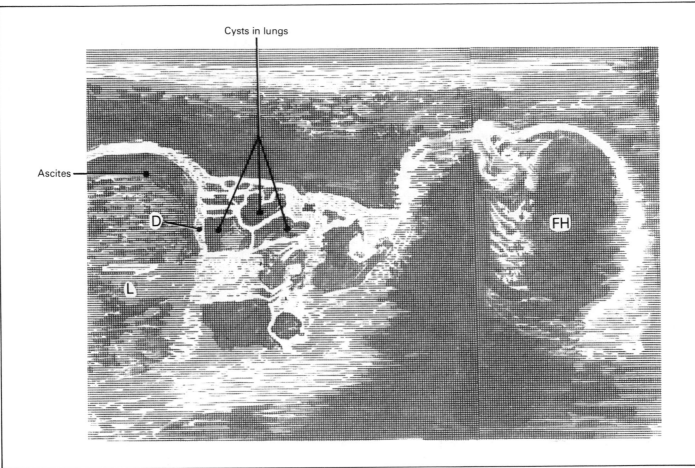

Cysts in lungs

Ascites

D

L

FH

FIGURE 31-7. In cystic adenomatoid malformation, the normally echogenic lungs are replaced by cysts, which vary in size and shape. Ascites is usually present.

LIMB SHAPE

In some forms of limb anomalies (e.g., Campomelic dwarfism), the limbs are bowed. Fractures in utero may occur in osteogenesis imperfecta with abrupt angulation of the limbs.

HEAD-TO-TRUNK RATIO

Some forms of dwarfism are associated with a narrow chest (e.g., thanatophoric dwarfism); therefore, a head-to-trunk ratio is an important measurement when dwarfism is possible. The ratio will be increased in dwarfism.

POLYHYDRAMNIOS

This sign is found with some types of dwarfism. A bewildering array of types of dwarfism exists, but because most are very rare, we will not list all of their distinctive features here.

Chest Anomalies

PLEURAL EFFUSION

Pleural effusions can easily be recognized surrounding the lungs at the level of the heart or above (see Fig. 28-2). Although they are usually associated with the changes of hydrops, they may be an isolated finding.

CYSTS

Cystic spaces occur in the lungs with cystic adenomatoid malformations (Fig. 31-7). Because the mediastinal structures are rudimentary, the entire chest may be filled with cysts, yet survival is possible.

HERNIA

In diaphragmatic hernia some portion of the diaphragm will be invisible, and tubular structures may be present within the chest owing to dilated loops of bowel. If the texture is evenly echogenic, liver herniation is suspect. All detectable chest conditions are likely to be associated with fetal ascites.

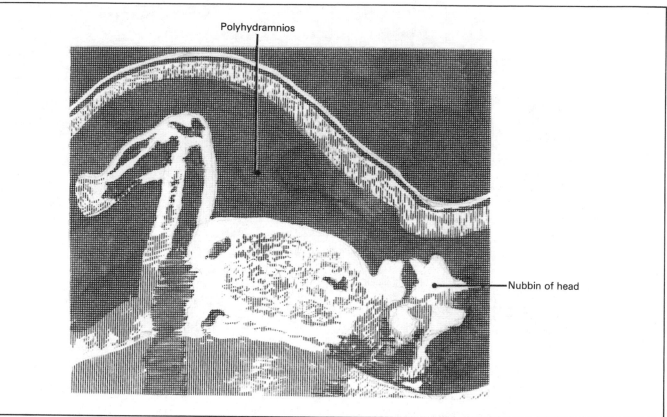

Polyhydramnios

Nubbin of head

FIGURE 31-8. With anencephalus the fetal head is replaced by a "nubbin" of tissue in which the bones of the base of the head can be made out.

Cardiac Anomalies

The fetal heart is a difficult organ to evaluate and has only recently been investigated in utero. The fetuses of patients with a family history of congenital heart disease are at a small increased risk of increased fetal cardiac anomalies, although the anomaly is usually not of the same type. Other groups at risk are fetuses of diabetic mothers and nonimmune hydrops fetuses. Only the grossest anomalies can be detected in utero.

PERICARDIAL EFFUSION

A sonolucent zone will be present around the fetal heart between the heart and the lungs.

HYPOPLASTIC LEFT HEART SYNDROME

The heart is enlarged, and the aortic arch is small and difficult to demonstrate.

RHYTHM PROBLEMS

Alterations in fetal rhythm with excessive speed (tachycardia) or excessive slowing (bradycardia) are easy to recognize (normal fetal pulse rate is 140 beats per minute). More difficult is the recognition of irregular rhythms with dropped beats. Videotaping is essential to recognize this anomaly. Most rhythm abnormalities in the third trimester are of no pathologic significance unless fetal ascites is seen.

Cerebral Anomalies

Most CNS anomalies are associated with polyhydramnios. Common anomalies are anencephalus, hydrocephalus, microcephalus, encephalocele, and spina bifida.

ANENCEPHALUS

A large segment of the brain is absent, and only the structures at the base of the brain are present. Sonographically, a nubbin of tissue is visible at the cranial end of the trunk (Fig. 31-8).

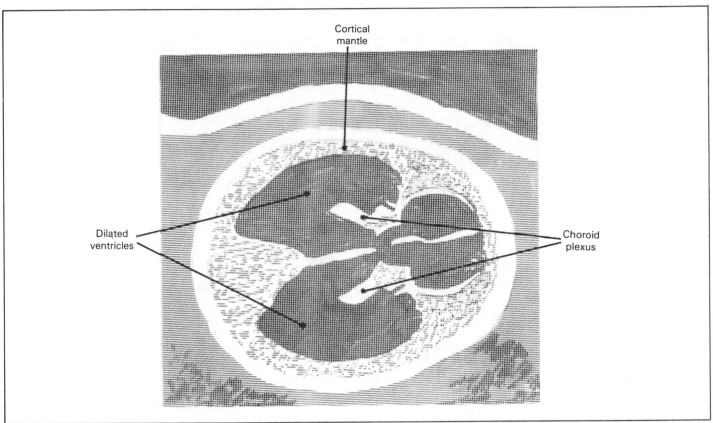

Cortical mantle

Dilated ventricles

Choroid plexus

FIGURE 31-9. In the usual type of hydrocephalus most of the skull is filled with two large fluid-filled structures—the lateral ventricles. The cortical mantle is the term used to describe the width of the remaining brain.

HYDROCEPHALUS

After 13 weeks' gestational age, the ventricles should be seen routinely. Normal ventriculohemispheric ratios are available, and early in gestation these values are surprisingly large. If hydrocephalus is present and the lateral ventricles are symmetrical (Fig. 31-9), try to visualize the third and fourth ventricles to establish the level of obstruction. If hydrocephalus is not generalized, consider the following possibilities:

1. *Porencephalic cyst.* A single sonolucent cystic area within the brain communicating with the ventricles (see Chapter 40).
2. *Holoprosencephaly.* Fused ventricles forming one large central cavity with distorted brain parenchyma elsewhere (see Chapter 40).
3. *Dandy Walker syndrome.* Bilateral ventricular enlargement with a large posterior fossa cyst occupying most of the site where the cerebellum normally lies (see Chapter 40).

4. *Arachnoid cyst.* Fluid-filled space within the brain substance not communicating with the ventricles.
5. *Vein of Galen aneurysm.* Fluid-filled space posterior to the third ventricle due to a dilated vein; usually associated with hydrocephalus (see Chapter 40).

Make sure to obtain a good view of the amount of cortex (the "mantle") around the ventricle because the width of the mantle has some relationship to whether or not the fetus has a worthwhile future.

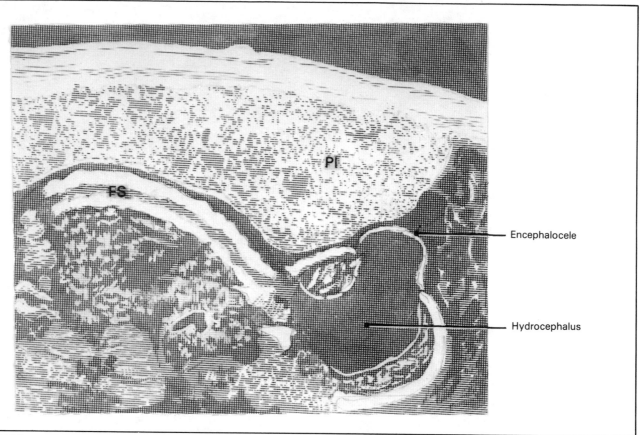

FIGURE 31-10. With an encephalocele hydrocephalic ventricles communicate with a fluid-filled brain-lined space that lies outside the skull, usually in an occipital location.

MICROCEPHALUS

The brain is too small, resulting in mental retardation. An abnormally low head-to-trunk ratio suggests that the head is microcephalic. Microcephaly is a more difficult diagnosis to make than hydrocephalus but is equally important. A decision has to be made about whether the trunk is too large or the head is too small. Serial sonograms will show decreased growth of the head with microcephaly.

ENCEPHALOCELE

A defect is present, usually in the posterior (but may be anterior) aspect of the head through which portions of the brain substance and ventricles prolapse (Fig. 31-10). Usually such structures contain cerebrospinal fluid, but they may contain brain tissue. Associated hydrocephalus is usual.

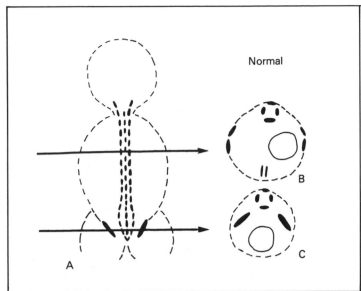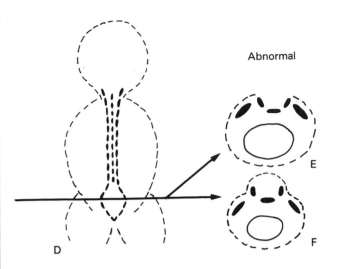

SPINA BIFIDA

This term encompasses masses that arise from the spinal cord (meningocele) and masses that are a combination of spinal cord protrusion and an adjacent cystic mass known as a meningomyelocele. Most such lesions occur in the lumbar spine area, but they may occur at any point in the spinal cord. They are slightly more common in the cervical area than in the thoracic spine. If a pure cord anomaly is present, the soft tissue mass is too small to be visualized, but a secondary bony deformity (absent lamina) and widening of the spinal canal will be demonstrable. Longitudinal sections will show widening at the involved level (Fig. 31-11)—but remember that the spine widens normally in the cervical area. A bend in the spine is often present at the level of deformity. The skin will be displaced over the spinal deformity. The widening is best seen on transverse sections, which should be performed at serial levels throughout the spine. A U-shaped deformity is seen (Fig. 31-11). In the lumbosacral area the spine bends forward normally, and lesions may be easily missed. One should be able to see a complete bony circle surrounding a normal spinal cord at all levels. At an affected level, the lamina are missing, and consequently the posterior border of the spinal canal will not be seen. However, if the fetus is not prone or supine, a decision about widening may be difficult. Putting the mother in a knee-elbow position or on her side may make the fetal spinal position more favorable.

FIGURE 31-11. Spina bifida. A. A longitudinal sonographic section of a normal spine has three components. The vertebral arches form two parallel series of echogenic dots. The width of the space between them widens slightly in the cervical and lumbar areas. In the center is another series of echogenic dots, which represents the spinous process. B. On transverse section a circle of echoes is formed in levels. C. Level of the bladder. D. Longitudinal section. In spina bifida the circle is incomplete with no posterior echo. The space between the arches is widened at the involved level and the spinous processes are absent. E. The spina bifida creates a U-shaped gap. F. A fluid-filled sac (a meningomyelocele) may be present.

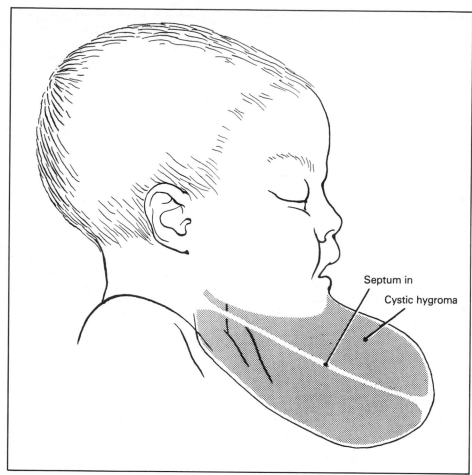

FIGURE 31-12. Diagram of typical location of a cystic hygroma. Septa are common.

Fetal Masses

Two mass lesions, teratoma and cystic hygroma, are common in utero.

TERATOMA

These tumors occur most often in the region anterior to the sacrum and are known as sacrococcygeal teratomas. They extend inferiorly beyond the spine and bladder. Although they may be cystic, many contain internal echoes with calcification and acoustic shadowing. Teratomas are possible in other locations, particularly around the head and neck.

CYSTIC HYGROMA (LYMPHANGIOMA)

Cystic hygromas usually occur anterior to the neck (Fig. 31-12). They are almost always fluid-filled, although occasionally they contain internal echoes. They can be very large, and septa are common. Polyhydramnios is usual with cystic hygromas.

PITFALLS

1. *Lumbosacral spina bifida.* Low lumbar spina bifida are easily missed because the spine normally bends forward at this point. Only transverse views show the abnormality.
2. *Neck area.* The neck area is confusing. One can get the impression of a tumorous mass in this area from normal structures.
3. *Microcephalus.* Microcephalus can be missed if a head-to-trunk ratio and femoral length are not performed as well as the biparietal diameter.
4. *Femoral length.* Apparent dwarfism can be created if the sonographer is not meticulous about making sure that the longest bone length views are obtained.
5. *Adrenal glands versus kidney.* The fetal adrenal glands have been mistaken for kidneys in cases of renal agenesis. Make absolutely sure that you can see a central echogenic sinus if renal agenesis is a possibility.
6. *Gut versus kidney.* Do not mistake gut dilatation for a renal cystic anomaly. Renal problems lie in contact with the spine, whereas gut problems lie at a more anterior level.
7. *Gut distention.* Do not mistake normal loops of bowel for pathologically dilated bowel. On some occasions the fetal bowel can reach a size of approximately 4 mm and yet not be pathologically enlarged. An examination on another day will probably show that the fluid-filled loops have disappeared.
8. *Pseudohydronephrosis due to distended bladder.* If the bladder is large, secondary dilatation of the pelvicalyceal system in the kidneys can occur transiently. This dilatation disappears when the fetus voids.

SELECTED READING

Athey, P. A., and Hadlock, F. P. *Ultrasound in Obstetrics and Gynecology.* St. Louis: Mosby, 1981.

Callen, P. W. (Ed.). *Ultrasonography in Obstetrics and Gynecology.* Philadelphia: Saunders, 1983.

Sanders, R. C., and James, A. E. (Eds.). *The Principles and Practice of Ultrasonography in Obstetrics and Gynecology.* New York: Appleton-Century-Crofts, 1980.

32. ADRENALS

IRMA L. WHEELOCK

SONOGRAM ABBREVIATIONS

Ad   Adrenal gland
Ao   Aorta

Ca   Celiac artery
Cr   Crus

D   Diaphragm

IVC   Inferior vena cava

K   Kidney

L   Liver
LRa   Left renal artery
LRv   Left renal vein

Pv   Portal vein

RRa   Right renal artery
RRv   Right renal vein

S   Spine
SMa   Superior mesenteric artery
Sp   Spleen
Spv   Splenic vein
St   Stomach

KEY WORDS

Adenoma. Tumor of the adrenal cortex that causes Cushing's syndrome; may be bilateral.

Cortex. Portion of adrenal tissue that secretes steroid hormones.

Cushing's Syndrome. Caused by hypersecretion of hormones from the adrenal cortex. An adrenal tumor or excess stimulation of the pituitary may be responsible.

Hyperplasia. Enlargement of adrenal glands.

Medulla. Central tissue of adrenal glands. It is under the control of the sympathetic nervous system.

Neuroblastoma. Malignant adrenal mass occurring in children.

Pheochromocytoma. Adrenal tumor that secretes hormones that elevate blood pressure.

THE CLINICAL PROBLEM

The adrenal glands are not easy to detect by ultrasound because they are small (4 × 2.5 × 0.5 cm) and have an acoustic structure that is similar to the surrounding fat. The left adrenal is partially surrounded by stomach and bowel, adding to the difficulty in imaging the gland. Children and small adults can be successfully examined, but in larger patients, the normal gland is usually difficult to visualize although masses may be detected. Adrenal pathology such as pheochromocytoma is usually suggested by laboratory studies. Ultrasound can help by detecting enlargement of the gland and in deciding whether one or both glands are enlarged.

Metastatic lesions from lung cancer to the adrenal are common and usually of little clinical significance.

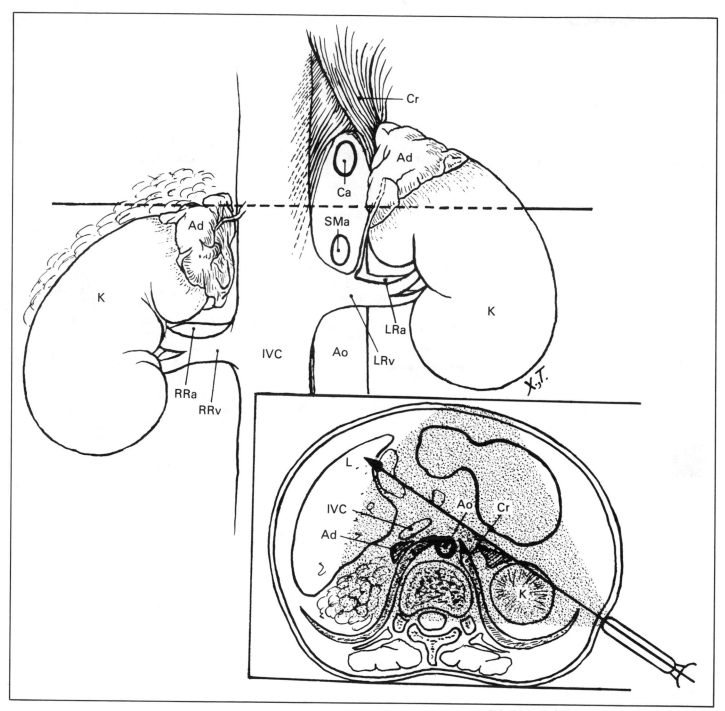

FIGURE 32-1. Adrenal glands. A. The adrenals are triangular glands located superior and antero-medial to the kidneys. B. The arrow shows the transducer angle used to show the left adrenal gland.

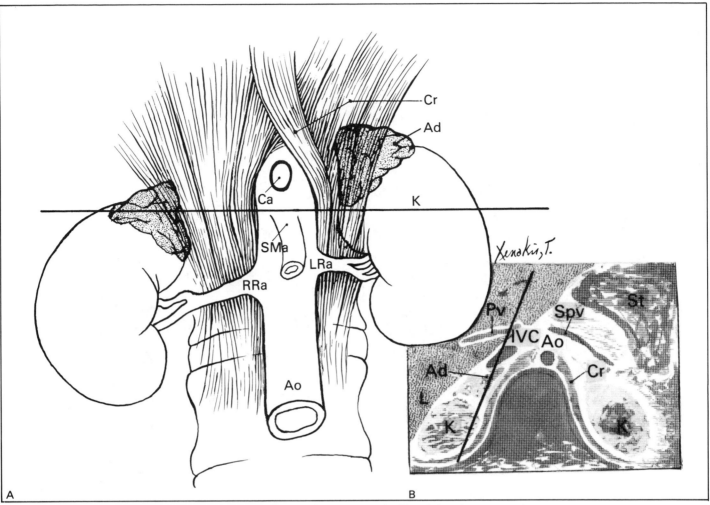

FIGURE 32-2. Right adrenal. A. The right adrenal lies posterior to the inferior vena cava and lateral to the crus of the diaphragm. B. Transverse view showing the appropriate transducer angle needed to show the right adrenal through the inferior vena cava.

ANATOMY

Both glands are normally triangular in shape (Fig. 32-1). They are located superior and antero-medial to the upper pole of the kidneys. The right gland lies posterior to the inferior vena cava and anterior to the crus of the diaphragm (Fig. 32-2). The left gland lies between the spleen, the upper pole of the kidney, and the aorta and behind the tail of the pancreas.

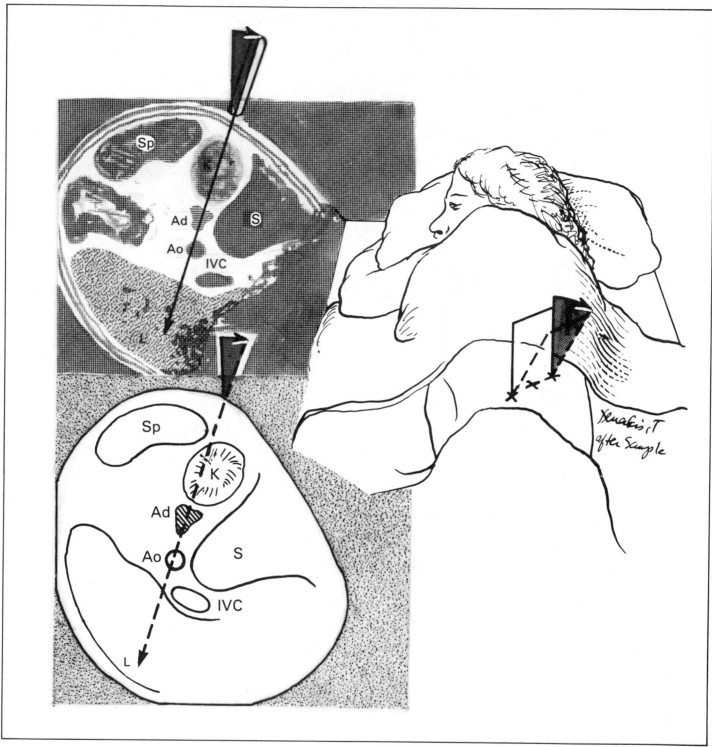

FIGURE 32-3. Technique used to show the left adrenal. Scanning transversely, show the aorta through the left kidney at three levels, marking the patient's skin. Align the scanning arm in a longitudinal axis to these marks, making sure to employ the same posterior-to-anterior angle.

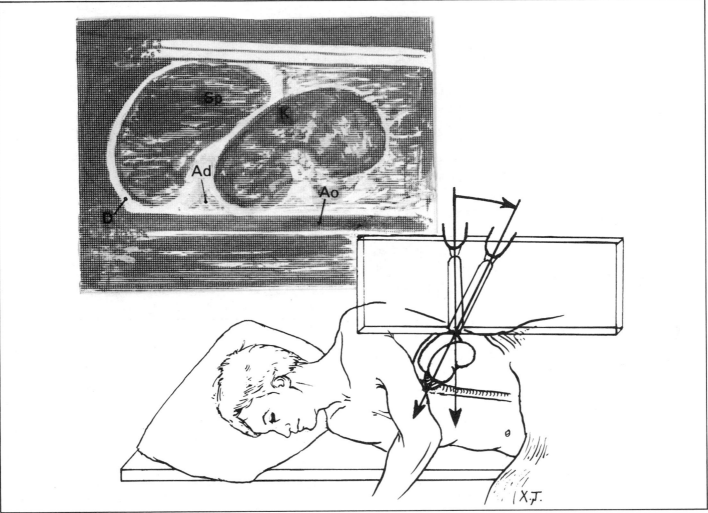

FIGURE 32-4. The resulting longitudinal section should show the adrenal at the junction of the spleen, aorta, and upper pole of the left kidney.

TECHNIQUE

Left Adrenal Gland

The left adrenal is best approached with the patient in the right lateral decubitus (left side up) position (Fig. 32-4). Longitudinal views are most helpful, but alignment must initially be determined in the transverse plane.

1. A 3.5-MHz medium focus transducer is usually satisfactory, but in thinner people a 5-MHz transducer can be used. You may wish to make adjustments in the gain setting depending on the texture of the spleen and the left kidney.

2. Start scanning transversely to show the aorta through the left kidney (Fig. 32-3). Mark the patient's skin with a grease pencil. Pay meticulous attention to the posterior-anterior angulation because this angle must be reproduced for the longitudinal approach. Repeat this step three times to obtain the long axis of the kidney.

3. Now change the scanning arm to the longitudinal position following the previously marked sites on the patient's skin.

4. Reproduce the posterior-to-anterior angulation needed to visualize the aorta through the kidney and spleen.

5. The left adrenal should appear as a triangular area where the spleen, upper pole of the left kidney, and the aorta meet. The normal gland will have concave or straight margins.

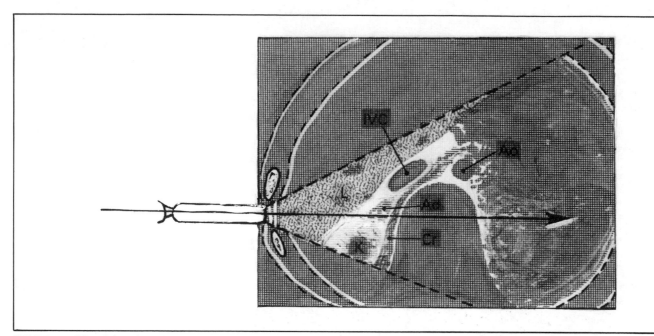

FIGURE 32-5. The right adrenal is most effectively imaged by scanning perpendicular to the right margin of the spine in an area bounded by the inferior vena cava, medial margin of the liver, and crus of the diaphragm.

Right Adrenal Gland

The right adrenal can usually be imaged in the traditional transverse and longitudinal views with the patient supine, using the liver as an acoustic window. If this is unsuccessful because of liver size or position, you may use the technique described for the left adrenal.

1. Initiate scanning transversely from the right side of the patient perpendicular to the medial borders of the liver and kidney and the right margin of the spine in an oblique axis (Fig. 32-5).
2. Enlarge the field size (usually 2 times or to a 20-cm field of view) to see small structures.
3. Select the highest frequency transducer possible for adequate penetration. Fine resolution is important, but you must be able to penetrate the liver well.
4. Adjust the gain or output controls so that there is uniform liver texture throughout the field.

5. Start scanning transversely in the region of the mid to upper pole of the kidney. Continuing in small increments superiorly, identify the pertinent normal anatomy (kidney, liver, crus of the diaphragm). The adrenal should become apparent just superior to the right kidney.
6. Try to confirm the presence or absence of pathology with longitudinal images. (The transverse scans will probably be more helpful.)
   a. Longitudinal sections angling slightly laterally to show an enlarged adrenal behind the inferior vena cava usually succeed (**Figs. 32-6 and 32-2**).
   b. Longitudinal sections with medial angulation (approximately 30°) aligning the right kidney and aorta may show the adrenal superior to the kidney. This technique is similar to that described for the left adrenal.

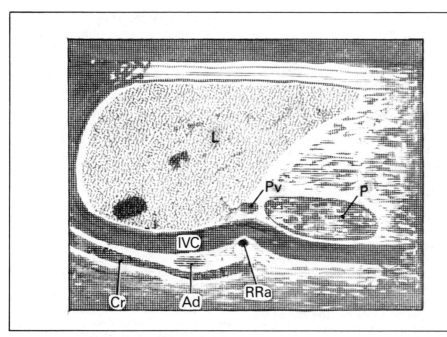

FIGURE 32-6. The right adrenal can be imaged longitudinally by using a lateral angulation through the inferior vena cava.

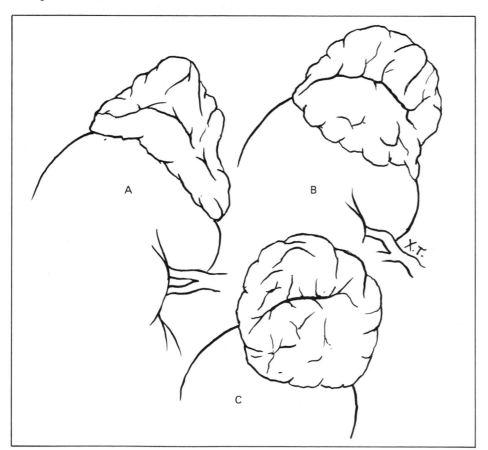

FIGURE 32-7. Progressive signs of adrenal enlargement are A, normal concave margins, B, convex margins of the slightly enlarged gland, and C, the larger the gland, the more rounded the contour.

PATHOLOGY

Early Signs of Adrenal Enlargement

The early signs of adrenal enlargement are

1. The normally concave margins become convex with masses.
2. The larger the gland, the more rounded the outline becomes (Fig. 32-7A–C).

Changes in Position of Adjacent Organs

The changes in position of adjacent organs may assist the sonographer in locating the organ of origin when a large mass is identified.

1. On the *right* are found
   a. The retroperitoneal fat line. Anterior displacement of the fat line that lies in front of the kidneys, adrenal, and behind the liver.
   b. Anterior displacement of the inferior vena cava by the mass.
   c. Postero-inferior displacement of the kidney.
   d. Draping of the right renal vein over the mass.
2. On the *left* are
   a. Anterior displacement of the splenic vein.
   b. Postero-inferior displacement of the kidney.

Causes of Enlargement

The possible causes of enlargement are

1. *Adenoma.* Smooth, rounded, homogeneous masses.
2. *Carcinoma.* Predominantly solid, irregular masses that may grow quite large.
3. *Cysts.* Must be distinguished from renal, pancreatic, or splenic cysts.
4. *Hemorrhage.* Seen in premature infants. The appearance will vary depending on the time elapsed since the bleed. A "fresh" bleed will appear echogenic, developing sonolucent areas after a few days. Later the borders may become calcified, causing a mass with very echogenic borders and perhaps shadowing (Chapter 14).
5. *Metastases.* Relatively common, usually arising from lung carcinoma. They vary in size and echogenicity. These masses may be very large (± 7 cm).
6. *Neuroblastoma.* A malignant adrenal mass seen in children. See Chapter 14.
7. *Pheochromocytoma.* A mass that causes uncontrollable hypertension, usually evenly echogenic. These masses may occur in locations other than the adrenal glands.

PITFALLS

1. Mimics of right adrenal
   a. *Liver metastases* may be mistaken for adrenal pathology. Note the position of the retroperitoneal fat line, which is displaced posteriorly by liver pathology.
   b. A *medially located right kidney.* Occasionally an enlarged liver may displace the right kidney medially, making it appear to be a mass displacing the inferior vena cava anteriorly on the longitudinal projection. Transverse views should make the position of the kidney apparent.
   c. The *crus of the diaphragm* may be misread as a normal adrenal. The crus is a tubular structure that lies medial to the adrenal location.
2. Mimics of left adrenal
   On the left many structures converge in the vicinity of the adrenal. The *esophagogastric junction,* the *tail of the pancreas, splenic vessels,* the *stomach,* and *lobulations of the spleen or kidney* can all mimic the adrenal. Always identify or rule out a normal structure before deciding that adrenal pathology is present.

WHERE ELSE TO LOOK

1. If adenocarcinoma is found, examine the liver for possible metastatic lesions.
2. Some adrenal masses produce biochemical and clinical findings that are similar to ovarian masses, particularly in small children. If nothing is found in the adrenals, examine the ovaries.
3. If a metastatic lesion is found on one side, examine the opposite side thoroughly. Look for accompanying adenopathy.

SELECTED READING

Sample, W. F., and Sarti, D. A. Computed tomography and gray scale ultrasonography of the adrenal gland: A comparative study. *Radiology* 128:377–383, 1978.

Renal, Adrenal, Retroperitoneal and Scrotal Ultrasonography. In D. A. Sarti and W. F. Sample (Eds.), *Diagnostic Ultrasound Text and Cases.* Boston: Hall, 1980.

Yeh, H. C. Sonography of the adrenal glands: Normal glands and small masses. *A.J.R.* 135:1167-1177, 1980.

Yeh, H. C. Ultrasound and CT of the adrenals. *Semin. Ultrasound* 3:97, 1982.

33. NECK MASS

IRMA L. WHEELOCK
ROGER C. SANDERS

SONOGRAM ABBREVIATIONS

CCa   Common carotid artery

IJv   Internal jugular vein

PTh   Parathyroid gland

Th   Thyroid gland

KEY WORDS

Adenoma. Benign solid tumor of the thyroid.

Branchial Cleft Cyst. Congenital cystic mass located close to the angle of the mandible.

Cervical Adenopathy. Enlargement of lymph glands in the neck.

Cold Nodule. A region of the thyroid where radioisotope has not been taken up on a nuclear study. The area of decreased uptake usually corresponds to a palpable mass.

Goiter. Diffuse enlargement of the thyroid gland due to iodine deficiency.

Halo Effect. A sonolucent zone surrounding a mass in the thyroid that is usually found with an adenoma (a benign tumor) but is rarely seen with carcinoma.

Hashimoto's Disease. Inflammatory disease of the thyroid gland usually characterized by diffuse enlargement and altered acoustic texture.

Major Neurovascular Bundle. A tubular structure that includes the common carotid artery, jugular vein, and vagus nerve.

Minor Neurovascular Bundle. A tubular structure that contains the inferior thyroid artery and the recurrent laryngeal nerve.

Photon Deficient Area. See Cold Nodule (above).

Traumatic Pseudocyst. A fluid collection that is a response to damage to the salivary duct.

Thyroglossal Duct Cyst. A developmental fluid-filled space variably extending from the base of the tongue to the isthmus of the thyroid.

THE CLINICAL PROBLEM

Thyroid Mass

A cold nodule on a nuclear medicine study indicates a nonfunctioning area within the thyroid gland. Because all cysts and most malignancies do not take up isotope, an ultrasound study is then performed to differentiate a solid from a cystic lesion. Of the lesions that are detected by nuclear scan approximately 20% are cysts, 60% are benign, and 20% are malignant.

Medical management is influenced by the ultrasonic separation of cysts from solid lesions. The diagnosis of a cystic lesion is followed by either observation or aspiration of the cyst, whereas the management of a solid mass involves either surgery or thyroid medication. If follow-up ultrasound studies or clinical examinations show that the lesion continues to enlarge, in spite of administration of thyroid extract to suppress thyroid activity, surgery is recommended. If no increase in size occurs, a conservative clinical approach may be appropriate (thyroid carcinomas are slow-growing neoplasms).

A small parts scanner (8- to 10-MHz) is useful because its fine resolution will show whether there are multiple rather than single nodules present. Multiple nodules usually carry a benign prognosis.

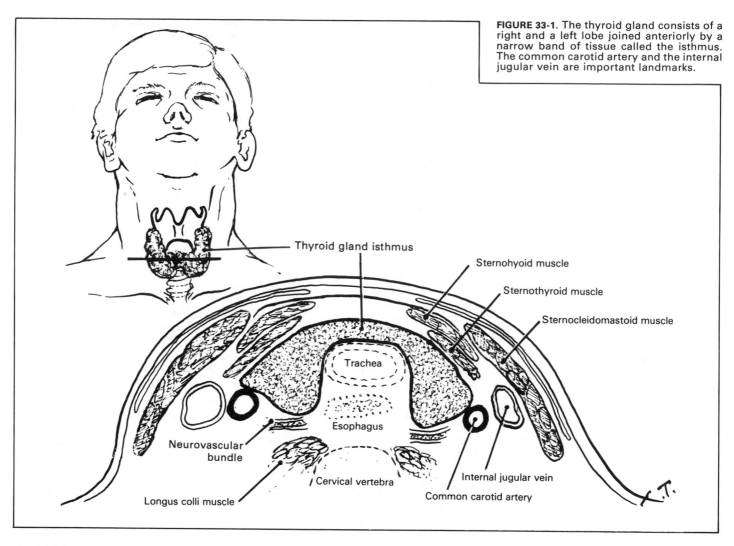

FIGURE 33-1. The thyroid gland consists of a right and a left lobe joined anteriorly by a narrow band of tissue called the isthmus. The common carotid artery and the internal jugular vein are important landmarks.

Thyroid gland isthmus

Sternohyoid muscle

Sternothyroid muscle

Sternocleidomastoid muscle

Trachea

Esophagus

Neurovascular bundle

Cervical vertebra

Internal jugular vein

Common carotid artery

Longus colli muscle

Parathyroid Mass

A persistently high blood calcium level may suggest a diagnosis of parathyroid adenoma or cancer even though the gland cannot be felt. Surgery is difficult in this area because of the small size of the abnormal gland and the overlying thyroid; thus surgery is greatly assisted by knowing which parathyroid gland or glands are enlarged.

Neck Mass

When a mass is found in the neck, the origin may not be obvious—that is, does it arise in the thyroid, nodes, or other structures adjacent to the thyroid? Masses in the region of the salivary glands can also be confusing. If the mass is extrathyroidal, a different spectrum of clinical possibilities such as nodes or abscesses must be considered. Two congenital anomalies, thyroglossal duct cyst and branchial cleft cyst, cause cystic masses outside the thyroid.

ANATOMY

Thyroid gland

The thyroid has two lobes connected anteriorly by a narrow bridge of tissue anterior to the trachea called the isthmus (Fig. 33-1). The common carotid artery and the internal jugular vein are important landmarks that lie posterior and lateral to the thyroid and define whether the mass is within the thyroid. These vessels should not be confused with cysts. The pyramidal lobe is a variant in which there is a superior extension of the thyroid from the isthmus. The "strap muscles" lie anterior to the lateral aspect of the thyroid.

Parathyroid glands

The four parathyroid glands lie posterior to the thyroid and usually adjacent to the carotid artery (Fig. 33-2), two on each side. The inferior gland lies at the lower border of the thyroid and may lie adjacent to the esophagus (Figs. 33-2, and 33-3). Other variant positions are within the thyroid gland and adjacent to the carotid lateral to the internal jugular vein (Fig. 33-3). The minor neurovascular bundle (a combination of the recurrent laryngeal nerve and the inferior thyroid artery) may be mistaken for the gland. The major neurovascular bundle (a combination of the common carotid artery, jugular vein, and vagus nerve) is usually a distinct structure. Parathyroid glands are normally less than 5 mm in size.

TECHNIQUE

Three competitive techniques exist for examining the thyroid and the structures around it.

Small Parts Scanner

The small parts scanner is a high-frequency real-time system using an 8- or 10-MHz transducer, which has a small field of view. This system allows the detection of many abnormal areas in the thyroid that cannot be seen with contact or water bath scanning techniques. Unfortunately, with this system it is difficult to document what is seen because the field of view is so small. Attempt to obtain an image that has some relevant associated part of the anatomy (e.g., the carotid) that provides a reference point. We perform additional static scans after a real-time small parts examination to show where the abnormality lies in reference to the surrounding anatomy.

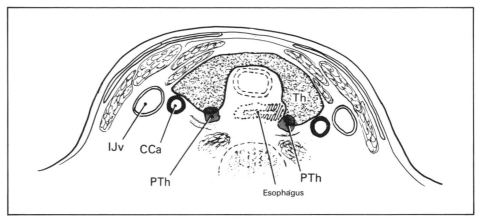

FIGURE 33-2. Four tiny parathyroid glands can be found posterior to the thyroid gland at its upper and lower poles. The esophagus often lies a little to the left. It can be mistaken for the parathyroid.

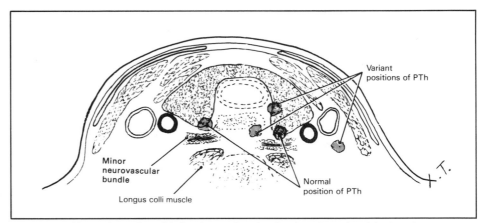

FIGURE 33-3. Normal parathyroid glands can develop in a number of variant locations. Locate the normal structures (minor neurovascular bundle and longus coli muscle) so that they will not be mistaken for parathyroid glands.

Contact Scanning or Water Bath Techniques

There are several factors common to both methods.

1. *Transducer choice.* The thyroid gland must fall within the focal range of the transducer. If the direct contact method is employed, a 5-MHz or higher *short* focus transducer would be appropriate. However, a 5-MHz or higher *medium* focus may be more suitable for the water bath technique because the distance between the transducer and the area of interest is increased.
2. *Patient position.* Place the patient supine with the head extended and a pillow or bolster under the shoulders. A pillow case or scarf around the patient's hair prevents water or oil contamination.
3. *Scanning technique.* Examine the patient before starting the procedure. If the mass is palpable, determine its location and approximate size. Also locate the mass by reviewing the nuclear medicine study.

    Scanning motions should be slow and deliberate. The gain curve should be nearly flat because the beam is passing through only a small amount of tissue that is very superficial.
4. *Image size.* The image should be enlarged as much as possible (preferably a 1 : 1 field size or a 10-cm field of view). Avoid zoom magnification because it degrades the image quality.
5. *Scan levels.* Starting slightly above the sternoclavicular junction (the sternal notch), scan at 5-mm increments through the gland (Fig. 33-4). Perform longitudinal scans along the longitudinal axis of the carotid artery (palpate to map it out). Obtain successive images at 5-mm intervals until the entire gland has been examined.

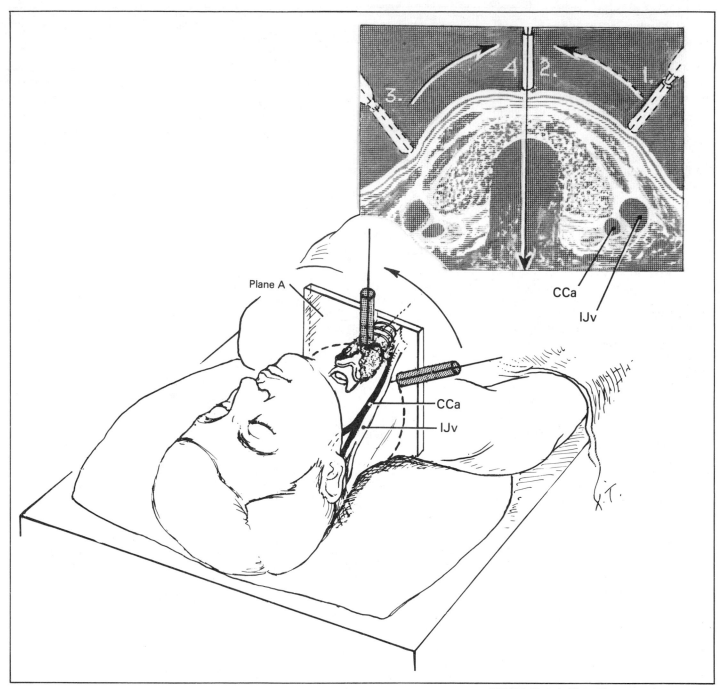

FIGURE 33-4. Initiate the scanning process transversely from lateral to medial on one side (1 to 2) then lateral to medial on the opposite side (3 to 4). The common carotid artery and the internal jugular vein should be demonstrated on each image.

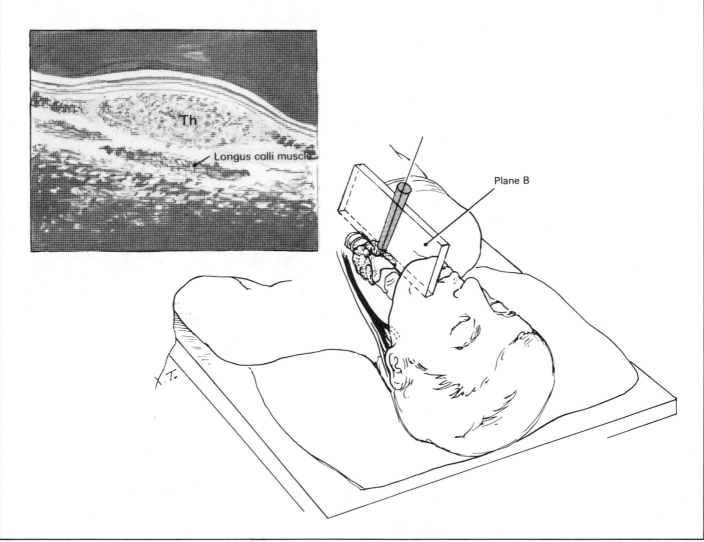

FIGURE 33-5. Longitudinal sections through the thyroid can best be obtained by using a 10° to 20° medial angle for maximum contact. Note the longus colli muscle posterior to the thyroid.

Direct Contact Technique

1. Apply acoustic couplant such as gel to the neck (gel dribbles less than mineral oil).
2. Set the approximate gain curve or output levels for visualizing the vessels and the homogeneous medium amplitude echoes of the normal thyroid.
3. Scan transversely (Fig. 33-4) in a lateral to medial fashion on one side. Stop at the midline and then scan lateral to medial on the opposite side. Care must be taken not to obliterate the texture of the isthmus, which may be very difficult to visualize. Proceed transversely in 5-mm increments through the gland.
4. Mark the site of any palpable mass with dots on the image so that the physician knows where it lies.
5. Follow with longitudinal scans at 5-mm intervals (Fig. 33-5). Locate the carotid artery on one side and scan medially. Usually a 10° to 20° medial angulation will allow good contact with the skin. Proceed in the same manner on the opposite side.

Water Bath Technique

This technique incorporates the use of a water interface between the transducer and the patient's skin, allowing placement of the focal zone of the transducer at the desired level. Difficulties encountered with this technique are reverberation artifacts due to the water bath membrane and difficulty in angling the transducer obliquely.

Any thin plastic bag or wide plastic wrap that can be supported on a frame can be utilized to contain the water bath (Fig. 33-6).

1. Apply couplant to the patient's neck.
2. Place the water bath over the patient's neck, allowing it to mold to the patient's skin.
3. Fill the water bath with water that has been allowed to settle to eliminate air bubbles, which hinder sound transmission.
4. Carefully smooth away air bubbles between the skin surface and the plastic material or creases in the plastic membrane.
5. Start scanning transversely in a lateral to medial fashion. The transducer tip should be just under the water surface. Do not submerge the transducer.
6. Use only enough water to permit the thyroid tissue to come within the focal range of the transducer—probably 3 to 6 cm.

PATHOLOGY

Intrathyroidal Masses

CYSTS

Thyroid cysts resemble those in other parts of the body except that their walls may be irregular and they may contain internal echoes (Fig. 33-7).

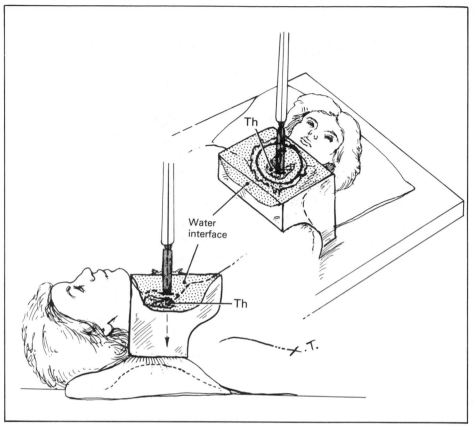

FIGURE 33-6. Both longitudinal and transverse images can be obtained by using a water bath technique. This technique is useful (1) if the neck contour is irregular or painful, making good contact impossible, or (2) to increase the distance between the transducer face and the gland so that the gland will fall within the focal range of the transducer.

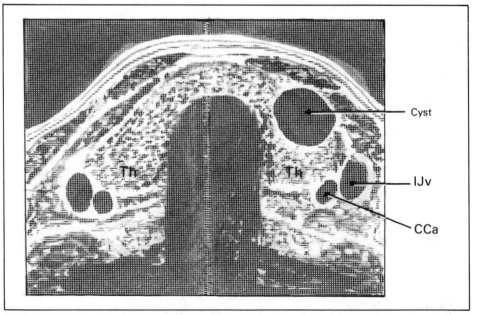

FIGURE 33-7. Thyroid cyst, showing the typical characteristics of smooth borders, lack of internal echoes, and increased through transmission.

ADENOMAS

The most common thyroid masses are adenomas. They have several sonographic manifestations. Typical appearances are (1) a halo of echopenic tissue surrounding a more echogenic mass (Fig. 33-8A), (2) a solid homogeneous mass with very few internal echoes that can easily be confused with a cyst, and (3) a densely echogenic lesion. Unlike carcinomas, adenomas are almost invariably multinodular.

CARCINOMAS

Carcinomas of the thyroid do not have any pathognomonic appearances, but suggestive features are (1) an irregular border (Fig. 33-8B), (2) both cystic and solid internal contents, (3) a single nodular lesion, and (4) adenopathy.

GOITERS

Goiters are a diffuse asymmetrical expansion of the thyroid with a coarse acoustic texture. Multiple nodules are present.

HASHIMOTO'S THYROIDITIS

In this inflammatory condition, there is diffuse mild enlargement of the thyroid with multiple nodules.

HEMORRHAGE

With hemorrhage there is sudden onset of pain with development of a mass associated with intrathyroidal clot. The clot appearances are similar to those in other parts of the body.

Extrathyroidal Masses

THYROGLOSSAL CYST

A thyroglossal cyst is an embryologic remnant. It has the typical appearance of a cyst and is found in the midline high in the neck.

BRANCHIAL CLEFT CYST

This congenital cyst is found lateral to the thyroid, usually at a higher level.

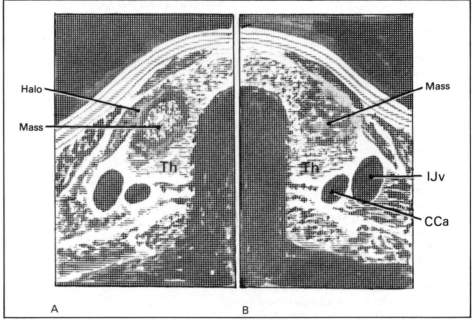

FIGURE 33-8. Thyroid masses. A. The "halo" effect, most often associated with an adenoma, is typified by an echogenic mass with an echo-free border. B. This solid thyroid mass, a carcinoma, contains echoes and exhibits little through transmission.

NODES

Lymph nodes occur quite commonly in the neck and can be difficult to distinguish clinically from the thyroid gland. They lie lateral to the major vessels.

ABSCESS

Abscesses may develop in the neck. They have the typical features of abscesses in other parts of the body.

CARCINOMATOUS INVASION

Carcinoma (e.g., of the tongue) may invade the neck; the extent of the tumor can be seen with ultrasound.

PARATHYROID ENLARGEMENT

The parathyroids are difficult to distinguish from an intrathyroidal mass; they appear as relatively sonolucent masses adjacent to the posterior aspect of the thyroid close to the carotid artery. If it is more than 5 mm in size, a parathyroid gland is abnormal.

PITFALLS

1. *Cyst versus solid lesion.* Small solid lesions may be difficult to distinguish from cysts. Solid lesions should fill with echoes more easily. Observe the through transmission.

2. *Identify the mass.* Small lesions may be displaced by the transducer with a direct scanning technique and may never actually be imaged. Therefore, try to use very light pressure on the neck while scanning to keep the mass under the transducer. If the mass is palpable, try to immobilize it with your fingers and scan over the area of interest.

3. *Isthmic mass.* An anterior mass may be overlooked because of the "main bang" artifact—reverberations and contact problems.

4. *Parathyroid adenoma.* This type of adenoma may be mimicked by

   a. The *minor neurovascular bundle.* This structure has a longitudinal axis, unlike the parathyroid (Fig. 33-3).

   b. The *left lateral border of the esophagus.* Giving the patient something to drink will show that the lesion is not really the parathyroid (Fig. 33-2).

   c. The *longus coli muscle.* This muscle will be seen on both sides of the neck.

   d. It may be impossible to distinguish an *intrathyroidal adenoma* from a parathyroid enlargement (Fig. 33-3).

WHERE ELSE TO LOOK

If a mass is shown to lie outside the thyroid, consider the possibility that it represents an enlarged lymph node, and look for adenopathy in the abdomen.

SELECTED READING

Austin, C. W. Ultrasound evaluation of thyroid and parathyroid disease. *Semin. Ultrasound* 3:250, 1982.

Barton, T. B. The thyroid gland: A review for sonographers. *Med. Ultrasound* 4:127–134, 1980.

Cole-Beuglet, C. Ultrasonography of thyroid and neck masses. In D. A. Sarti and W. F. Sample (Eds.), *Diagnostic Ultrasound Text and Cases.* Boston: Hall, 1980.

Simeone, J. F., Meuller, P. R., Ferrucci, J. T., Jr., et al. High resolution real-time sonography of the parathyroid. *Radiology* 141:745, 1981.

Wicks, J. D., Ball, W., Mettler, F. A., et al. The ultrasonic spectrum of the "cold" thyroid nodule. *Med. Ultrasound* 5:4, 1981.

34. POSSIBLE CAROTID ARTERY PLAQUE

ROGER C. SANDERS
IRMA L. WHEELOCK

KEY WORDS

Atheroma. Abnormal tissue laid down on the inner wall of arteries such as the aorta.

Bruit. A buzzing sound heard over the carotid artery, usually indicating arterial narrowing.

Ectasia. Tortuosity and enlargement of the carotid artery.

Emboli. Fragments of plaque responsible for transient ischemic attacks.

Intima. Arterial walls have three components—adventia, media, and intima; the intima is the innermost segment.

Plaque. A localized area of atheroma on the borders of the carotid artery. Such a plaque may be ulcerated, giving rise to emboli composed of blood clot and platelets, which are conveyed into the brain.

Stroke. Neurologic state due to brain infarct or hemorrhage; usually there is paralysis of some part of the body.

Transient Ischemic Attack (TIA). A brief period (less than 24 hours) of unconsciousness or other abnormal neurologic state, for example, paralysis. Evaluation is of great importance because TIA often precedes a stroke. Such patients usually require carotid artery surgery.

THE CLINICAL PROBLEM

Patients in whom a stroke is likely to occur owing to narrowing of the carotid artery are treated surgically. Investigation of such cases is difficult because the most accurate method of detecting whether a plaque is present is a carotid arteriogram, which carries serious potential hazards. Ultrasound can noninvasively assess the regularity of the lumen of the carotid artery and show whether plaques are present. Flow can be to some extent quantitated by the use of concurrent Doppler.

In some patients a carotid artery aneurysm may be clinically suspected. The pulsatile mass usually turns out to be a very tortuous subclavian artery, which rises above the clavicle to an abnormal position.

ANATOMY

The carotid arteries can be traced (Fig. 34-1) from a point just above the clavicle toward the skull. At approximately the angle of the jaw the common carotid artery bifurcates into the internal and external carotid arteries. The internal carotid artery lies posterior and lateral to the external carotid. The external carotid has several small extracranial branches near the angle of the jaw, whereas the internal carotid has none. Usually the carotid vessels cannot be followed with ultrasound more than 2 to 3 cm above the bifurcation.

TECHNIQUE

1. A high-frequency real-time scanner should be used (e.g., 5- or 7-MHz linear array).
2. The artery is traced on a transverse axis from the clavicle moving superiorly, taking sections at approximately 1-cm intervals. When the bifurcation is discovered, try to obtain views of both vessels together, tracing them as far superiorly as you can.
3. Repeat these sections on a longitudinal axis, documenting the entire length of the common carotid artery up to the site of the bifurcation. At that level, attempt to obtain views that show both the external and internal carotids simultaneously.
4. Angling the patient's jaw medially away from the transducer can help; the transducer often has to be angled from a steep lateral approach to show the bifurcation.
5. Be sure to label the images very carefully so that the two arteries can be distinguished at a later review. Ideally, a physician should be present at this examination because it is so difficult to recognize structures at a later date.
6. The use of simultaneous Doppler is of value because typical sounds are heard over the common internal and external carotids. Usually Doppler will establish that the vessel is completely occluded, which may otherwise be difficult to determine.

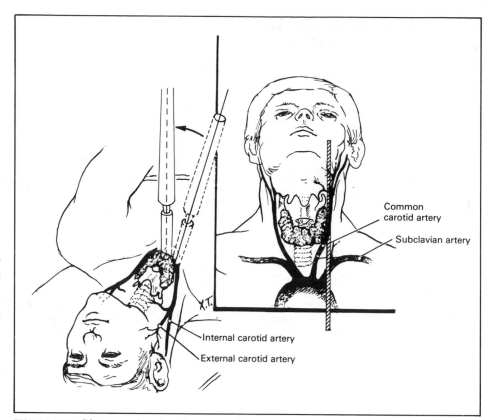

Common carotid artery

Subclavian artery

Internal carotid artery

External carotid artery

FIGURE 34-1. Diagram showing the normal arteries in the neck with the appropriate transducer angulation.

PATHOLOGY

Atheromatous Plaques

Atheromatous plaques (Fig. 34-2A,B) are irregular echogenic areas that impinge on the normally smooth border of the carotid artery. They are echogenic and may be associated with acoustic shadowing. An attempt to estimate the amount of carotid artery narrowing by the plaque should be made. Show its location in relation to the bifurcation of the common carotid.

Aneurysm

An aneurysm is a widening of the carotid artery similar to that seen in the abdomen and is sometimes associated with intraluminal clot.

Glomus Tumor

A rare, highly vascular tumor located at the bifurcation, a glomus tumor will pulsate on real-time but will show the features of a mass lesion.

PITFALLS

1. Do not mistake the intima of the normal carotid artery wall for plaque. With high-quality imaging systems, a narrow line can be seen to border the carotid lumen.
2. Total occlusion of the internal carotid artery may be missed if absence of pulsation within the vessel is not noted.

SELECTED READING

Blasberg, D. J. Duplex sonography for carotid artery disease: An accurate technique. *AJNR* 3:609–614, 1982.

Wolverson, M. K., Heilberg, E., Sundaram, M., et al. Carotid atherosclerosis: High-resolution real-time sonography correlated with angiography. *AJNR* 3:601-607, 1982.

Zwiebel, W. J. (Ed.). *Introduction to Vascular Ultrasonography.* New York: Grune & Stratton, 1982.

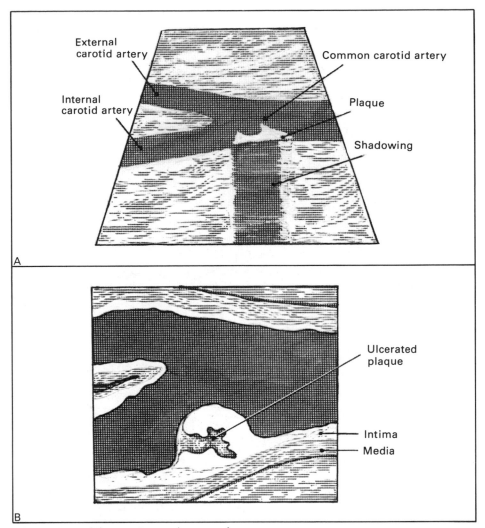

FIGURE 34-2. Atheromatous plaques. A. Sonogram of a partially calcified carotid artery plaque. Shadowing is seen behind the calcified segment. B. Diagram showing the pathologic appearance of an ulcerated atheromatous plaque.

35. BREAST

KEY WORDS

Areola. Brown area around the nipple.

Cooper's Suspensory Ligaments. Fibrous strands forming a lobular network within the breast.

Cystosarcoma Phylloides (Giant Myxoma). Huge mass similar in nature to a fibroadenoma; occasionally can be malignant.

Fibroadenoma. Benign mobile breast mass seen in young women; commonly called a "breast mouse."

Galactocele. Milk collection within the breast.

Galactorrhea. Milky discharge from nipple not associated with pregnancy.

Invasive Ductal Carcinoma (Squamous Cell Carcinoma). Most common neoplasm in the breast. It has a distinctive ultrasonic pattern.

Medullary Cancer. Unusual type of breast cancer that has a sonographic appearance resembling a fibroadenoma.

Sclerosing Adenosis. Benign condition affecting much of the glandular portion of the breast; occurs in menstruating women.

Fibrocystic Disease. Multiple small cysts with fibrosis are common in young women. This condition is benign but is not necessarily easy to distinguish clinically from carcinoma.

THE CLINICAL PROBLEM

Ultrasound has recently been shown to be almost the equal of mammography in the investigation of breast masses. Any palpable mass can be accurately categorized as cystic or solid, and, to some extent, benign solid masses can be separated from malignant. Ultrasound is of particular value in (1) examining young glandular breasts for which mammography is less valuable, (2) confirming the presence of a possible mass found by palpation or seen on mammography, and (3) separating cysts from solid lesions. Ultrasound is also a valuable follow-up examination for patients who are at risk for breast cancer, such as those with a maternal family history of breast cancer or a previous cancer in the other breast.

ANATOMY

The breast undergoes fatty replacement with age, and after the menopause the breast is virtually all fat. This type of breast is not easy to examine with ultrasound, in contrast to mammography. On the other hand, in the menstruating woman, the breast consists of a large, central glandular element with a small fatty component in a subcutaneous location. These patients are easy to examine ultrasonically but difficult on mammography.

Quite a bit of anatomic information can be obtained with ultrasound. Some of the ducts leading to the breast can be visualized. The rib cage and muscles beneath the breast are visible. Cooper's ligaments (fibrous strands) are sometimes delineated by fat (Fig. 35-1).

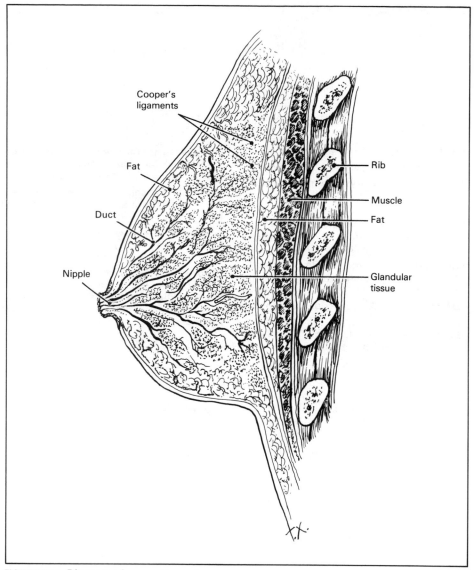

FIGURE 35-1. Diagram of normal breast structures visible on a sonogram.

TECHNIQUE

Numerous competing techniques are available for ultrasonic breast examination. None has yet clearly demonstrated its superiority. Prior to any breast ultrasonic examination, examine the breasts to get a clear idea where the mass is and obtain a clinical history. Enquire about the rapidity of onset, any recent pregnancy, where the lesion is painful, and whether there has been any nipple discharge.

Contact Scanning

The breast mass is located and fixed between the fingers. Single pass scans are performed using a high-frequency transducer. This type of examination is usually limited to a study of a specific mass.

Water Bath

A water bath is draped over the breast so that the mass is immobilized beneath the water bath. Serial sections are performed at 0.5-cm intervals using a contact scanner or, taking care not to damage the transducer by water, a real-time scanner. This technique has the virtue of immobilizing the breast but makes a secondary sign of malignancy, skin thickening, difficult to assess.

Linear Array Real-Time

A linear array real-time system with a 3.5- or 5-MHz transducer can also be used. A clockwise approach is employed, using the nipple as a reference point (Fig. 35-2). A high-frequency transducer is desirable to obtain detailed views of the mass. The mass is palpated and fixed between the fingers while the patient is examined. The erect position helps to immobilize large breasts.

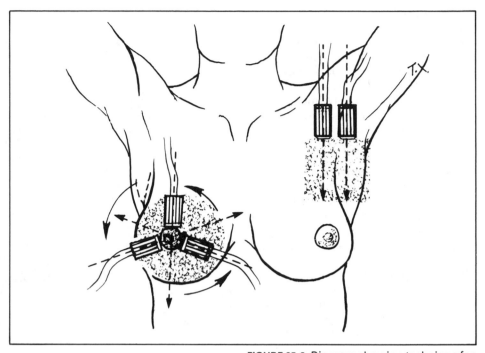

FIGURE 35-2. Diagram showing technique for examining the breast with real-time using a clockwise approach for the breast and parallel views for the axilla.

Automated Scanning

Several expensive automated scanners exist. The woman lowers her breast into a water bath. An automated transducer scans from below. These systems suffer from the disadvantage that the site of the possible lesion is not accurately known at the time the study is interpreted because it cannot be simultaneously palpated, but they do not require as skilled an operator and are quite rapid. Accuracy rates are no better with this technique than with cheaper systems. Skin thickening is well seen, and a global view of the breast is obtained, so it is simpler to follow breast appearances on consecutive examinations with these systems rather than with real-time or contact scanning.

PATHOLOGY

Cysts

Cysts are common in menstruating women and may resemble a solid mass on mammography. They have the sonographic features of cysts elsewhere in the body (i.e., relatively smooth walls, good through transmission, and a relative absence of internal echoes).

Fibroadenomas

These masses are usually ovoid in shape with poor through transmission, even internal echoes, and a regular border (Fig. 35-3). Cystosarcoma phylloides, another benign lesion, has a similar appearance, but the mass is much larger.

Ductal Carcinoma

These carcinomas lead to an increase in duct size. Dilated ducts can be traced to the site of the mass. However, the mass itself may be quite small (Fig. 35-4).

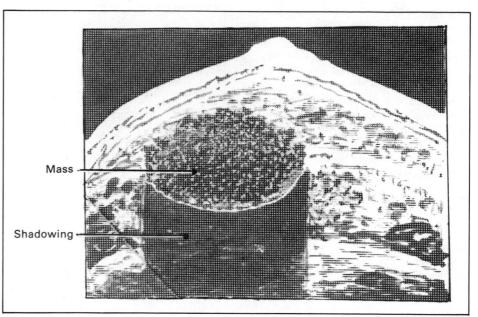

FIGURE 35-3. Relatively smooth bordered mass with a few internal echoes and some shadowing—fibroadenoma.

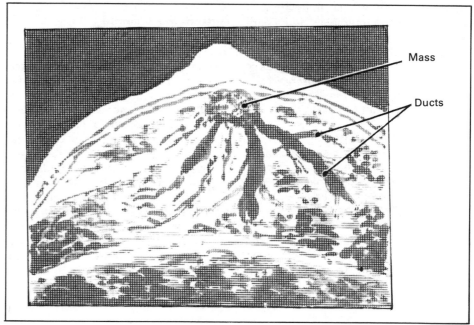

FIGURE 35-4. Ductal carcinoma with dilated ducts distal to a relatively small mass.

Invasive Ductal Carcinoma (Squamous Carcinoma)

These masses are acoustically absorbent and show very poor through transmission. They have a ragged border and an irregular internal echo pattern (Fig. 35-5). Secondary signs of malignancy can be seen, including skin thickening and retraction.

Medullary Carcinoma

This mass is hard to separate from a fibroadenoma, but it is said that there are a few more internal echoes and a slightly more irregular border.

Abscesses

Abscesses are fluid-filled but may contain some internal echoes. They have a well-defined border, which is thick and irregular, and tend to occur in the periareolar area.

Fat Necrosis

Fat necrosis can be a close mimic of a cancer in the older patient; it has poor through transmission and a ragged border.

Galactoceles

This rare milk collection is seen as a poorly outlined, relatively echo-free area with a few internal echoes.

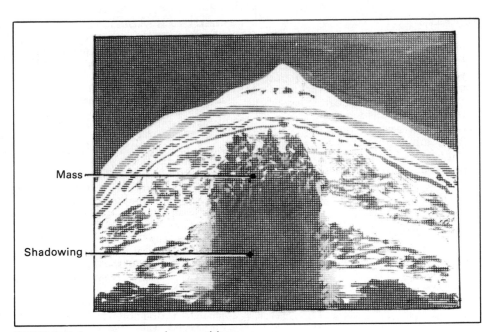

FIGURE 35-5. A squamous carcinoma with an irregular outline and acoustic shadowing.

PITFALLS

1. Large, floppy breasts are difficult to examine, and the mass may get lost if the breast is not immobilized by a water bath technique or examined in the erect position with real-time so that the breast tissue can be swept in front of the transducer.

2. Lactating breasts normally contain large tubular structures corresponding to milk-filled ducts.

3. Interpretation of a breast sonogram is difficult and requires considerable experience. Pseudolesions can be easily invented.

SELECTED READING

Coel-Beuglet, C., Goldberg, B. B., Kurtz, A. B., et al. Ultrasound mammography: A comparison with radiographic mammography. *Radiology* 139:693-698, 1981.

Croll, J., Kotevich, J., and Tabrett, M. The diagnosis of benign disease and the exclusion of malignancy in patients with breast symptoms. *Semin. Ultrasound* 3:38–50, 1982.

Kurtz, A. B., Rubin, C. S., and Goldberg, B. B. Ultrasound mammography. *Radiol. Clin. North Am.* 18:133–143, 1980.

Maturo, V. G., Zusmer, N. R., Gilson, A. J., et al. Ultrasonic appearance of mammary carcinoma with a dedicated whole-breast scanner. *Radiology* 142:713–718, 1982.

Picker, R. H., and Fulton, A. J. Maturational and physiological changes in the female breast. *Semin. Ultrasound* 3:34-37, 1982.

Schneck, C. D., and Lehman, D. A. Sonographic anatomy of the breast. *Semin. Ultrasound* 3:13–32, 1982.

Zusmer, N. R., Goddard, J., and Maturo, V. G. Automated water bath techniques for breast sonography. *Semin. Ultrasound* 3:63–71, 1982.

36. RULE OUT LOWER LIMB MASS AND BAKER'S CYST

Possible Popliteal Aneurysm

ROGER C. SANDERS

KEY WORDS

Baker's Cyst (Popliteal Cyst). Synovial fluid collection adjacent and posterior to the knee joint due to trauma or rheumatoid arthritis.

Deep Venous Thrombosis (DVT). Clot in the deep leg veins; causes swelling of the calf and thigh pain.

Popliteum. Area posterior to the knee joints.

Synovium. The lining of the joint. It produces the fluid that occupies the joint space and a Baker's cyst.

THE CLINICAL PROBLEM

Masses or collections in limbs are easy to demonstrate with ultrasound but usually do not cause much clinical confusion except when located near the knee joint. Baker's cysts are synovial fluid collections that develop posterior to the knee joint. They are common in people with rheumatoid arthritis and when they rupture can have the same clinical features as deep vein thrombosis. Popliteal artery aneurysms occur in the same location. Clinically, other confusing masses such as abscesses, hematomas, and tumors, recognizable by ultrasound, may occur around the knee joint or at any other site in the limbs (Fig. 36-1).

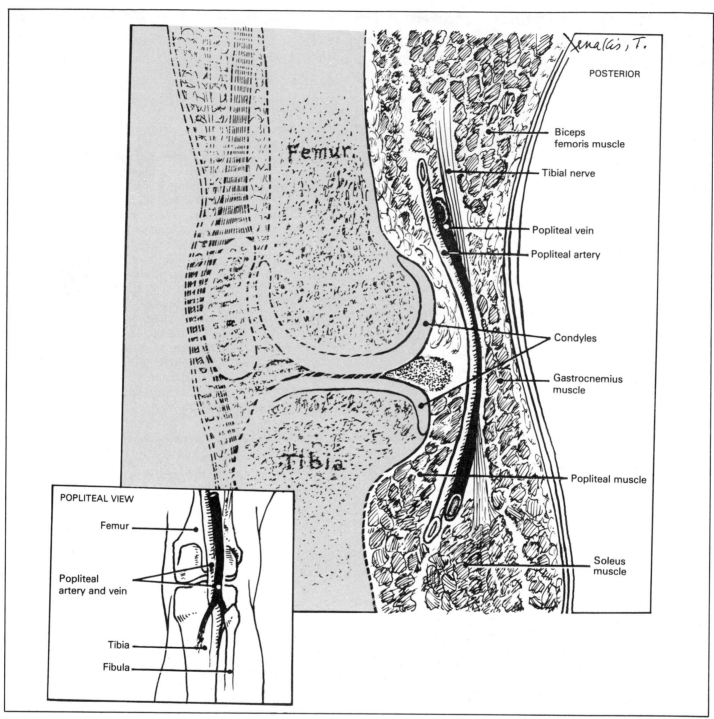

Xenakis, T.

POSTERIOR

Biceps femoris muscle

Tibial nerve

Popliteal vein

Popliteal artery

Femur

Condyles

Gastrocnemius muscle

Tibia

Popliteal muscle

Soleus muscle

POPLITEAL VIEW

Femur

Popliteal artery and vein

Tibia

Fibula

FIGURE 36-1. Diagram showing the normal structures visible in the popliteal fossa and the course of the popliteal artery and vein in relation to the knee joint.

ANATOMY

The popliteal artery runs posterior to the knee joint. The vein that runs alongside the artery may be visible. The bones around the knee joint can be recognized posterior to the artery. Groups of muscles are seen in the adjacent lower thigh and upper calf.

TECHNIQUE

Real-time should be used to determine the popliteal artery's long axis. A static scan along the axis as predetermined by real-time is valuable. The same procedure should be followed on the opposite extremity for comparison. The study is best performed with the patient prone and the knee slightly flexed so that fluid associated with the knee joint is not pinched back into the joint.

PATHOLOGY

Baker's Cyst

Baker's cyst is a fluid-filled collection posterior to the joint that may extend into the calf or, rarely, into the thigh. The collection may contain internal echoes and may have an irregular outline (Fig. 36-2).

Popliteal Aneurysm

A focal expansion of the popliteal artery, which shows pulsation on real-time and may contain clot, is a popliteal aneurysm. The walls may be partially calcified (Fig. 36-3).

Abscesses

Abscesses, tumors, and hematomas may occur in this area but have no specific features.

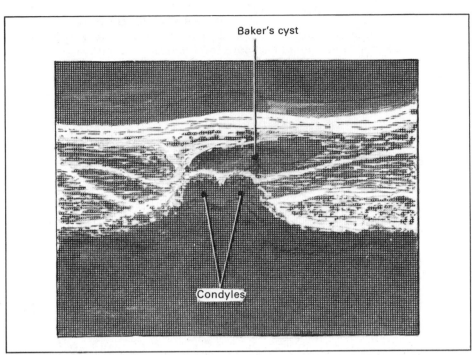

FIGURE 36-2. A Baker's cyst is a fluid-filled structure extending into the calf that usually communicates with the knee joint.

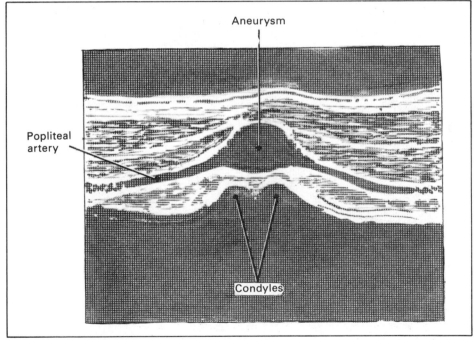

FIGURE 36-3. A popliteal artery aneurysm expands the popliteal artery posterior to the knee joint.

PITFALLS

Undue extension of the leg will obliterate a Baker's cyst that communicates with the knee joint because the fluid will return into the knee joint proper.

WHERE ELSE TO LOOK

If a popliteal aneurysm is found, the aorta and the opposite popliteal artery should be examined; abdominal aortic aneurysms are often present in association with popliteal artery aneurysms.

SELECTED READING

Bluth, E. I., Merritt, C. R. B., and Sullivan, M. A. Gray-scale ultrasound evaluation of the lower extremities. *J.A.M.A.* 247:3127–3129, 1982.

Braunstein, E. M., Silver, T. M., and Martel, W. Ultrasonographic diagnosis of extremity masses. *Skeletal Radiol.* 6:157–163, 1981.

Cooperberg, P. L., Tsang, I., Truelove, L., et al. Gray scale ultrasound in the evaluation of rheumatoid arthritis of the knee. *Radiology* 126:759–763, 1978.

Hermann, G., Yeh, H. C., Lehr-Janue, C., et al. Diagnosis of popliteal cyst: Double-contrast arthrography and sonography. *A.J.R.* 137:369–372, 1981.

Lenkey, J., Skolnick, M. L., Slasky, B.S., et al. Evaluation of the lower extremities. *J. Clin. Ultrasound* 9:413–416, 1981.

Yeh, H. C., and Rabinowitz, J. G. Ultrasonography of the extremities and pelvic girdle and correlation with computed tomography. *Radiology* 143:519–525, 1982.

37. POSSIBLE TESTICULAR MASS

ROGER C. SANDERS

SONOGRAM ABBREVIATIONS

AEp Appendix epididymis

E Endometrium

Ep Epididymis

MT Mediastinum testis

T Testis

KEY WORDS

Appendix Epididymis. Portion of the epididymis that lies in a superior location just above the testicle and is larger than the remainder of the epidiymis.

Epididymis. Organ that lies posterior to the testicle in which the spermatozoa accumulate.

Epididymitis. Inflammation of the epidiymis.

Hematocele. Blood filling the sac that surrounds the testicle.

Hydrocele. Distention of the sac that encloses the testicle by straw-colored fluid.

Mediastinum Testes. Linear fibrous structure in the center of the testicle.

Pampiniform Plexus. Group of veins that drain the testicle. They dilate and become tortuous when a varicocele is present.

Scrotum. Sac in which the testicle and epididymis lie.

Spermatic Cyst (Spermatocele). Cyst along the course of the vas deferens containing sperm.

Testicle (Testes). Male gonad enclosed within the scrotum; it produces hormones that induce masculine features and spermatozoa.

Varicocele. Dilated veins caused by obstruction of the venous return from the testicle. Varicoceles may be associated with infertility or tumor.

Vas Deferens. Tube that connects the epididymis to the seminal vesicle.

Seminal Vesicles. Reservoirs for sperm located posterior to the bladder.

Serous. Term used to describe the thin, straw-colored fluid present within a cyst regardless of location (e.g., renal, thyroid, or ovarian cysts or hydrocele).

Cryptorchidism (Undescended Testicle). Condition in which the testicles have not descended and lie either in the abdomen or in the groin. The latter is the site in 95% of cases. Such a testicle has an increased chance of becoming malignant.

THE CLINICAL PROBLEM

The testicle is superficial and therefore easily examined with high-frequency ultrasound. The detection of a small mass within the testicle is important because this is an early sign of malignancy. Although fluid within the scrotal sac is usually detected easily clinically, identification is difficult if the scrotal wall is thickened.

When the clinical differentiation of an epididymal from a testicular mass is difficult, the ultrasonic decision is simple, and the findings of epididymitis, whether acute or chronic, by sonography may be the first clue to the diagnosis of this condition.

ANATOMY

The testicle is an ovoid, homogeneous, mildly echogenic structure (Fig. 37-1A,B). A central line within it is termed the mediastinum testis. The linear tubular, slightly sonolucent structure posterior to the testes is the epididymis.

The epididymis expands focally and superiorly to form the appendix epididymis. The two testicles are normally symmetrical in size. The testicular artery and the veins of the pampiniform plexus run along the posterior aspect of the testicle in the region of the epididymis and are not normally visible.

TECHNIQUE

Although water bath scanning has been advocated by some, we feel that manual techniques are superior unless an automated system is used.

Contact Scanner

The testicle and the scrotum are supported by the examiner's hand or by a towel under the scrotum. Using a towel, the patient can retract the penis. The transducer is moved smoothly and slowly along the anterior aspect of the scrotum, first in the longitudinal axis and then in the transverse axis. This examination should be performed by two examiners or by the sonographer and a cooperative patient because satisfactory use of controls is difficult to attain when both hands are occupied with scanning and holding the testicle. Do not use a heavy towel or the testicle will be distorted. Use a 5- or 7-MHz transducer.

Small Parts Scanner

A small parts scanner is used in the same way as the contact scanner, wielding the instrument in one hand while supporting the testicle in the other.

Automated Scanners

With some automated scanners it is possible to suspend the testicles in the water bath and obtain automated scans.

FIGURE 37-1A,B. Diagram showing the normal structures visible within the scrotum. The mediastinum testes is only occasionally seen as an echogenic line.

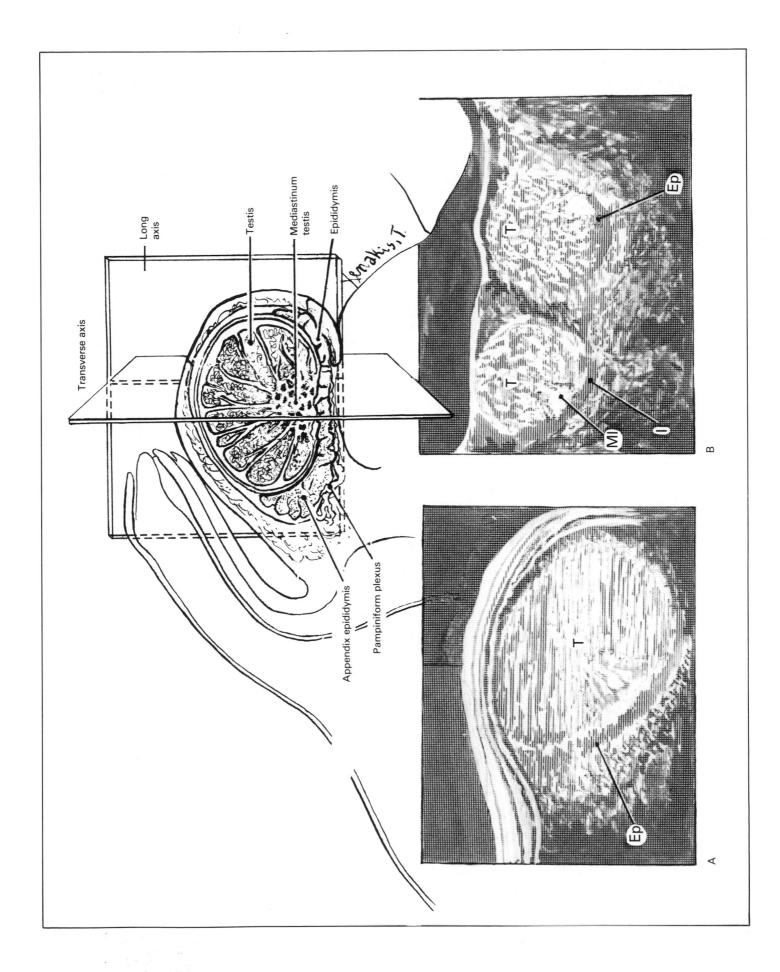

Long axis

Transverse axis

Testis

Mediastinum testis

Epididymis

Appendix epididymis

Pampiniform plexus

PATHOLOGY

Tumors

Normally, the testicle is evenly echo-genic. The most common testicular tumor, seminoma, is usually echopenic compared with the remaining testicular parenchyma. The tumor can be as small as 2 to 3 mm in size (Fig. 37-2). Teratomas and embryonal cell tumors are often patchily echogenic.

Epididymitis

ACUTE

The epididymis in acute epididymitis is enlarged and more sonolucent than usual.

CHRONIC

A chronically inflamed epididymis be-comes thickened and focally echogenic and may contain calcification (Fig. 37-3).

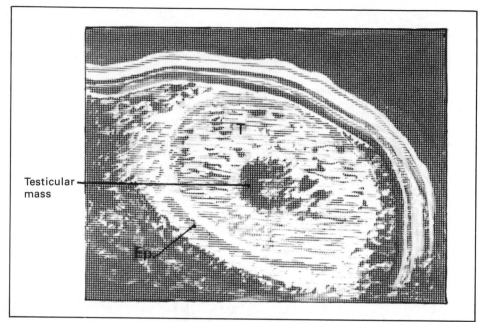

FIGURE 37-2. Intertesticular mass due to seminoma.

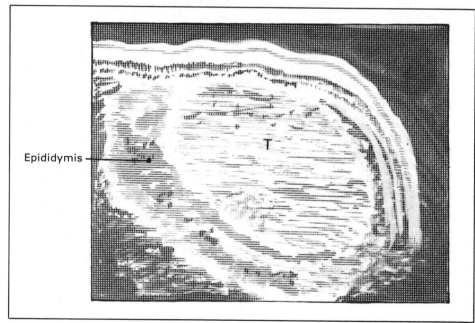

FIGURE 37-3. Enlargement and coarse echogenic texture of epidymis with chronic epididymitis.

Varicocele

Varicoceles are numerous tortuous curvilinear structures in the region of the epididymis and extending superiorly with respect to the testicle toward the pubic symphysis (Fig. 37-4).

Hydrocele

In hydrocele the testicle and the appendix epididymis are surrounded by fluid, which is usually sonolucent unless blood (hematocele) is present (Fig. 37-5).

Undescended Testicles

During the embryologic development of the genitourinary tract, the testicles descend from the region of the kidneys into a normal location. Arrested development may occur at any point. However, the usual "sticking point" occurs when the testicles are in the region of the inguinal ligament and pubic symphysis in an extra-abdominal location. At this site, undescended testicles can be visualized by ultrasound.

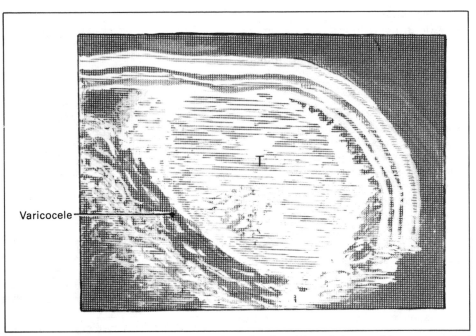

FIGURE 37-4. A varicocele can be seen to be pulsatile with real-time and is composed of numerous veins.

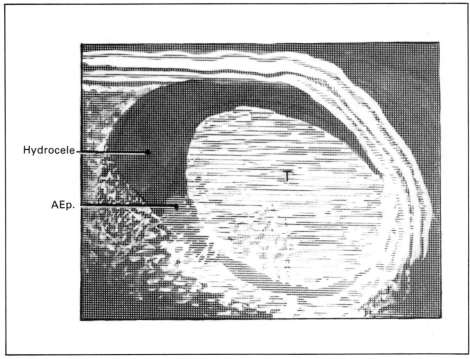

FIGURE 37-5. Hydrocele surrounding the testes.

Spermatocele

A cystic structure found along the course of the vas deferens superior to the testicle, a spermatocele is of little pathologic significance (Fig. 37-6). Epididymal cysts may be seen but are of no clinical significance.

Infarcted Testicle (Following Testicular Torsion)

The testicles are less echogenic than usual because the blood supply has been interrupted. The sonographic appearance may be indistinguishable from that of a sonolucent tumor occupying the entire organ. The clinical presentation is usually quite different. In the long run an infarcted testicle will become small and more echogenic.

Abscess

Abscesses may develop in the testicle or epididymis and are sonolucent with an echogenic irregular border.

PITFALLS

1. Scanning the testicle evenly and symmetrically can be difficult. Be sure that an apparent diminution in testicular size is not due to poor scanning technique.
2. Do not mistake the mediastinum testes for an echogenic mass.

WHERE ELSE TO LOOK

If a testicular tumor is found, look in the abdomen around the region of the renal hilum for possible nodal metastases.

SELECTED READING

Blei, L., Sihelnik, S., Blood, M. D., et al. Ultrasonographic analysis of chronic intratesticular pathology. *J. Ultrasound Med.* 2:17–23, 1983.

DiGiacinto, T. M., Patten, D., Willscher, M., et al. Sonography of the scrotum. *Med. Ultrasound* 6:95–101, 1982.

Madrazo, B. L., Klugo, R. C., and Parks, J. A. Ultrasonographic demonstration of undescended testes. *Radiology* 133:181–183, 1979.

Phillips, G. N., Schneider, M., Goodman, J. D., et al. Ultrasonic evaluation of the scrotum. *Urol. Radiol.* 1:157–163, 1980.

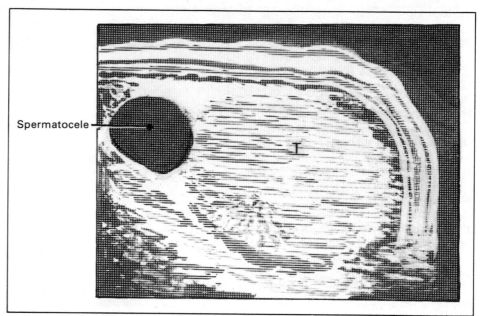

Spermatocele

FIGURE 37-6. Spermatocele lying superior to the testicle.

38. RULE OUT PLEURAL EFFUSION AND CHEST MASS

NANCY A. SMITH

SONOGRAM ABBREVIATIONS

Ao Aorta

D   Diaphragm

K   Kidney

L   Liver

S   Spine
Sp Spleen

KEY WORDS

Consolidation. An infected segment of the lung filled with fluid.

Empyema (Pyothorax). Pus in the pleural cavity.

Hemothorax. Blood in the pleural cavity.

Pneumothorax. Air within the pleural cavity outside the lung—a possible complication of thoracentesis.

Pleura. A serous membrane that lines the thorax and diaphragm and surrounds the lungs.

Pleural Cavity. The space between the layers of the pleura.

Pleural Fibrosis. Fibrous tissue thickening the pleura; results from chronic inflammatory diseases of the lungs such as tuberculosis.

Subpulmonic. A fluid collection located inferior to the lungs above the diaphragm.

Thoracentesis. Puncture of the chest to obtain pleural fluid.

THE CLINICAL PROBLEM

Ultrasound has a limited role in the chest because sound is not conducted by air. Its role is confined to the following conditions:

1. *Pleural effusion.* The presence of a pleural effusion can be confirmed and its site delineated. Pleural effusions are a nonspecific reaction to an underlying pulmonary or cardiac process or a systemic disease such as cirrhosis. Obtaining fluid for analysis may allow a more specific diagnosis. For details of technique, see Chapter 41.
2. *Pleural-based mass.* The nature of a mass that abuts the pleura can be determined (i.e., whether it is a loculated pleural effusion or a tumorous mass).
3. *Opaque hemithorax.* The nature of an opaque hemithorax on the chest radiograph can be determined. Such a "white lung" may indicate:
   a. Tumor
   b. Fluid
   c. Lung collapse
   d. A combination of the above

ANATOMY

Normal Chest

When no fluid or mass is present, the tissues within the chest do not conduct sound. There will be alternating bands of echogenicity due to reverberations from bone and echo-free areas due to air (Fig. 38-1).

Diaphragm

The diaphragm is seen as an echogenic line above the liver and spleen. The diaphragm is difficult to demonstrate, especially on the left, because it lies along virtually the same axis as the ultrasonic beam. The spleen provides less of a window to angle through than the liver.

TECHNIQUES

Upright Position

The patient is scanned upright sitting on a stool without a back, thus affording ready access from all sides (Fig. 38-1). A 3.5-MHz transducer with a 13-mm face usually has a low enough frequency to display the chest wall and a small enough face to be used between ribs.

Demonstration of Diaphragm

The diaphragm must be shown well. This can be difficult, especially on the left side where there is no liver to act as an acoustic window. Angling up through the liver and spleen helps to show the diaphragm. The spleen may be mistaken for an effusion if the diaphragm is not demonstrated. Showing the left kidney establishes the location of the spleen and diaphragm.

Pleural Effusion

Pleural effusions (Fig. 38-1) usually pool above the diaphragm along the posterior chest wall. It is sometimes necessary to scan along the axillary line to check for fluid laterally. Loculated effusions can be found in any location. Plan the search by examining the lateral chest radiograph.

Real-Time

Real-time, especially a linear array, is surprisingly successful in the chest and will show movement of a pleural effusion, confirming the presence of fluid.

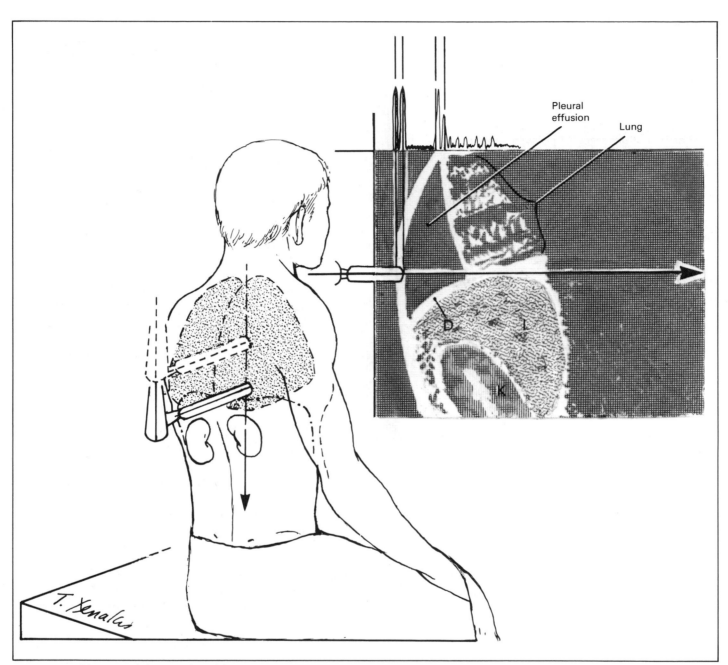

FIGURE 38-1. Diagram of the usual position used when scanning a pleural effusion. The ultrasonic appearance of a pleural effusion and lung are shown in the inset.

Supine Views

Right-sided pleural effusions can be easily assessed on a supine view looking through the diaphragm and liver (Fig. 38-2A,B). Effusions on the left are more difficult to see in the supine position but can sometimes be seen with an oblique scan through the spleen. The upright position is not necessary if no evidence of fluid shift is seen on a decubitus radiograph.

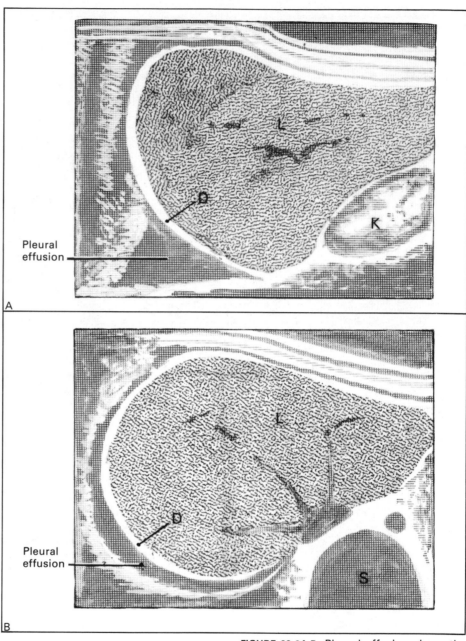

Pleural effusion

Pleural effusion

FIGURE 38-2A,B. Pleural effusion above the diaphragm on a supine longitudinal view, A, and supine transverse view, B.

PATHOLOGY
Pleural effusion

Pleural effusions (Figs. 38-1, 38-2) are usually echo-free, wedge-shaped areas that lie along the postero-lateral inferior aspect of the lung. Occasionally they contain internal echoes, sometimes indicating the presence of a neoplasm. These echoes may be due to blood or pus (empyema), especially when the collection is loculated. Loculated effusions do not necessarily lie adjacent to the diaphragm and may be located anywhere on the chest wall. Some effusions lie between the lung and the diaphragm and are known as subpulmonic.

Pleural Fibrosis

Unlike an effusion, which is wider inferiorly, fibrosis tends to be the same width at any site along the chest wall (Fig. 38-3). Fibrotic areas contain low-level echoes, but these are all too easily suppressed by an incorrect time gain compensation curve or too little gain. True fluid remains echo-free at settings that are good for the liver and spleen.

Solid Mass

If there are numerous internal echoes within a mass compared with a known fluid-filled structure such as the heart, one can be fairly confident that the lesion is a mass. Solid homogeneous masses with few internal echoes are more difficult to distinguish from fluid because they simulate a cystic collection. They may have strong back walls and appear to have no echoes at low gain settings. Because the lung lies beyond the lesion and does not conduct sound, through transmission is not easy to evaluate.

Consolidation

A consolidated lung contains a lot of fluid and may conduct sound even though there will be a number of internal echoes due to small pockets of air.

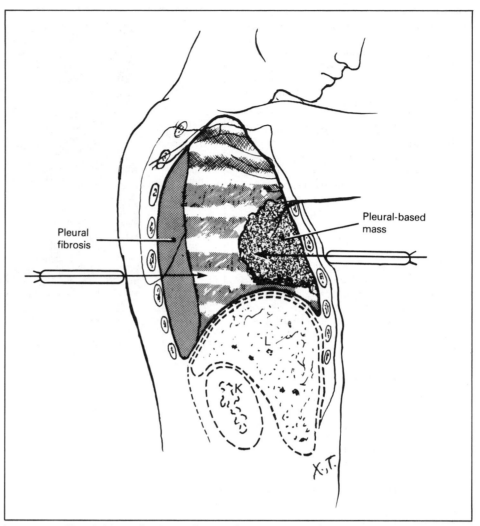

FIGURE 38-3. Usual shape of a pleural fibrosis (posterior lesion). There will be some internal echoes. A pleural-based solid mass is shown on the anterior aspect of the chest.

PITFALLS

1. *Reverberation versus effusion.* At times there may be doubt about whether an "effusion" is real on decubitus or supine views or just a mirror artifact (Fig. 38-4; see also Chapter 45). Placing the patient in a sitting position and scanning to look for fluid will place the transducer at another angle to the area in question and will eliminate this artifact.

2. *Spleen versus effusion.* The spleen may be mistaken for an effusion if the position of the kidney in relation to the spleen is not documented and the diaphragm is not seen adequately.

3. *Mass versus effusion.* A solid mass may be mistaken for a loculated effusion if the mass contains few or no internal echoes because the soft tissue—lung interface creates a strong "back wall" echo. Usually soft tissue masses adjacent to the pleura do contain internal echoes, and therefore a distinction can be made.

SELECTED READING

Cunningham, J. J. Gray scale echography of the lung and pleural space: Current applications of oncologic interest. *Cancer* 41:1329–1339, 1978.

Doust, B.D., Baum, J. K., Maklad, N. F., et al. Ultrasonic evaluation of pleural opacities. *Radiology* 114:135, 1975

Goldenberg, N. J. , Spitz, H. B., and Mitchell, S. E. Gray scale ultrasonography of the chest. *Semin. Ultrasound* 3:263, 1982.

Hirsch, J. H., Rogers, J. V., and Mack, L. A. Real-time sonography of pleural opacities. *A.J.R.* 136:297–301, 1981.

Marks, W. M. Filly, R. A., and Callen, P. W. Real-time evaluation of pleural lesions: New observations regarding the probability of obtaining free fluid. *Radiology* 142:163–164, 1982.

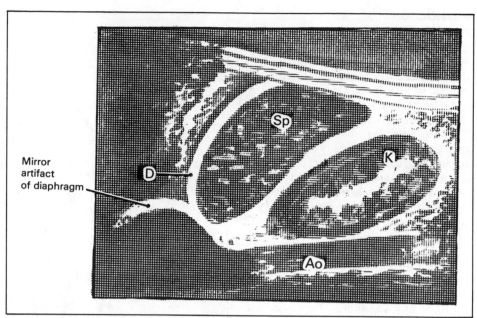

FIGURE 38-4. Mirror artifact of the diaphragm above the spleen. This artifact is seen when the patient is scanned from an oblique axis through the spleen.

39. A-MODE ECHOENCEPHALOGRAPHY

MIMI MAGGIO

SONOGRAM ABBREVIATIONS

AM   Acoustic midline

EEC   End echo complex

FC   Falx cerebri

IEC   Initial echo complex

LtH   Left side of head
LV   Lateral ventricle

RtH   Right side of head

3V   Third ventricle

KEY WORDS

Echoencephalography. Technique using A-mode to obtain a midline echo from the brain to show a midline shift.

THE CLINICAL PROBLEM

One of the few remaining clinical uses of A-mode is examination of the brain. The detection of midline shift is important in victims of trauma or in patients who have a possible intracranial tumor. In the absence of a calcified pineal gland on skull radiograph, expensive or slightly hazardous techniques are required to make the diagnosis. These techniques, such as computerized tomography (CT) or angiography, are found only in the larger medical centers. In addition, A-mode can be used to follow and diagnose hydrocephalus because the walls of the ventricles are visible. Other uses of echoencephalography, such as diagnosis of tumor, have been rendered obsolete with the development of CT.

ANATOMY

Five sizable echoes are seen along the A-mode display (Fig. 39-1).

1. The *initial echo complex (IEC)* results from the reflection from the face of the probe and the patient's scalp, skull, and dura mater.
2. The *end-echo complex (EEC)* is composed of reflections from the opposite side of the internal table of the skull.
3. The *midline echo* originates from the third ventricle. It appears as a prominent single or double high-amplitude echo with an M shape (AM). At a higher level, the falx cerebri is the midline structure.
4. *Two echoes* from the *lateral ventricles,* about 2 cm from the falx, are visible (Fig. 39-2).

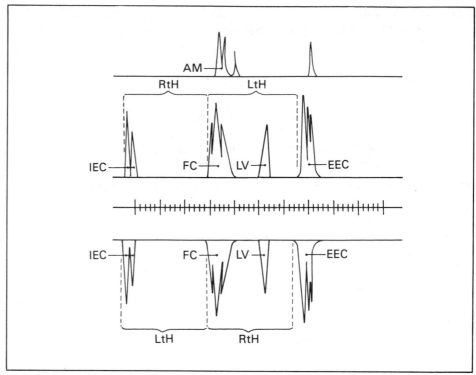

FIGURE 39-2. Moving the transducer higher up on the head from the 3V position, the midline structure will be the falx cerebri (FC). The walls of the lateral ventricle (LV) can be demonstrated lateral to the FC.

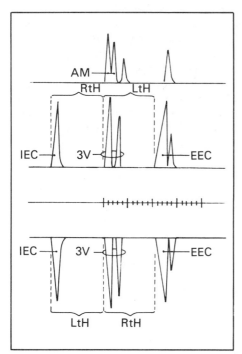

FIGURE 39-1. Echoencephalogram made with the transducer over the temporoparietal suture. The initial echo complex (IEC) is due to reflections from the probe and the patient's scalp; the end-echo complex (EEC) results from reflections from the opposite side of the internal table of the skull. The third ventricle (3V) is a midline structure, which should be lined up with the acoustic midline (AM), a stationary midline echo.

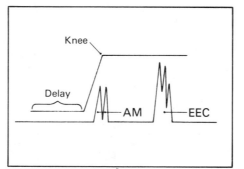

FIGURE 39-3. Only the far hemisphere can be demonstrated owing to excessive reverberations in the near field. The TGC curve should be set so that the near field echoes are suppressed by the delay. The knee should be placed just before the acoustic midline (AM).

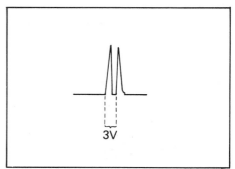

FIGURE 39-4. To determine the size of a dilated ventricle, the measurement is taken from the initial break of the proximal wall to the initial break of the distal wall.

TECHNIQUE

1. Due to the attenuation of the sound beam as it travels through the skull, two transducers can be used, one for transmitting and one for receiving.

2. The head should be supported in an upright position with plenty of coupling gel between the transducer and the skull.

3. To determine the midline shift, examinations from both temporal regions must be compared. A millimeter scale should be displayed on the screen. Place the transducer on the right side of the head 3 cm above the external auditory meatus (ear) to visualize the third ventricle. The face of the transducer should be as parallel to the sagittal plane as possible. Line up the third ventricle with the acoustic midline (Fig. 39-1).

4. When setting the TGC curve, place the delay curve slightly in front of the acoustic midline (Fig. 39-3). Attenuate the echoes maximally in the near hemisphere because of the many reverberations that occur in this area.

5. Place the transducer on the left side of the head. Line up the midline echo complex to the third ventricle. If one complex lies in the midline, the other complex must also; otherwise, one of these reflections does not belong to the third ventricle.

6. *Measurements.* If the third ventricle is truly shifted, both complexes will be displaced an equal distance in both directions. To determine the size of the ventricle, measure from the initial break of the proximal wall to the initial break of the distal wall (Fig. 39-4). The normal third ventricle does not exceed 8 mm in size (less in babies).

7. Place the transducer on the right side of the head 6 to 7 cm above the external auditory meatus. The midline echo seen here is the falx cerebri, with the lateral ventricles 2 cm from the falx (Fig. 39-2). Follow the same procedure on the left side.

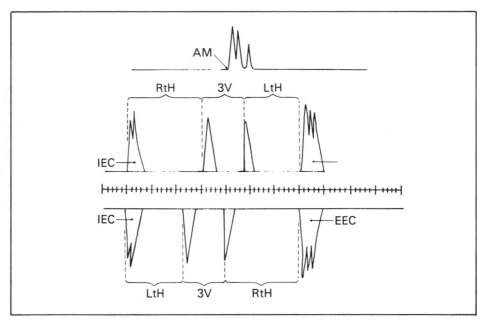

FIGURE 39-5. When there is dilatation of the third ventricle (3V), both complexes will be displaced an equal distance in both directions. Some midline shift is also present.

PATHOLOGY

1. If the *midline shift* is displaced more than 33 mm, it is considered abnormal.

2. *Lateral ventricular dilatation* with a third ventricle of more than 10 mm in width is abnormal (Fig. 39-5). The lateral ventricles can be seen at a higher level, and if the distance is more than 2 cm from the falx midline echo to the internal table, there is lateral ventricular enlargement.

PITFALLS

Both false positives and false negatives can occur. Because the technique in practice is rather difficult to perform, A-mode examination is becoming less and less common.

SELECTED READING

Tenner, M. S., and Wodraska, G. M. (Eds.). *Diagnostic Ultrasound in Neurology.* New York: Wiley, 1975.

40. NEONATAL INTRACRANIAL PROBLEMS

MIMI MAGGIO

SONOGRAM ABBREVIATIONS

A   Anterior horn
AS   Aqueduct of Sylvius

B   Body of lateral ventricle
BS   Brainstem

Cb   Cerebrum
CC   Corpus callosum
CN   Caudate nucleus
CP   Choroid plexus

FM   Foramen of Monro

IF   Interhemispheric fissure

Me   Medulla
MI   Massa intermedia

O   Occipital horn

PF   Posterior fontanelle
Po   Pons

SP   Cavum septi pellucidi
Su   Sulci

Te   Temporal
Ten   Tentorium
Thl   Thalamus
Tr   Trigone

VC   Vermis of cerebellum
3V   Third ventricle
4V   Fourth ventricle

KEY WORDS

Arnold-Chiari Malformation. Congenital anomaly associated with spina bifida in which the cerebellum and brainstem are pulled toward the spinal cord and secondary hydrocephalus develops.

Asphyxia. Difficulty in breathing in the first few minutes of life. Often associated with intracranial hemorrhage.

Atrium (Trigone) (of Lateral Ventricles). Site where the anterior, occipital, and temporal horns join.

Axial. Refers to a scan taken from a lateral approach through the temporal bone.

Brainstem. Part of the brain connecting the forebrain and the spinal cord; consists of the midbrain, pons, and medulla oblongata.

Caudate Nucleus. Portion of the brain that forms the lateral borders of the frontal horns of the lateral ventricles and lies anterior to the thalamus.

Cavum Septi Pellucidi. (See Fig. 40-28,A–C). A thin, triangular hole filled with cerebrospinal fluid that lies between the anterior horn of the lateral ventricles; it is particularly prominent in the neonate. It may appear as three different portions. If located posteriorly, it is termed a cavum vergi.

Cerebellum. Portion of the brain that lies posterior to the pons and medulla oblongata below the tentorium.

Cerebrum. The largest part of the brain, consisting of two hemispheres.

Choroid Plexus. Mass of special cells located in the atrium of the lateral ventricles. These cells regulate the intraventricular pressure by secretion or absorption of cerebrospinal fluid.

Cisterna. Enclosed space serving as a reservoir for cerebrospinal fluid.

Coronal View. Scan taken along the axis of the coronal suture (transverse in the skull).

Corpus Callosum. Forms the roof of the lateral ventricles.

Dandy-Walker Syndrome. Congenital anomaly in which a huge fourth ventricle cyst occupies the area where the cerebellum usually lies, with secondary dilatation of the third and lateral ventricles.

Encephalocele. Congenital anomaly in which a portion of the brain protrudes through a posterior (or rarely, anterior) defect in the skull.

Ependyma. The membrane lining the cerebral ventricles.

Falx Cerebri (Interhemispheric Fissure). A fibrous structure separating the two cerebral hemispheres.

Fontanelle. Spaces between the bones of the skull. Ultrasound can be directed through the anterior fontanelle to examine the brain until about the age of 1½ years.

Germinal Matrix. Periventricular tissue, including the caudate nucleus, which prior to about 32 weeks' gestation is fragile and bleeds easily.

Gyri. Convolutions on the surface of the brain caused by infolding of the cortex.

Horns. The recesses of the lateral ventricles; there are three horns of importance sonographically—frontal, temporal, and occipital horns.

Hematocrit. The volume percentage of red blood cells in whole blood.

Holoprosencephaly. Grossly abnormal brain in which there is a common large central ventricle.

Hydranencephaly. Congenital anomaly in which the cortical brain structures are absent. The midbrain and brainstem tissues are present.

Hydrocephalus. Dilatation of the ventricles with accumulation of cerebrospinal fluid, usually due to blockage of cerebrospinal fluid drainage.

Interhemispheric Fissure. The area in which the falx cerebri sits that separates the two cerebral hemispheres.

Meninges. The brain coverings.

Neonate. Newborn infant.

Parenchyma. Overall term for tissues of the cortex.

Porencephalic Cyst. Cyst arising from a ventricle that develops as a consequence of a parenchymal hemorrhage.

Sagittal View. Scan taken along the axis of the sagittal suture (longitudinal in the skull).

Seizure. A sudden episode of altered consciousness (known also as an epileptic fit).

Subependyma. The area immediately beneath the ependyma. In the caudate nucleus this area is the site of hemorrhage from the germinal matrix.

Sulcus. A groove or depression on the surface of the brain, separating the gyri.

Tentorium. V-shaped echogenic structure separating the cerebrum and the cerebellum; it is an extension of the falx cerebri.

Thalamus. Two ovoid brain structures situated on either side of the third ventricle superior to the brainstem

Trigone. See Atrium above.

Ventricle. A cavity within the brain containing cerebrospinal fluid.

THE CLINICAL PROBLEM
Intracranial Hemorrhage

Intracranial ultrasound examination in the neonate is mainly concerned with the diagnosis of hemorrhage, hydrocephalus, and congenital malformations. Clinical symptoms that make the pediatrician suspicious of intracranial hemorrhage include respiratory distress syndrome (RDS), a drop in hematocrit, a low birth weight (under 1500 g), and problems at delivery. It has been shown that most intracranial bleeds occur between 24 and 48 hours after birth. Diagnosis of these hemorrhages is important because although they are untreatable, a search for alternative treatable lesions in other parts of the body can be ended. Later complications of the hemorrhage such as hydrocephalus may need treatment, so follow-up by sonography is helpful. Some hemorrhages occur without symptoms in infants under 32 weeks' gestational age.

Intracranial hemorrhages develop in premature infants in the immature subependymal germinal matrix of the caudate nucleus, in the choroid plexus, and, rarely, in the cerebellum. If the subependymal bleed is severe, it can rupture into the ventricular system or the surrounding cortical tissue. A bleed into the cortical parenchyma is a serious complication that usually results in a porencephalic cyst. Intracranial hemorrhages and their complications in the neonate are graded as follows:

Grade I. Subependymal bleed without hydrocephalus

Grade II. Subependymal and intraventricular bleed without hydrocephalus

Grade III. Subependymal and intraventricular bleed with hydrocephalus

Grade IV. Subependymal and intraventricular bleed with hydrocephalus and a parenchymal bleed

Hydrocephalus

Hydrocephalus can be monitored by ultrasound through the anterior fontanelle until the age of 1 to 1½ years, so that severe ventricular dilatation requiring a shunt can be recognized. Following shunt placement, blockage of the shunt with consequent hydrocephalus sometimes occurs, and therefore postoperative ultrasound follow-up is important. Hydrocephalus can be followed until the child is 6 or 7 years old using an axial approach after the anterior fontanelle has closed.

Congenital Malformations

Congenital malformations with ventricular dilatation can be diagnosed with ultrasound—for example, hydranencephaly, Dandy-Walker syndrome, and holoprosencephaly. These malformations are compatible with life for a short time. Encephaloceles can be examined usefully with ultrasound because one can see how much remaining brain tissue exists within the portion of the meninges that has prolapsed out of the skull.

ANATOMY

The anatomy in the neonatal brain is complex and will be considered from three angles—the longitudinal (sagittal) (Figs. 40-1, 40-2), the transverse (coronal) using the anterior fontanelle as a window (Figs. 40-3, 40-4, and 40-5), and the axial (from the lateral side of the head).

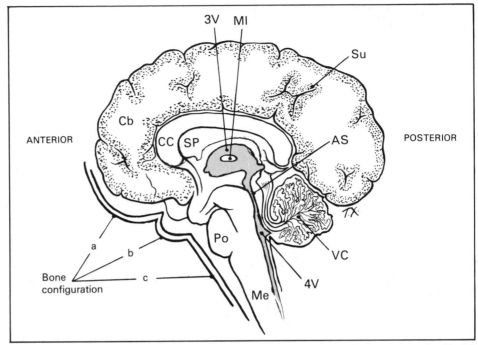

FIGURE 40-1. Normal midline sagittal view. Important structures are the cavum septi pellucidi (SP), the third ventricle (3V), the fourth ventricle (4V), and the vermis of the cerebellum (VC). Note the bone configuration of a midline section: (a) sphenoid, (b) pituitary fossa, (c) clivus.

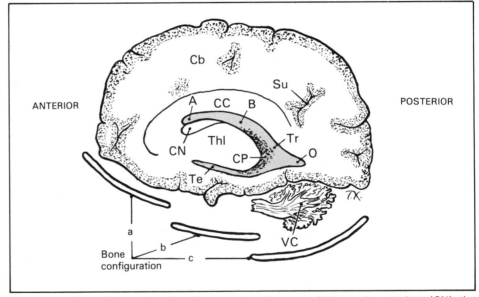

FIGURE 40-2. Normal lateral sagittal view showing the area of the caudate nucleus (CN), the thalamus (Thl), and the occipital horn (O). Note the different bone configurations: (a) anterior sphenoid, (b) middle sphenoid, (c) occipital fossa.

FIGURE 40-3. Normal anterior coronal view. The curvilinear darkened slits are the anterior horns; the caudate nucleus (CN) is adjacent.

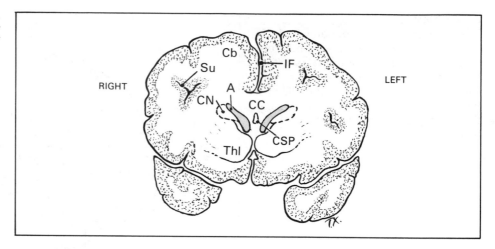

FIGURE 40-4. Normal midcoronal view, showing the body of the lateral ventricles (B) and the third ventricular area. The thin slit of the third ventricle may not be seen unless it is slightly dilated.

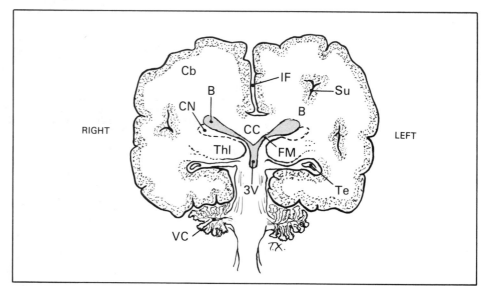

FIGURE 40-5. Normal posterior coronal view. Emphasis should be placed on seeing the choroid plexus (CP) in the trigone (Tr) of the lateral ventricles.

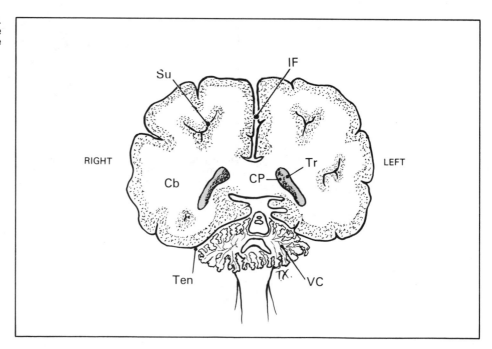

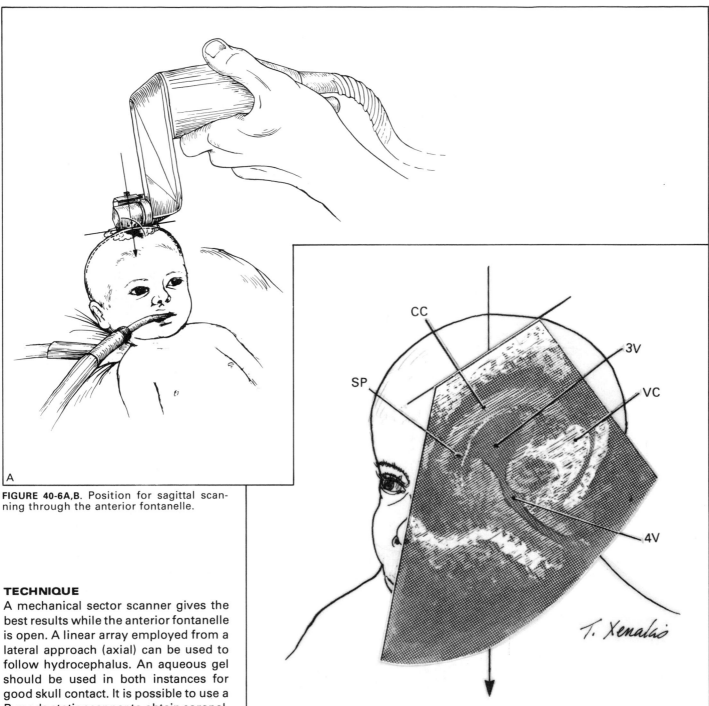

FIGURE 40-6A,B. Position for sagittal scanning through the anterior fontanelle.

TECHNIQUE

A mechanical sector scanner gives the best results while the anterior fontanelle is open. A linear array employed from a lateral approach (axial) can be used to follow hydrocephalus. An aqueous gel should be used in both instances for good skull contact. It is possible to use a B-mode static scanner to obtain coronal, sagittal, or axial images, but this technique is inherently more difficult and less efficient and involves transport of the infant to the ultrasound department.

Mechanical Sector Scanner Sagittal View

A 5.0-MHz transducer will offer better detail for infants with a large anterior fontanelle and a small head. Use a 3.5-MHz transducer for infants with a small fontanelle or a medium to large head.

MIDLINE

Start with sagittal scans with the baby's head in either the supine or the lateral position. Place the transducer on the anterior fontanelle along the plane of the sagittal suture (Fig. 40-6). Scan along the midline, making sure to identify the cavum septum pellucidum, the brainstem, and the area of the third ventricle (midline sagittal view).

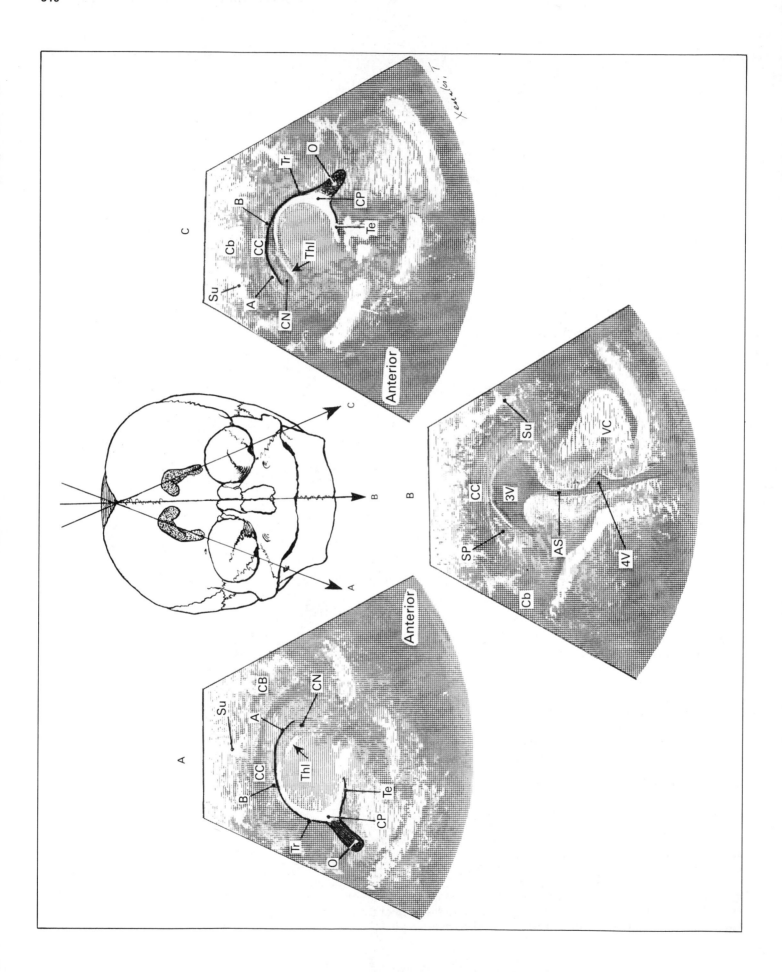

PARASAGITTAL

Staying in the same position, angle out slightly to the left and right sides (parasagittal view, Fig. 40-7A–C). The brain parenchyma can be seen by angling further laterally. Make sure to demonstrate the interface (bright line) between the caudate nucleus (CN) and the thalamus (T)—a common site for a bleed (Fig. 40-8). Take particular care to show the occipital horn because this is where blood frequently collects. The TGC curve should be set to identify the occipital horns properly. They cannot always be seen if the anterior fontanelle is small.

LABELING

To distinguish the left and right sagittal views, we use the following convention: left sagittal view anterior faces the sonographer's left; right sagittal view anterior faces the sonographer's right.

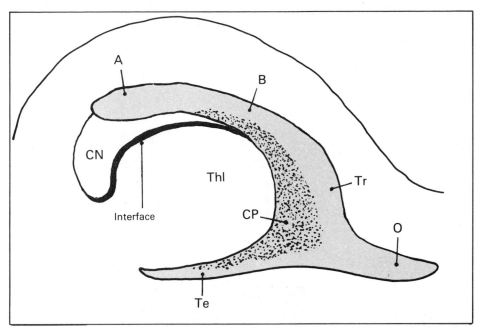

FIGURE 40-8. Lateral sagittal view demonstrating the lateral ventricle and the interface between the caudate nucleus (CN) and the thalamus (Thl). The caudate nucleus is the area where subependymal hemorrhages occur.

FIGURE 40-7. Sagittal views. A. Normal right lateral sagittal view. Note that the anterior of the section is facing toward the right. B. Midline sagittal view. The third ventricle (3V), the aqueduct of sylvius (AS), and, if possible, the fourth ventricle (4V) should be visualized. The vermis of the cerebellum (VC) will have bright level echoes. C. Normal left lateral sagittal view. Note that the anterior is facing toward the left. The entire lateral ventricular system should be demonstrated. It will appear normally as a black slit. The choroid plexus (CP) will appear as bright level echoes surrounding the thalamus (Thl). The sulci (Su) are the bright wiggly lines in the cerebrum (Cb).

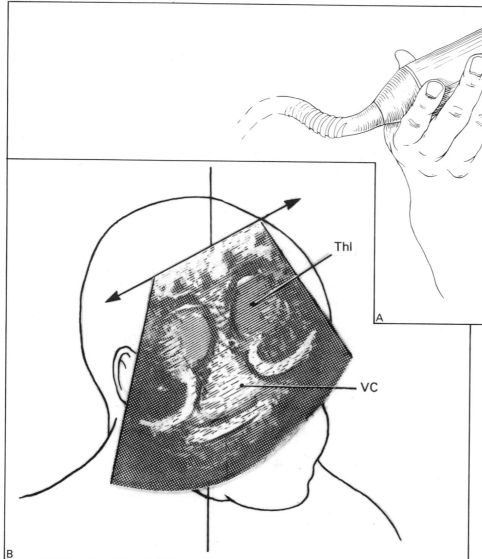

FIGURE 40-9A,B. Position for scanning the coronal views. It is important to make the images symmetrical.

Thl

VC

A

B

CORONAL (TRANSVERSE) VIEWS

The following views are routine:

POSTERIOR. Place the transducer on the anterior fontanelle along the plane of the coronal suture (Fig. 40-9); angling posteriorly, identify the choroid plexus in the atrium of the lateral ventricles (posterior view, Fig. 40-10A).

MIDCORONAL. Slowly sweep anteriorly toward the body of the lateral ventricles until the foramen of Monro can be seen entering the third ventricle (Fig. 40-10B).

ANTERIOR CORONAL. Angle more anteriorly toward the frontal horns (Fig. 40-10C). Make sure that the orientation is correct on the coronal views. The right ventricle should be on your left as you look at the picture.

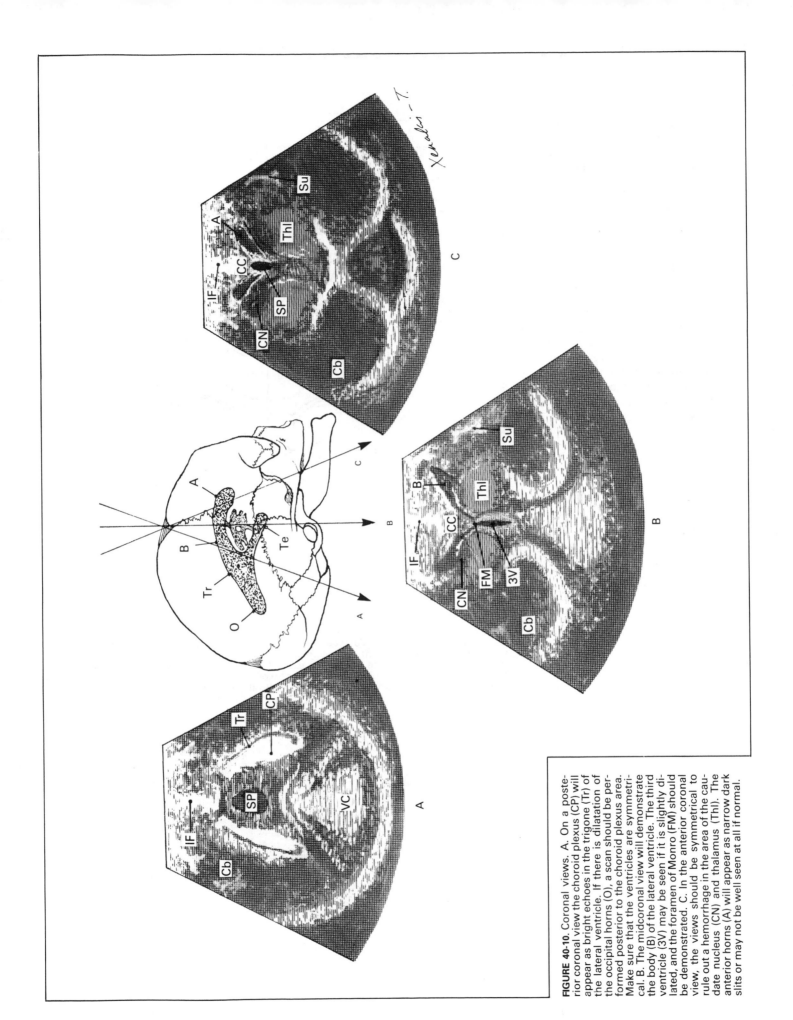

FIGURE 40-10. Coronal views. A. On a posterior coronal view the choroid plexus (CP) will appear as bright echoes in the trigone (Tr) of the lateral ventricle. If there is dilatation of the occipital horns (O), a scan should be performed posterior to the choroid plexus area. Make sure that the ventricles are symmetrical. B. The midcoronal view will demonstrate the body (B) of the lateral ventricle. The third ventricle (3V) may be seen if it is slightly dilated, and the foramen of Monro (FM) should be demonstrated. C. In the anterior coronal view, the views should be symmetrical to rule out a hemorrhage in the area of the caudate nucleus (CN) and thalamus (Thl). The anterior horns (A) will appear as narrow dark slits or may not be well seen at all if normal.

MEASUREMENTS. Comparison with previous sonographic measurements can be made by measuring the occipital horn on the sagittal views (Fig. 40-11A, the most sensitive measurements) and of the biventricular distance on the coronal views. Mild dilatation can be measured in an oblique fashion in the region of the ventricular body (Fig. 40-11B). The third ventricle can be measured on coronal views (Fig. 40-11B).

ADDITIONAL TECHNIQUES

In selected cases when the occipital horns are difficult to see, angle through the posterior fontanelle to obtain better detail of the occipital horns (Fig. 40-12). Examining the patient in the erect position helps to see the occipital horns better and to demonstrate a fluid-fluid level caused by blood.

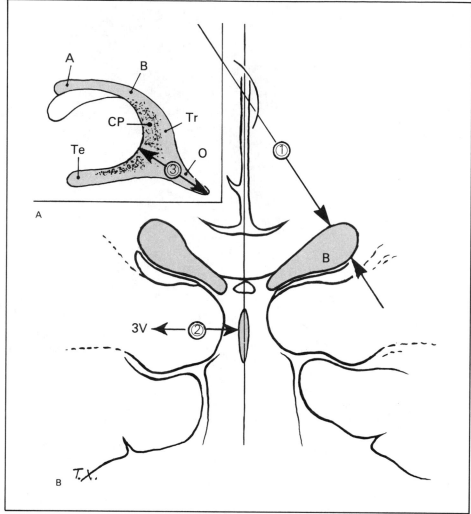

FIGURE 40-11. Measurements of lateral ventricles. A. A lateral sagittal view measurement ③ taken at an oblique axis at the occipital horn (O) is an early indication of ventricular enlargement. This distance should not exceed 16 mm. B. On the coronal view a measurement ①, which should not exceed 3 mm, is taken at the body of the lateral ventricle (B). The third ventricle (3V) width measurement ② should not exceed 2 mm.

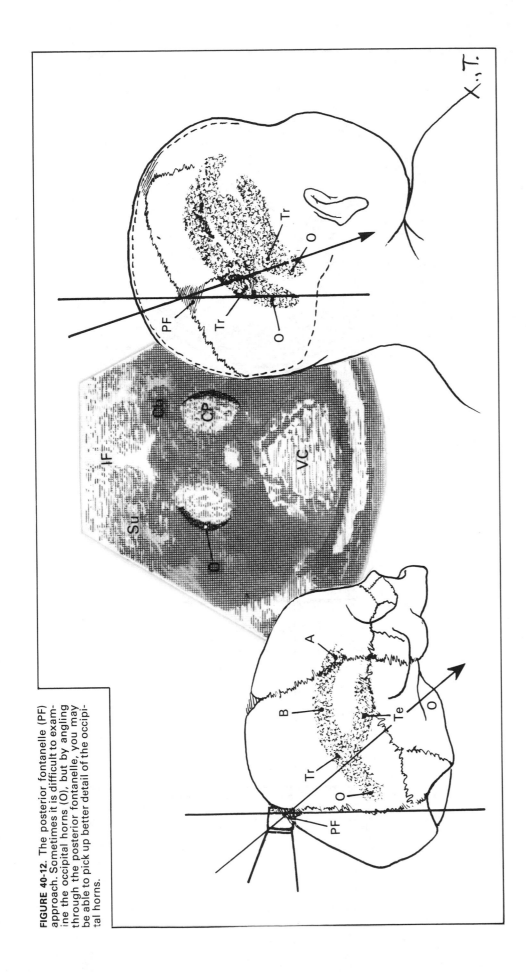

FIGURE 40-12. The posterior fontanelle (PF) approach. Sometimes it is difficult to examine the occipital horns (O), but by angling through the posterior fontanelle, you may be able to pick up better detail of the occipital horns.

Axial Views

An axial view (Fig. 40-13) is obtained by placing the transducer on the lateral aspect of the neonatal head with either a mechanical sector scanner or a linear array; it is useful for following ventricular size.

Linear Array Techniques

Linear array techniques are helpful in follow-up studies of hydrocephalus (that is, in babies with hydrocephalus whose anterior fontanelle has closed).

With the baby's head in the lateral position, place the probe along the temporoparietal region to demonstrate the lateral ventricular area and angle it toward the face, the area of the thalamus, and the third ventricle. The lateral ventricle measurement can then be made on the side facing down (Fig. 40-13A).

Lateral ventricular ratio

$$= \frac{\text{Lateral ventricle width (a)}}{\text{Hemispheric width (b)}}$$

The ventricle nearest the transducer is usually impossible to measure owing to reverberation artifacts, so scan the other side of the skull for the second ventricular measurement.

Linear arrays using the lateral approach are less easy to use because of difficulty in seeing small bleeds and the similarity of the choroid plexus to hemorrhage, especially when the ventricle is not dilated.

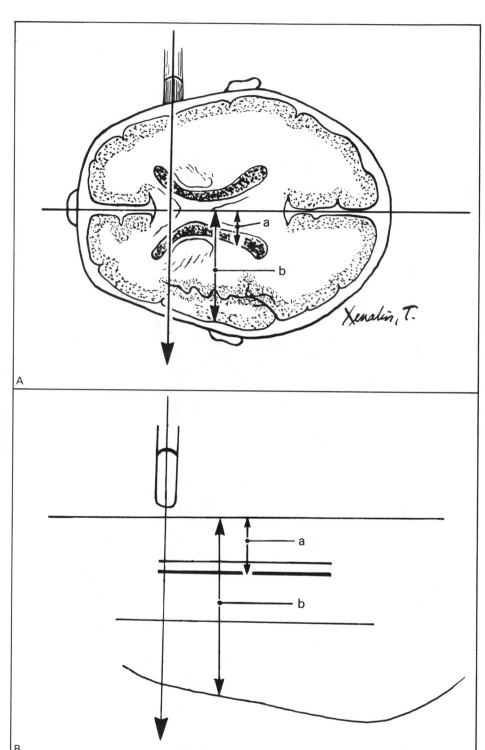

FIGURE 40-13A,B. When scanning with an axial approach, the downside lateral ventricle should be measured because there is too much artifact in the near field. The progress of hydrocephalus is followed by monitoring the ventricular-hemispheric ratio. Appropriate sites for measurement of the "hemisphere," b, and ventricle, a, are shown.

PATHOLOGY

The appearance of intracranial hemorrhage changes with time. Early hemorrhages are echogenic. Within a couple of weeks, the increased echogenicity decreases, leaving relatively sonolucent areas.

Subependymal Hemorrhages

Increased echogenicity in the caudate nucleus can be seen on the coronal view inferior to the floor of the lateral ventricles (Fig. 40-15). On the sagittal view the head of the caudate nucleus is echogenic (Fig. 40-14). An affected caudate nucleus may bulge into the ventricle.

It may be difficult to differentiate between a subependymal hemorrhage extending around the ventricle and an intraventricular hemorrhage or clot. Such hemorrhages may not be associated with hydrocephalus initially. Occasional hemorrhages occur in the thalamus (Fig. 40-15).

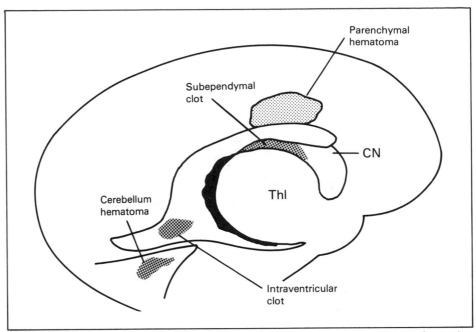

FIGURE 40-14. Lateral sagittal view. The various sites where hemorrhage and clot formation may occur are shown.

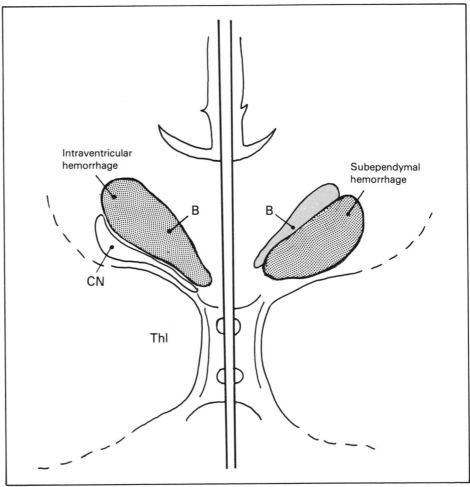

FIGURE 40-15. Sometimes it is difficult to decide if a hemorrhage is subependymal or intraventricular. The midcoronal view is helpful for distinguishing the two lesions.

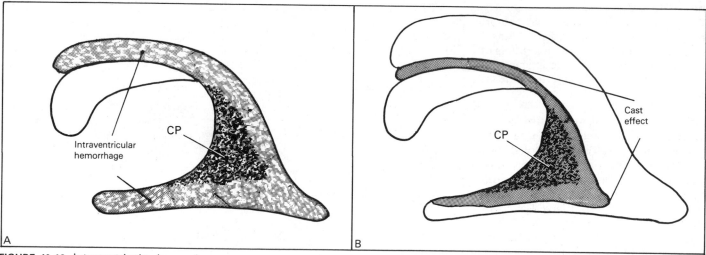

FIGURE 40-16. Intraventricular hemorrhage. A. Lateral sagittal view. An intraventricular hemorrhage fills the entire lateral ventricle. The choroid plexus (CP) is difficult to distinguish from the hemorrhage. B. With time, the hemorrhage will take on a cast effect and adopt the shape of the ventricle as the blood resolves. The choroid plexus (CP) is still difficult to distinguish from the clot.

Ventricular Hemorrhage

A hemorrhage has to be distinguished from the choroid plexus, which rarely extends into the occipital horn (Figs. 40-14, 40-16A). Therefore, detection of echoes in the occipital horn usually indicates hemorrhage. In older hemorrhages, clot will be more easily discerned because hydrocephalus will occur and the clot will be more compact (Fig. 40-16B) and will be surrounded by cerebrospinal fluid. Blood may completely fill the ventricles, forming a "cast," in which case it may be difficult to distinguish a ventricular blood clot from a large subependymal bleed and choroid plexus (Fig. 40-16A).

Parenchymal Hemorrhage (Bleeding into the Brain Substance)

A dense echogenic area occurs in the brain substance at a site usually near the caudate nucleus and lateral to the ventricles (Figs. 40-14, 40-17). This hemorrhage resolves slowly with the formation of a porencephalic cyst (a fluid-filled cavity within the brain substance, Fig. 40-17A–C). Dilatation of the lateral ventricles is often associated with parenchymal hemorrhage.

Choroid and Cerebellar Bleeds

These bleeds are very difficult to detect because they occur within echogenic structures—the choroid and cerebellum. Irregularity of the choroid outline and increased echogenicity suggest a bleed.

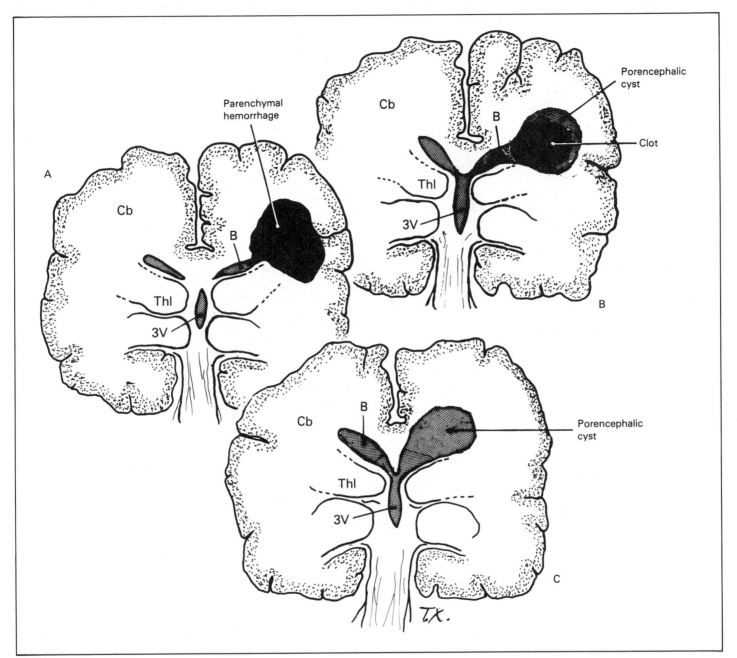

FIGURE 40-17. Parenchymal hemorrhage. A. Midcoronal view of parenchymal hemorrhage. At first the parenchymal hemorrhage will appear as a bright echogenic area in the cerebrum (Cb). B. The hemorrhage will begin to resolve and communicate with the lateral ventricle. The parenchymal hemorrhage becomes a porencephalic cyst with a clot within. C. The clot will resolve completely, leaving a porencephalic cyst with lateral ventricular dilatation.

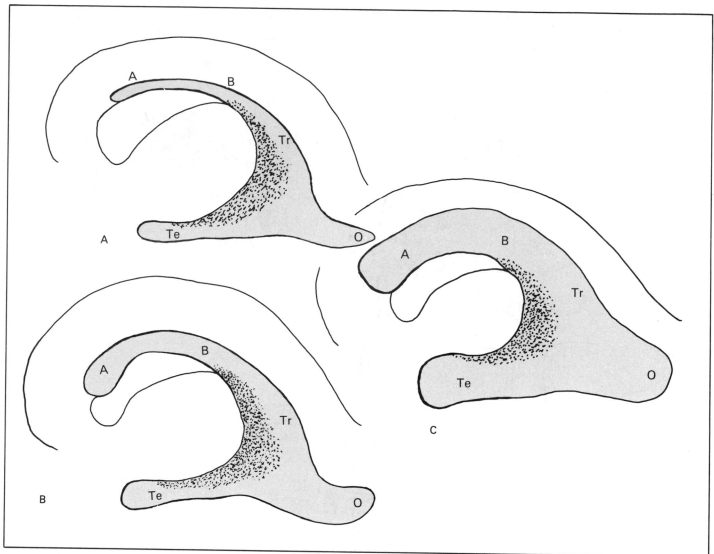

FIGURE 40-18. Lateral sagittal views with varying degrees of lateral ventricular dilatation. A. Minimal ventricular dilatation. B. Moderate ventricular dilatation. C. Marked ventricular dilatation.

Ventricular Dilatation

LATERAL VENTRICLES

Normal ventricles in the neonate usually appear as tiny, barely visible slits (Fig. 40-3). Usually the first indication of ventricular dilatation appears in the occipital horn; the body and anterior horn dilate subsequently. Ventricular dilatation of minimal, moderate, and marked degree is easy to judge on sagittal views (Fig. 40-18A–C). The coronal views offer another plane for assessing ventricular enlargement (Fig. 40-19A–C). Third and fourth ventricular dilatation can be seen on the sagittal midline section. Usually these structures are barely visible, so evidence of enlargement is easy to see (Fig. 40-20A,B).

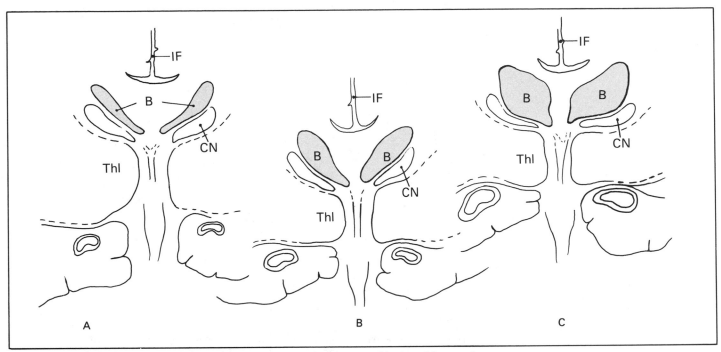

FIGURE 40-19. Varying degrees of ventricular dilatation are also measured in the midcoronal view. A. Minimal ventricular dilatation. B. Moderate ventricular dilatation. C. Marked ventricular dilatation.

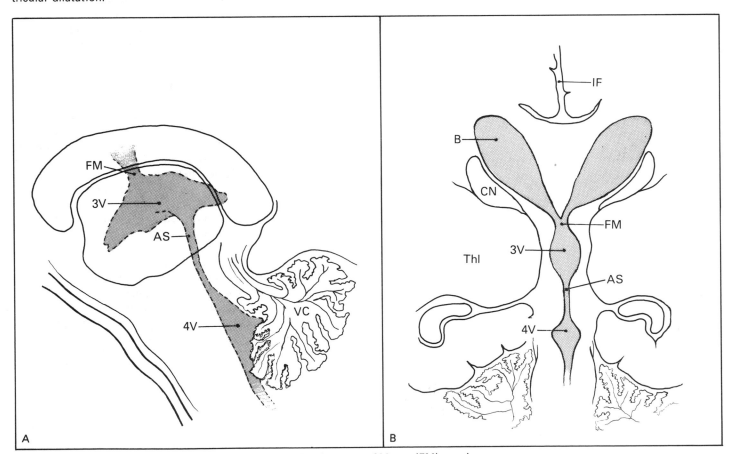

FIGURE 40-20. Midline sagittal (A) and coronal (B) views. The foramen of Monro (FM) may be seen. There may also be third (3V) and fourth (4V) ventricular dilatation.

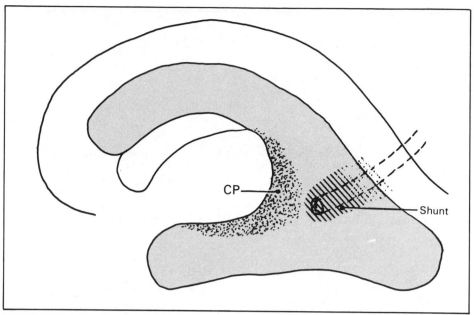

FIGURE 40-21. Lateral sagittal view. A shunt in the lateral ventricle appears as a dense group of echoes. The sonographer should demonstrate carefully where the shunt ends.

Shunt Tube Placement

Shunts appear as dense echogenic lines. The shunt tip location should be visualized. Sometimes a shunt tip lies in the brain parenchyma or in the choroid plexus or crosses the midline (Figs. 40-21 and 40-29)—less than ideal locations.

Congenital Anomalies

There are many congenital anomalies of the brain, and only the common types will be described here. Some anomalies are incompatible with long-term survival. The role of the sonographer is to show the nature of the anomaly so that a decision can be made about whether resuscitation attempts are worthwhile or whether surgery (usually shunting) needs to be performed.

DANDY-WALKER SYNDROME

In Dandy-Walker Syndrome a large cystic cavity occupies the occipital infratentorial area with symmetrical dilatation of the lateral ventricles and enlargement of the third ventricle (Fig. 40-22). The cerebellum is small. The malformation is considered an expansion of the fourth ventricle.

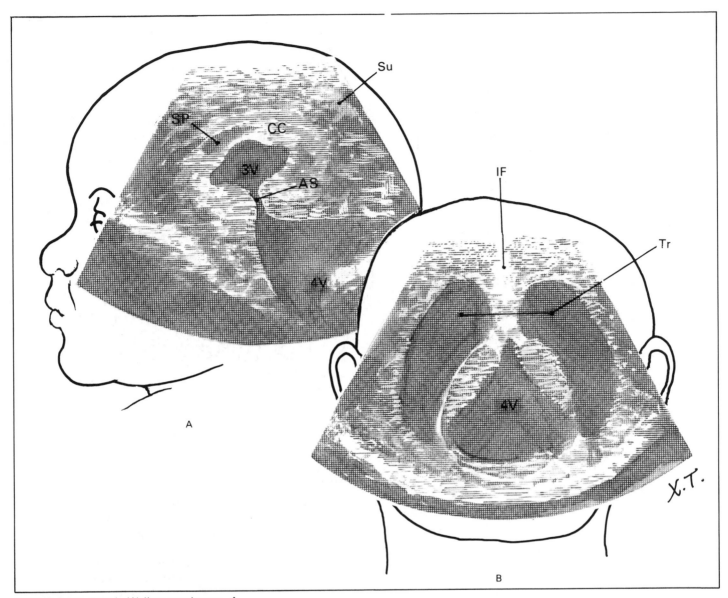

FIGURE 40-22. Dandy-Walker syndrome. A. Midline sagittal view. With the Dandy-Walker syndrome there is cystic dilatation of the fourth ventricle (4V); the third ventricle (3V) and aqueduct of Sylvius are dilated to a lesser degree. B. Posterior coronal view. Massive fourth ventricular (4V) enlargement and secondary lateral ventricular enlargement.

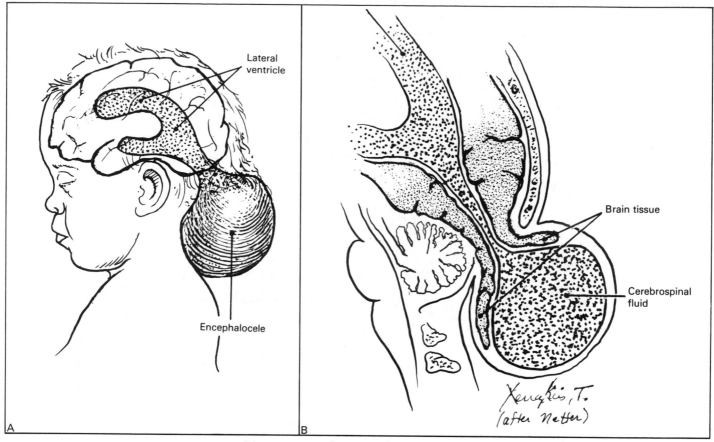

FIGURE 40-23A,B. Encephalocele. There is an extension of the lateral ventricle and of brain substance into the encephalocele.

ENCEPHALOCELE

A portion of the brain prolapses through a hole in the midline of the skull (Fig. 40-23A,B). The hole is usually located occipitally but may be located in the nasal region. In many instances the mass is almost entirely fluid-filled. The amount of brain tissue in the defect varies and affects the surgical management and survival.

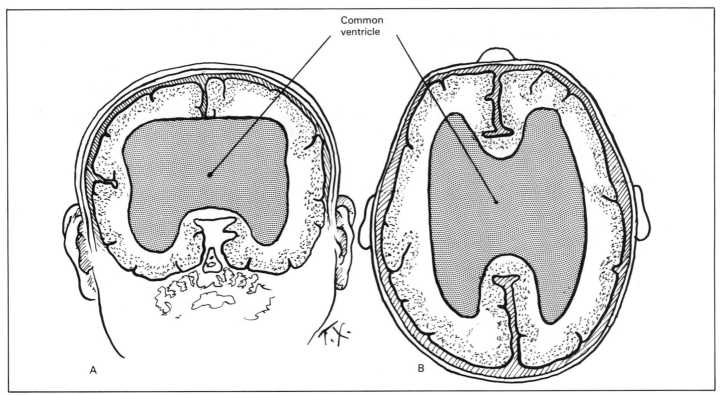

FIGURE 40-24A,B. Holoprosencephaly. Anterior coronal and axial views. A single misshaped ventricle is present.

HOLOPROSENCEPHALY

In this anomaly the brain is grossly disorganized and the ventricular pattern is markedly abnormal with one large ventricle (Fig. 40-24A,B). Holoprosencephaly is not compatible with long-term survival.

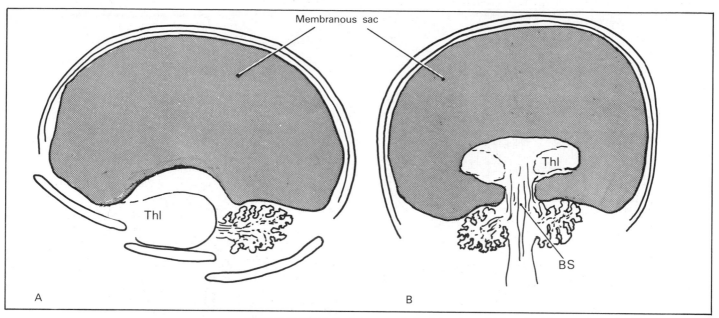

FIGURE 40-25A,B. Hydranencephaly, lateral sagittal and midcoronal views. There is no evidence of cortical tissue. A membranous fluid-filled sac replaces the brain. Only the brainstem (BS) and midbrain are present.

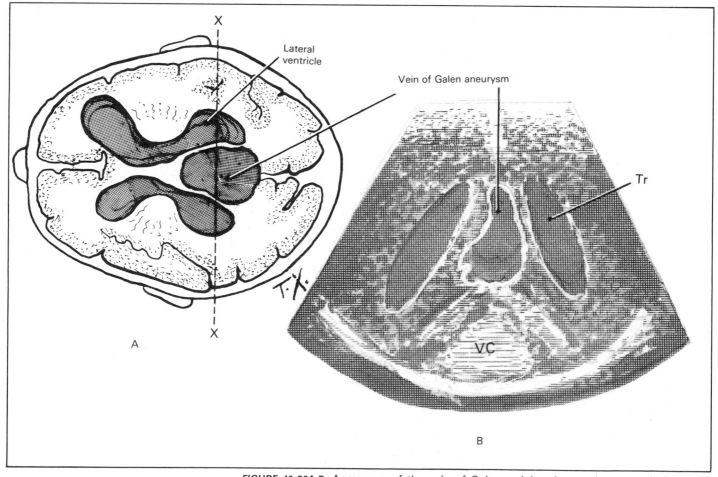

FIGURE 40-26A,B. Aneurysm of the vein of Galen, axial and posterior coronal views. An aneurysm of the vein of Galen is usually associated with lateral ventricular dilatation. The posterior coronal view was performed along line x–x.

HYDRANENCEPHALY

Absence of the cerebral hemispheres of the brain is called hydranencephaly; the condition is not compatible with survival. It is often mistaken for severe hydrocephalus. Only the midbrain and brainstem are present. No midline echo is seen (Fig. 40-25A,B).

VEIN OF GALEN MALFORMATION

There is aneurysmal dilatation of the vein of Galen—a large midline vein—with secondary hydrocephalus (Fig. 40-26A,B). Because so much blood is entering the head, there is often associated heart failure. Sonographically, one sees a large eccentrically shaped midline cystic space with lateral ventricular dilatation. The cystic space is superior to the tentorium and posterior to the third ventricle.

ARNOLD-CHIARI MALFORMATION

This relatively common syndrome is thought to be a consequence of a spina bifida tethering the spinal cord so that the brain structures cannot rise into the head to their normal site. The cerebellum is pulled inferiorly. Secondary hydrocephalus develops. The sonographic findings are

1. Superior and inferior sharp angles to the lateral ventricles
2. Possible absence of the septum pellucidum
3. Enlarged asymmetrical ventricles
4. Inferior placement of the tentorium

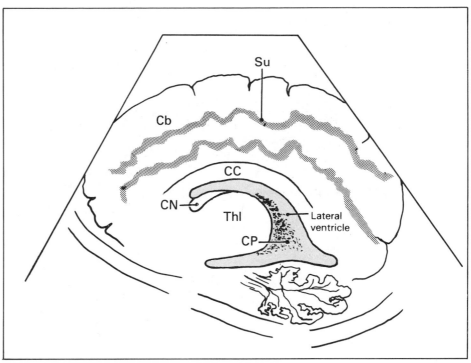

FIGURE 40-27. Lateral sagittal view. The sulci (Su) may appear as very prominent, bright lines. This is a normal variant.

PITFALLS

Normal Variants

1. *Sulci.* The sulci may appear more echogenic than usual. This finding is of no pathologic significance and is seen in older children (Fig. 40-27).

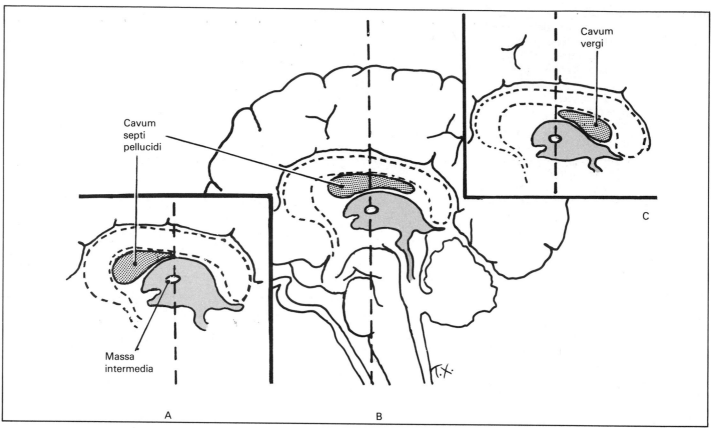

FIGURE 40-28. Cavum septi pellucidi. If the scanning angle is incorrect, this normal variant may be mistaken for a dilated ventricle. It may appear as one of three different patterns. A. Cavum septi pellucidi. B. Cavum septi pellucidi and cavum vergi. C. Cavum vergi.

2. *Cavum septum pellucidum.* A midline sonolucent space inferior to the corpus callosum is termed a cavum septum pellucidum (Fig. 40-28A–C). In the midline sagittal view a very prominent cavum septum pellucidum may be present, and if the positioning is incorrect, it may be mistaken for a dilated ventricle.

The posterior segment of this midline cavity is termed the *cavum vergi.* Only the anterior portion may be visible (Fig. 40-28). All of these cavities are normal variants.

3. *Massa intermedia.* The massa intermedia appears as an echogenic mass in the center of the third ventricle (Fig. 40-28).

4. *Shunts.* A shunt tube should not be mistaken for a bleed. These tubes often cause the ventricle to collapse around them (Fig. 40-29).

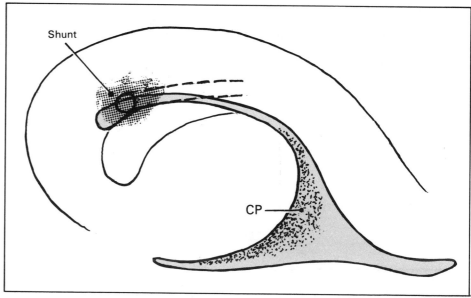

FIGURE 40-29. Clinical information is essential when scanning infants. In this lateral sagittal view, the bright echoes from a shunt could be mistaken for a hemorrhage. The wall of the ventricle collapsed around the shunt.

5. *Orientation.* Be sure that the orientation is correct to avoid confusion about which side has a bleed or is hydrocephalic. Wrong labeling will confuse follow-up studies and could have serious clinical consequences.

6. *Choroid plexus versus bleed.* The choroid plexus may extend into the occipital horn, mimicking a bleed (Fig. 40-30). Placing the patient in the erect position may help by showing that the blood moved and formed a fluid-fluid level (Fig. 40-31), whereas the choroid plexus will not.

7. *Choroid bleeds.* Choroid plexus bleeds may be overlooked. Compare both the choroid plexuses to see if they have the same echogenicity and outline. A lumpy outline suggests the presence of a bleed.

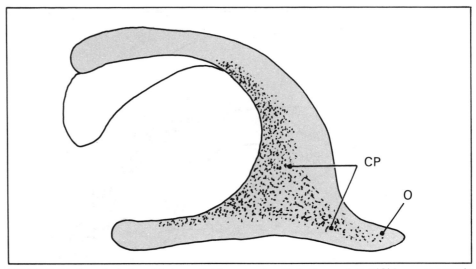

FIGURE 40-30. A variant choroid plexus (CP) may extend into the occipital (O) horn, as seen in this lateral sagittal view.

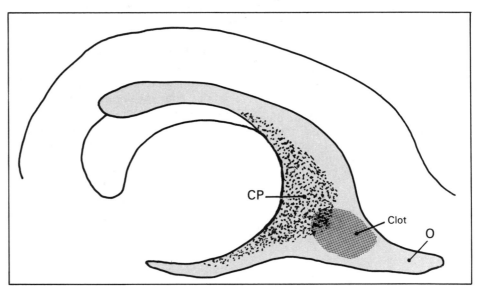

FIGURE 40-31. At times it is difficult to distinguish clot in the occipital horn (O) from an extension of the choroid plexus (CP), a rare variant. Positioning the patient's head erect helps to identify the clot.

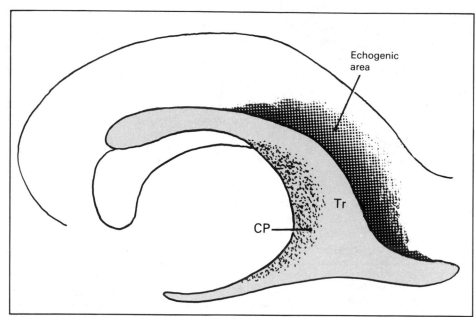

Echogenic area

Tr

CP

FIGURE 40-32. Sometimes there is an echogenic (bright) area behind the trigone (Tr) of the lateral ventricle, as seen in this lateral sagittal view. This should not be mistaken for a bleed. Note the mild dilatation of the lateral ventricle.

8. *Cerebellar bleeds.* Cerebellar bleeds may be overlooked because the cerebellum is normally densely echogenic. Look for asymmetry on coronal views.

9. *Occipital echogenic area.* There can be a very echogenic area in the brain tissue adjacent and posterior to the atrium of the lateral ventricles (Fig. 40-32). It is a normal variant.

WHERE ELSE TO LOOK
Arnold-Chiari Malformation
This condition is associated with spina bifida and myelomeningocele. In a neonate the spinal canal should be examined to make sure that no intraspinal mass is present and the cord does not extend too low.

Possible Hemorrhage
If a possible but not definite hemorrhage is detected, follow-up studies should be performed.

SELECTED READING

Babcock, D. S., Bove, K. E., and Han, B. K. Intracranial hemorrhage in premature infants: Sonographic-pathologic correlation. *A.J.N.R.* 3:309–317, 1982.

Babcock, D. S. *Cranial Ultrasound of Infants.* Baltimore: Williams & Wilkins, 1981.

Binder, G. A., Haughton, V. M., and Ho, K.-C. (Eds.). *Computed Tomography of the Brain in Axial, Coronal, and Sagittal Planes.* Boston: Little, Brown, 1979.

Grant, E. G., Kerner, M., Schellinger, D., et al. Evolution of porencephalic cysts from intraparenchymal hemorrhage in neonates: Sonographic evidence. *A.J.N.R.* 3:47–50, 1982.

Johnson, M. L., Rumack, C. M., Mannes, E. J., et al. Detection of neonatal intracranial hemorrhage utilizing real-time and static ultrasound. *J. Clin. Ultrasound* 9:427–433, 1981.

Leech, R., and Kohnen, P. Subependymal and intraventricular hemorrhages in the newborn. *Am. J. Pathol.* 77:3, 1974.

Shuman, W. P., Rogers, J. V., Mack, L.A., et al. Real-time sonographic sector scanning of the neonatal cranium: Technique and normal anatomy. *A.J.R.* 137:821–828, 1981.

Wilson, M. (Ed.). *The Anatomic Foundation of Neuroradiology of the Brain* (2nd ed.). Boston: Little, Brown, 1972.

41. PUNCTURE PROCEDURES WITH ULTRASOUND

NANCY A. SMITH
ROGER C. SANDERS

Ultrasound is now being used to guide a variety of invasive procedures that previously employed fluoroscopic localization or experienced guesswork. Ultrasonic localization should take place immediately before fluid aspiration or biopsy. Punctures can be done in the following situations:

1. After ultrasound shows the site direction without the use of a sterile transducer
2. With an A-mode transducer with a central hole
3. With a real-time transducer optionally with a central slot or guidance lever aspiration attachment—either a linear array or a mechanical sector scanner

Do not autoclave puncture transducers or they will be irreversibly damaged. Either gas-sterilize aspiration transducers or immerse them in an antiseptic solution.

PRACTICAL STEPS

Find the Puncture Site

Demonstrate

1. Where the mass or collection is
2. How deep it is
3. What lies between the patient's skin and the mass

Determine the Optimum Needle Depth

Move the patient so that as few structures as possible lie in the path of the needle. Piercing the liver or bowel is undesirable if it can be avoided by changing the angulation of the patient or the needle.

Mark the Site

The puncture site must be marked in such a way that the mark will not be scrubbed away when the patient's skin is cleaned. A simple but effective method is to imprint the skin by pressing on it with a "localizer." Among the many possible "scientific puncture site localizers" that are used are ballpoint pens, plastic needle caps, and caps from a Magic Marker. Anything will do that is not too sharp to cause the patient discomfort. Press on the skin just before the skin is cleansed, and a small red circle will remain.

Once the lesion is found and the puncture site has been marked, leave an image on the screen with a set of scale markers along the path of the needle. This can serve as a reference during the procedure, enabling the doctor to match the angle of the needle with that of the markers on the screen.

If the best approach demands two different angles, the scanning arm can be left in position (although not directly over the sterile field, of course) and used as a reference for the second angle (Fig. 41-1).

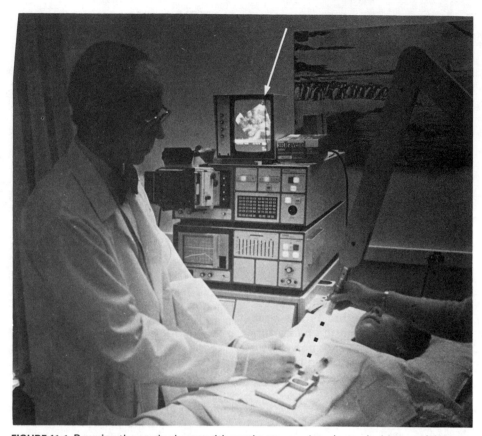

FIGURE 41-1. By using the angle shown with centimeter markers (arrow) a biopsy of the mass in the pancreas can be taken. The sonographer duplicates the angle of the scanning arm for the physician, allowing him to match it just before pushing the needle in.

Obtain Consent Forms

Punctures of any kind carry potential risks, and a full explanation must be given to the patient of the risks and benefits of the procedure, and the alternative diagnostic and therapeutic maneuvers that are available. The patient must then sign a consent form prior to the puncture. Consent forms are obtained by the physician performing the procedure, but such matters can be overlooked in any busy laboratory. The sonographer should therefore double-check that the form has been signed. The sonographer usually acts as a witness of the consent procedure.

Remove Oil

If oil has been used in performing the scan, it must be thoroughly removed or the iodine-prepping solution will bead up and roll off. Alcohol does not work well, but wiping the skin with acetone has proved to be effective.

Document the Puncture Site

Make sure that the actual puncture site has been photographed and is part of the patient's record. No matter how carefully a procedure is carried out, tissue or fluid is not always obtained, and documentation of an appropriate approach is therefore important. For example, an apparent collection may in fact be an organized hematoma, and nothing can be aspirated even though the needle is correctly placed.

PUNCTURE EQUIPMENT

The following sterile supplies should be available either as a basic tray or assembled (Fig. 41-2).

Sterile drapes (one with a hole for access to the puncture site)

Two containers (for antiseptic solutions)

Glass tubes (for collecting specimens)

10-ml syringe, 25- and 22-g needles (for local anesthetic)

Cleansing sponges

To be added:

Needle of choice

Syringe of choice (depends on the size of the collection)

Extension tubing (desirable for targets that move with respiration, for example, kidney)

Sterile ruler (to measure the correct depth on the needle)

Needle stop (to screw on the needle at the correct depth. A bandaid can be used)

Local anesthetic (usually lidocaine; may be 1% or 2%)

Alcohol wipes (for cleaning off the rubber stopper on any bottles, for example, lidocaine, Renografin, anaerobic culture bottles)

Sterile gloves

A-mode or real-time aspiration transducer

Sterile plastic bag to cover the transducer

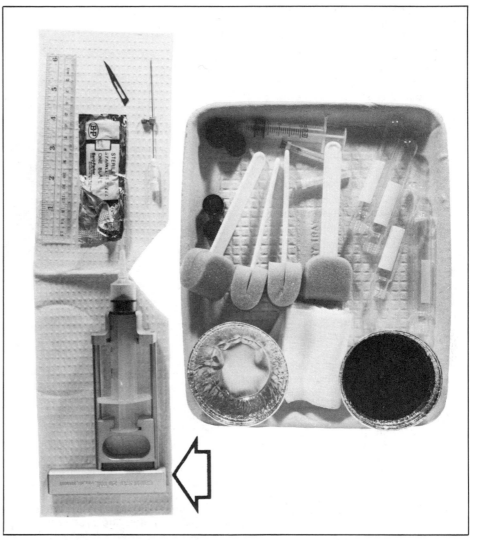

FIGURE 41-2. Supplies needed for a basic tray for a sterile procedure include containers for iodine and alcohol, prep sponges, a 5-ml syringe, 19-gauge and 25-gauge needles for drawing up local anesthetic, glass culture tubes, some 3 by 4 gauze pads and sterile drapes (at least one fenestrated). A sterile ruler, a scalpel blade, and the appropriate needle and sterile needle stop must be added. The black arrow points to an aspiration device that can be attached to a 20-ml syringe to help apply more negative pressure during biopsies.

SPECIFIC PUNCTURE PROBLEMS

Amniocentesis

When amniocentesis is performed in the second trimester, the site is easily localized. Second trimester amniocentesis is generally performed to rule out congenital defects at a stage early enough to give the parents the option of abortion if a fetal defect is found. In the third trimester amniocentesis is performed to see if the fetal lungs are mature. There is relative oligohydramnios in the third trimester, and the procedure can be difficult to perform.

There are several important points to be remembered when choosing a site.

1. *Avoid the placenta (Fig. 41-3).* This may be impossible if the placenta covers the entire anterior surface of the uterus. It is especially important to avoid the placenta if Rh incompatibility is the diagnosis because penetrating the placenta will aggravate the basic condition.
2. *Avoid the fetus.* The chances of striking the fetus are slim; however, do not photograph a puncture site with a baby in the field of view.
3. *Avoid the umbilical cord.* The cord can easily be seen floating in the fluid. If the puncture has to be performed through the placenta, be sure to avoid the site of the cord entrance.
4. *Avoid a site that is too lateral.* The uterine arteries run along the lateral walls of the uterus. Fortunately, these arteries are generally visible on the sonogram as large sonolucent areas (Fig. 41-3).
5. *Document the site.* The site should be recorded on the image with centimeter markers to show the path of the needle and to give the correct depth. If only a small site is available, the use of A-mode may be helpful.

    A-mode transducers can be obtained with a central hole through which a needle can be placed. Used in the fashion described for detection of ascites (see Chapter 15), they show the fluid depth and direction. A 20-gauge needle can be seen in fluid with a 3.5-MHz transducer. If the physician pushes the fetal head out of the pelvis, a small amount of fluid not previously seen may be demonstrated.

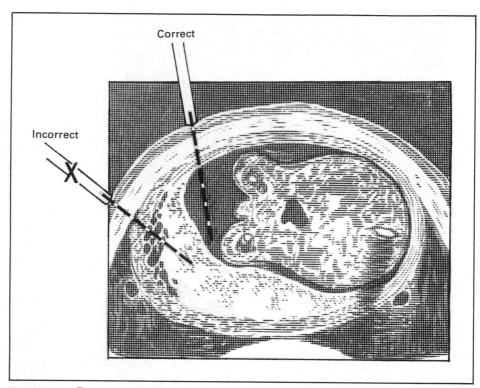

FIGURE 41-3. Transverse section through a pregnant uterus. A small area of amniotic fluid is present. The correct angle for obtaining fluid from this site is shown. Avoid the large vascular sinuses that would be punctured if a lateral approach were used.

6. *Check fetal heart motion.* Before and after amniocentesis, check that fetal heart motion is seen. It is reassuring for the parents to see that the fetus is unharmed after the procedure is finished.
7. *Twenty-two-gauge needles.* These needles are used to avoid complications.

    Opaque tubes are necessary to keep light from reaching fluid samples and breaking down the bilirubin pigments if an Rh problem is being investigated.

Fetal Transfusion

This procedure is performed to insert blood percutaneously through a needle into the peritoneum of a fetus affected by Rh incompatibility. A linear array transducer is placed at right angles to the needle in order to see the needle throughout its course.

1. Plot the correct site, which should lie just superior to the fetal bladder below the level of the liver.
2. Watch as the needle is introduced. The fetal abdominal wall will be indented by the needle, and at the same time its location can be checked.
3. After the needle has been inserted into the fetal abdomen, watch as blood is injected. You should be able to see small bubbles and fetal ascites develop as the fluid is introduced. If blood is introduced incorrectly into the amniotic fluid, bubbles will be seen within the amniotic fluid outside the fetus. As the transfusion progresses, monitor the fetal heart to be certain that the fetal pulse is not slowing. The normal rate is about 140 beats per minute.
4. After the procedure is over, perform a scan to assess the amount of fluid that has been placed in the fetal abdomen.

Pleural Effusions

Obtaining fluid by percutaneous puncture is necessary either to determine the nature of the fluid or to relieve shortness of breath. Thoracentesis, when not performed in the ultrasound suite, is customarily done in the patient's room. A site is chosen after percussing the chest and listening for dullness. A short needle is routinely used. This technique is not infallible; the effusion may be in a different location or may not be present at all. In an obese or muscular patient, more depth than is afforded by a short needle is often required. If a tap is unsuccessful when attempted "blindly," the patient is often referred to allow the puncture to be performed with the aid of ultrasound.

Mobile pleural effusions will fall to a dependent site at the back of the patient so if an effusion is freely mobile, the patient must sit upright even if assistance is needed. If the effusion does not shift on the chest radiograph (loculation), a prone or supine position is feasible. There are several points to remember when choosing a site.

1. *Demonstrate the diaphragm.* This is particularly important on the left side where the spleen can look "cystic."
2. *Check the A-mode.* There are two reasons for this rule. (a) Pleural fibrosis can look very much like pleural fluid. However, fibrosis does contain low-level echoes and does not have such pronounced through transmission. (b) Ribs interfere, and the transducer must be angled around them. Sometimes the best path to the fluid is not directly perpendicular to the patient's back. When the fluid pocket shows well on the A-mode (it has the same characteristics as a cyst), put centimeter markers on the screen and use that angle for the needle (see Chapter 38).
3. *Use a needle stop.* This is especially important in the chest. If the needle enters too deeply, the lungs may be pierced and pneumothorax will result. Document the needle side with a Polaroid for the chart if the puncture is to be performed elsewhere.
4. *Watch respiration.* If the pocket is small, watch the A-mode to see what phase of respiration best shows the effusion. Duplicate this phase of respiration for the puncture. If necessary, use an A-mode aspiration transducer.
5. *Laboratory tests.* The most commonly ordered laboratory tests for pleural effusions require the following fluid containers: *glass tubes* (for culture), *cytopathology tubes, heparinized tubes* (if tap is bloody), *anaerobic culture bottle* (one can use a sealed syringe instead.)

Cyst Puncture

Cysts occur throughout the abdomen, but the technique for localizing them is basically the same in all organs. A renal cyst is the most common target for cyst puncture.

There are three steps to follow for cyst puncture.

1. *Make sure that the patient is comfortable.* This is important because the patient must lie still for about half an hour during the procedure. However, the position should give the physician easy access to the cyst.
2. *Watch respiration.* Scanning and locating the site during quiet breathing is best. Kidneys move with respiration, so the needle will swing a little during the procedure.
3. *Make a site preferably below the ribs as close to the cyst as possible.* The patient should be in a prone or decubitus position. Use a similar needle insertion technique as that already described for pleural effusions.

Mass Biopsy

This simple procedure is best performed using a real-time system with a needle guide attachment, for example, a linear array with a slot or a mechanical sector scanner with a transducer guide. However, a B-scan transducer may also be used as a guide. The depth and direction should be chosen, and a 22-gauge needle is used. Essential equipment includes a needle stop, a sterile ruler, cytopathology bottles, and culture bottles. In an alternative technique a linear array transducer is used within a sterile plastic bag. Gel is placed within the bag, and then the transducer is dropped into place. More gel is required between the plastic bag and the patient's skin. Used at a 45° angle, such a transducer can also guide a needle at a 90° angle to the transducer.

If no real-time aspiration transducer is available, biopsy of lesions in the liver can be performed satisfactorily if a real time transducer is placed at right angles to the needle insertion site. Otherwise, the needle cannot be seen at the time the study is being performed. Even with real-time transducers, the needle tip may be difficult to see, but evidence that the needle is within the mass can be obtained by moving the needle. The larger the needle, the easier it is to see. The higher the frequency, the smaller the needle that can be used, for example, a 20-gauge needle with a 3.5-MHz transducer or a 22-gauge needle with a 5-MHz transducer.

Abscess Puncture

Puncture of an abscess involves the insertion under ultrasonic control of a large catheter to drain a collection of fluid. Because the procedure is hazardous, full precautions to detect bleeding should be undertaken, and blood pressure and pulse values should be obtained at 15-minute intervals. The main difference from the other puncture techniques described here is that different catheters are required. Abscess puncture is best performed with a real-time system on the fluoroscopy table because guidewire and catheter placement can be visualized by x-rays. Common systems used for abscess drainage are (1) a percutaneous nephrostomy set, (2) a trocar with associated catheter, sometimes with a terminal balloon, and (3) a Van Sonnenburg sump—a special catheter that has side holes and a second lumen to decompress an abscess. Because the procedure is painful, premedication should be given.

Percutaneous Nephrostomy

This procedure is similar to abscess drainage; however, because the catheter is often left in for a very long period of time, full sterile precautions, including masks, gowns, and hats, must be maintained. This procedure is also potentially hazardous and painful, and therefore, premedication should be given (obtain a consent form first). Make sure that there is no evidence of bleeding by watching the patient's pulse and blood pressure.

SELECTED READING

Chang, R. Ultrasonic Puncture Techniques. In R. C. Sanders (Ed.), *Ultrasound Annual.* New York: Raven, 1982.

Gerzof, S. G., Berkett, D. H., Pugatch, R. D., et al. Percutaneous catheter drainage of abdominal abscesses guided by ultrasound and computed tomography. *A.J.R.* 133:1–8, 1979.

42. SPECIALIZED TECHNIQUES

NANCY A. SMITH

LOCALIZATION FOR RADIOTHERAPY

Localization of a mass or organ for radiotherapy is helpful in several areas of the body, notably the prostate and the kidneys. The radiotherapist outlines the approximate location of the mass or organs with marks on the skin. Usually purple lines within a square field show the area that will be subjected to radiotherapy. In some instances a radiotherapist marks organs that should be excluded from the therapy field such as the kidneys. The sonographer outlines the target organ or the organ to be excluded from the therapy field. Make sure the patient's position is identical to that used for radiotherapy. If the plotted radiotherapy field does not correspond with the site of the mass or organ, a revised field is marked on the skin by the sonographer using indelible ink (carbolfuchsin [Fig. 19-7]). This can be applied only after the mineral oil or gel has been thoroughly wiped off with acetone.

PATIENTS IN ISOLATION

Isolated patients should be scheduled last in the day so that the equipment can be wiped down with an iodine solution after the examination is completed. After scanning patients on hepatitis isolation, 0.5% sodium hypochlorite solution should be used to clean the equipment. The sonographer should wear a special gown, gloves, mask, and hat, depending on the type of isolation ordered. (It should be routine to wipe off the transducer with alcohol between patients to preserve sterility.)

EMERGENCIES AND PORTABLE STUDIES

Because real-time units are portable, there is an increasing demand for portable studies in intensive care units. Emergency studies are also becoming common. Some studies that are well accepted as emergencies are (1) acute renal failure, to rule out hydronephrosis, (2) acute right upper quadrant pain, to rule out cholecystitis, (3) possible fetal death, (4) premature rupture of membranes to establish fetal weight, and (5) possible placenta previa.

Equipment that must be taken with the portable system includes

1. *Film.* Film is needed to document the case.
2. *Gel or Oil.* Gel may be preferable because oil may run off the patient onto the bed sheets.
3. *Alcohol wipes.* Wipes are necessary to clean off the transducer.
4. *Plastic bag.* A plastic bag is needed to fasten over the transducer in case the patient has an open wound. Gel is essential in such a case. Rubber bands hold the bag firmly and keep the gel against the transducer.
5. *Extension cord.* This is sometimes necessary in intensive care units where many sockets are being used for other equipment.

OPERATIVE ULTRASOUND

The use of ultrasound in the operating room requires the use of a small-headed transducer such as a sector scanner or a high-frequency linear array. A linear array device can be used in the liver and the kidney. Sector scanners are needed for bile duct and neurosonography work where only a small incision is made.

Insertion of a neonatal intracranial shunt is possible without a sterile transducer using the anterior fontanelle as described in Chapter 40.

For use in other body regions the transducer must be placed within a sterile bag, and the sonographer must put on sterile garb. It is therefore essential to be informed about an operative procedure at least 15 minutes beforehand. Sterile tube gauze is placed over the transducer cable, and the transducer head is dropped into a sterile plastic bag, which has already had acoustic gel placed within it. The sonographer must use the transducer within the limited area of the operative incision. Orientation is often difficult, and practice is required.

SELECTED READING

Blake, D. Use of Ultrasound in Radiotherapy. In M. F. Resnick and R. C. Sanders (Eds.), *Ultrasound in Urology*. Baltimore: Williams & Wilkins, 1979.

Brascho, D. J. Radiation therapy planning with ultrasound. *Radiol. Clin. North Am.* 13:505, 1975.

43. EQUIPMENT CARE AND QUALITY CONTROL

ROGER C. SANDERS
IRMA L. WHEELOCK

KEY WORDS

X-Y Axis. Transverse axis.

Azimuth. Depth axis.

Misregistration. System failure to plot the echo pattern accurately. For a compound scan this means superimposition of the image and incorrect calculation of the distance the echo has traveled.

Registration. The superimposition of a two-dimensional image on the TV screen in the X-Y and azimuth axes.

Resolution. Ability of a system to distinguish closely spaced targets. Lateral resolution is transverse to the beam (width), axial resolution is along the beam axis (depth).

SUAR. Phantom-sensitivity Uniformity Axial Resolution phantom (obtainable from R.M.I., Middleton, Wisconsin).

THE CLINICAL PROBLEM

Ultrasound systems are like people. They don't respond well to rough treatment or lack of attention. Certain day-to-day practical equipment checks decrease the downtime and increase the quality of the image.

Preventive Maintenance

1. Be careful if you must store oil or couplant on equipment. Spills may cause serious equipment problems.
2. Cables and transducers should be inspected visually for worn areas or cracks. These may be potential safety hazards or the causes of intermittent malfunctions.
3. Air filters should be cleaned periodically (weekly). They can usually be removed, cleaned with soap and water, and replaced. Neglect may cause equipment to overheat owing to decreased airflow.

Warm Up

When a multiformat camera, B-scanner, or real-time system is first turned on, there is a period during which images vary in brightness. Most systems require approximately a half hour to become stable. Many practitioners recommend leaving the systems on all the time so that problems with warm-up time do not occur. However, we suggest turning the systems off each night as well as over weekends because an unexpected breakdown in the air conditioning could give rise to major overheating problems. Analog scan converters should be turned off every evening because leaving them on shortens life expectancy.

Transducers

Transducers require careful handling. Dropping them sometimes damages the crystal or the backing used to damp the unwanted vibrations. Transducers should be cleaned between uses for different patients with an alcohol sponge, particularly if the patient has an open wound or a skin problem. Do not submerse transducers in liquid, especially if they are real-time transducers; most have to be gas-sterilized if used for sterile procedures.

Contact Agents

Use mineral oil as a couplant to ensure good acoustic contact between transducer and patient for B-scan studies. With real-time systems, use one of the commercial gels because some real-time transducers are damaged by mineral oil. In addition, if the patient is examined in a sitting or erect position, mineral oil does not adhere adequately. It is desirable to heat mineral oil or gel in a commercially available heating device. However, make sure that there is enough oil or gel in the container because oil can be overheated if only a small amount is present. Do not leave oil warmers on indefinitely because these pose a potential fire hazard. Use disposable gloves to place oil or gel on the patient to avoid the risk of infection and the possibility of oil getting into the electronic mechanism if oil-covered hands are used to alter the controls.

Quality Assurance

Quality assurance is a nuisance and is tedious to perform but is worthwhile because it is difficult or even impossible to detect major calibration and measurement distortions from examination of the image alone. Clearly, major clinical problems can occur if erroneous measurement data are produced. Incipient component breakdown can be detected before it occurs in some instances. Quality assurance checks should be performed on a weekly to monthly basis.

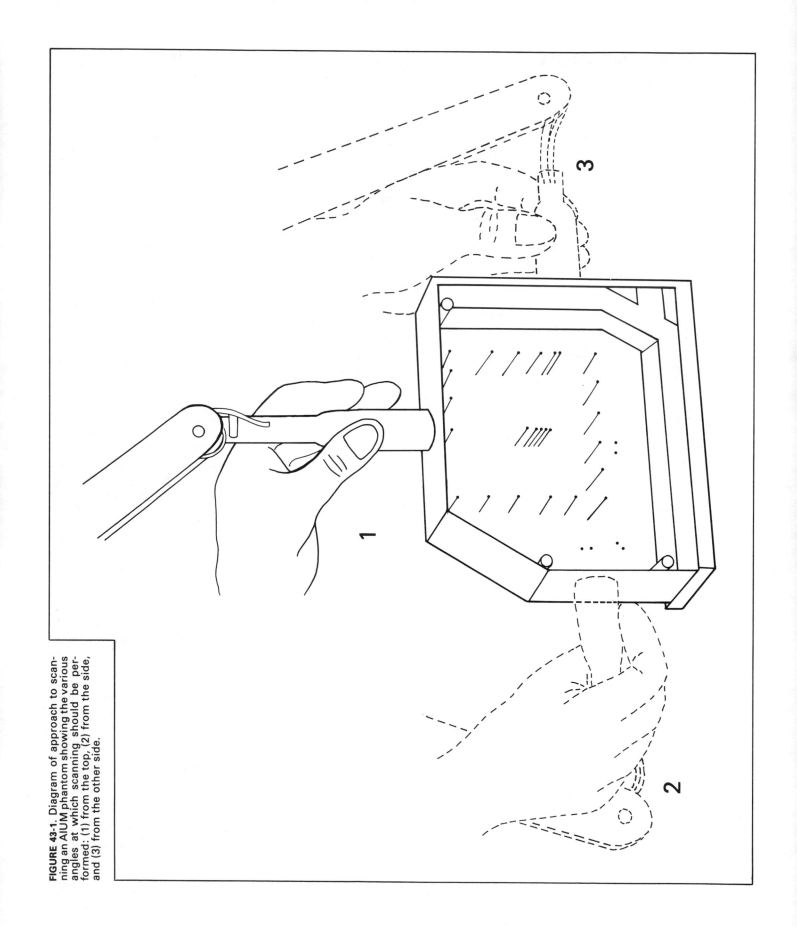

FIGURE 43-1. Diagram of approach to scanning an AIUM phantom showing the various angles at which scanning should be performed: (1) from the top, (2) from the side, and (3) from the other side.

Practical Use of a Test Object (AIUM Phantom)

1. Place the test object on flat surface.
2. Adjust the position of the test object so that you can easily scan all four surfaces.
3. Apply gel to surfaces; oil is ineffective on a flat, hard surface.
4. Use reproducible equipment settings (i.e., gain, TGC, transducer) for comparison with previous or future testing. Gain (output) should be as low as possible in order to visualize the pins well without reverberations. Use the largest field-of-view that will allow you to image the whole test object. Scan across the top surface (Fig. 43-1).

Superimpose the image of the pins seen from the top surface scan with those viewed from the other sides of the object (Fig. 43-2). The echoes recorded from the pins in all planes should form an asterisk (*). If there is more than a 5-mm separation between cross points, the system should be serviced to adjust the registration (Fig. 43-3).

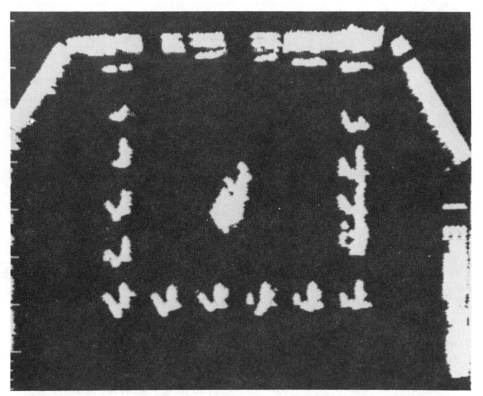

FIGURE 43-2. Diagram of the AIUM phantom showing adequate calibration. The sections performed from all angles intersect to form a cross.

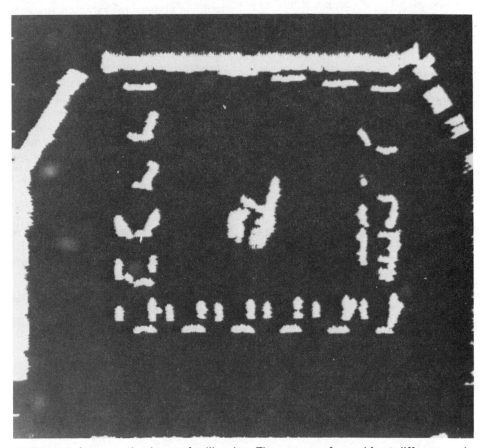

FIGURE 43-3. A system that is out of calibration. The scans performed from different angles do not intersect.

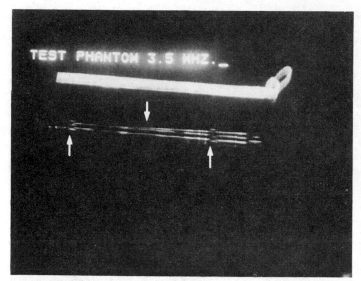

FIGURE 43-4. Scan obtained on a SUAR phantom. The bumps that mark the two ends of the scale can be seen (arrows). The two lines intersect half way along (middle arrow) in a normal fashion.

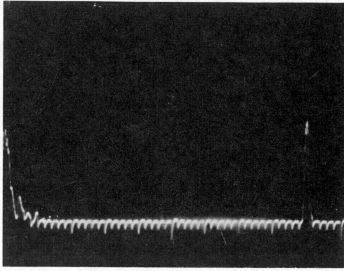

FIGURE 43-5. A-mode study showing the level of db at which an A-mode echo can be seen.

Calibration Tests for Scaling

1. Project depth markers (centimeter markers) *down* the center of the field and *across* the center of the field in the form of a cross on a 1 : 1 scale.
2. Take a photograph (multi-image or Polaroid). Place calipers on the photograph and measure the distance between the 1-to-1 dots along vertical and horizontal planes at many locations.
3. Place the caliper measurement against a centimeter ruler or scale. The measurements for all locations should be between 0.65 and 0.70 cm for the 1-to-1 scale.
4. Repeat the depth marker projections, photographs, and caliper measurements for 2 : 1, 3 : 1, and 4 : 1 scales.
5. Record all the data and verify that all scaling distances are correct. If they are not, the screen of the photographic system is out of proportion and needs adjustment.

Axial Resolution

Scan the ramp pattern of the SUAR test phantom with a 3.5-MHz transducer. The results of this scan will check the axial resolution of the system. Use the minimum output power needed to see the lower edge of the ramp clearly with no reverberations (Fig. 43-4). Axial resolution is the ability to see two closely spaced objects as the walls of the ramp merge together. The limit of the spacing will determine the point of separation. This point will be defined as the limit of axial resolution. Take a picture of this display and measure and record the smallest vertical area that is clearly seen.

The ramp spacing is 2.25 mm at the bump on the right and zero at the left bump. The distance between bumps is 10 cm (Fig. 43-4). If the spacing between the upper area of the ramp and the lower area merges halfway between these bumps, the axial resolution is about 1.1 mm. If it merges two thirds of the way toward the zero bump, the axial resolution is about 0.7 mm.

Equipment Sensitivity Test

1. With a 2.25-MHz transducer, scan the 16-cm direction of the SUAR test phantom.
2. Adjust the output (db output) and, using minimum TGC correction, establish when the echo from the far side (16-cm depth) is just barely displayed on the A-mode display (Fig. 43-5).
3. Record the db output.

This test establishes equipment sensitivity. Take an A-mode Polaroid picture to verify the results and mark the db output number on this picture for recordkeeping (Fig. 43-5).

SELECTED READING

Goldstein, A. Quality Assurance and Routine Preventive Maintenance. In Wells, P. N. T. and Ziskin, M. (Eds.), *New Techniques and Instrumentation in Ultrasonography.* New York: Churchill Livingstone, 1980.

Kremkau, F. *Diagnostic Ultrasound: Physical Principles and Exercises.* New York: Grune & Stratton, 1980.

44. PHOTOGRAPHY

ROGER C. SANDERS
MIMI MAGGIO

KEY WORDS

Brightness. Controls the degree of intensity of the CRT background

Cathode Ray Tube (CRT). The sonographic image is displayed on the screen of a cathode ray tube. A second CRT is used to display the A-mode. A third CRT displays the image for the multiformat camera.

Contrast. Controls the amount of gray level echoes seen, that is, how many medium- and low-level echoes are visible.

F-Stop. Controls the aperture of the lens; the wider it is, the more light is presented to the film, but the lower the F-stop number.

T (time). Sets the time interval of exposure (i.e., 0.5 second, 1 second, and so on).

SETTING UP THE CAMERA

Setting the photographic controls on the ultrasound system is one of the most important and difficult parts of obtaining a satisfactory long-term record of the examination. Subtle changes in brightness and contrast will greatly alter the image. Although observation of the graybars helps in setting up the image, a clinical scan showing an area such as the liver and kidney, where there are both high and low-level echoes, is of more value. A tissue-equivalent phantom that has pseudo metastatic and cystic lesions within it can also be used. Ideally, only one variable should be changed at a time (i.e., the background is adjusted for optimum brightness and the contrast is then varied for proper echo levels superimposed on this brightness level), but this is not entirely practical. The adjustment of either brightness or contrast could change the background. Adjust the camera CRT to display an acceptable image and then vary the F-stop and time to capture the proper image on film.

Practical Maneuvers

MULTIFORMAT CAMERA

1. Lower the background and contrast all the way. Select the mode (black or white background) that you wish to display.
2. Find the optimal background display by changing the brightness level. Small variations in settings are made with no image on the screen until an acceptable background for white or black is seen. Note the setting on the light meter; take films at various settings around this point.
3. Put graybars on the screen, and adjust the brightness until the light meter reads equivalent to the background.
4. Move the contrast to a level at which all graybars can be seen at the same time, keeping the background brightness at an optimal level, perhaps by reducing the brightness slightly.
5. Obtain a good quality image of the liver and right kidney on a longitudinal view.
6. Now vary the contrast and compensate with the brightness until you achieve an optimal setting. Photograph each setting and record the different levels. Unfortunately, both controls usually need to be varied at the same time.
7. Once the ideal photographic settings have been obtained, lock and record them (Fig. 44-1A–C). It takes time to set up a camera correctly, and a casual knob-fiddler can destroy an hour's work.

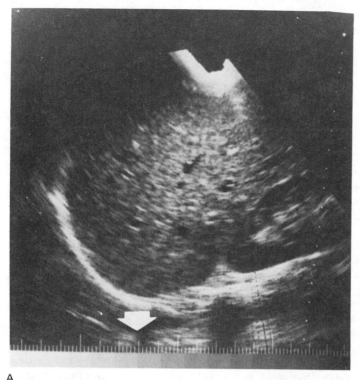

A

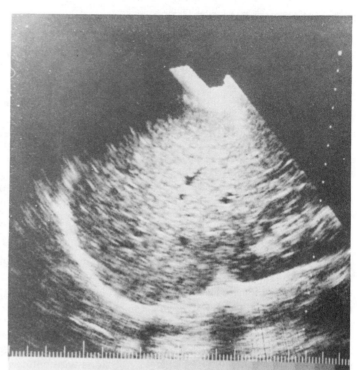

B

FIGURE 44-1. Obtaining correct photographic settings. A. A satisfactory photographic image. Note the gray scale bars (arrow). B. Excessive brightness. Compare the gray scale bars with those in A. C. Incorrect contrast settings with suboptimal graybar display.

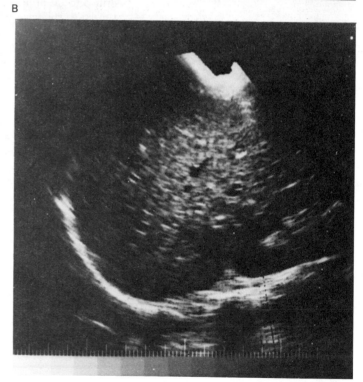

C

WARM-UP PROBLEMS

With analog scan converters, there may be some drift in the brightness and contrast during the course of the day, which makes it difficult to fix the settings. This is less of a problem with digital scan converters. Warm-up time adjustments should be avoided by making sure that the scanner and multiformat camera have been turned on a half hour before they are adjusted or used.

POLAROID CAMERA

Technique is different on Polaroid cameras; the F-stop and time must be adjusted (shutter speed). The F-stop on Polaroid cameras has an opposite effect on film from that in a multi-format camera because it is a positive image. A decrease in the F-stop number brightens the picture.

PHOTOGRAPHIC SYSTEMS

Several different methods of recording the image are in use; each has its virtues and disadvantages.

Polaroid Camera

Polaroid has the following advantages: The camera is cheap and easy to use, film development is rapid, and resolution is almost as good as that with the CRT image. However, the film is costly, it fades with time, and is difficult to store. Camera settings are not easy to maintain. With approximately three patients a day and an average number of films, one can save the price of a multiformat camera during the course of a year by not using Polaroid film.

Multiformat Cameras

Multiformat cameras have the following advantages: They use relatively cheap film, the film is easy to store and view, and exposures are relatively easy to set. However, the initial purchase of a multiformat camera is expensive, a processor is required, and personnel are needed to handle the film, chemicals, and so on.

Multiformat cameras come with various features, some of which are well worth having. The smaller and more compact versions are as cheap as the larger systems and are preferable because they can be placed on a portable real-time system. One feature that is unimportant is whether the system is "on axis" (i.e., whether the lens lines up with the CRT image directly), nor is a variable format system of much practical importance because the sonographer almost always uses the same settings (usually six on one film). This format displays an image of satisfactory size, but nine images on one film will provide optimum cost savings.

There are several important features in the choice of a multiformat camera.

1. Rapid exposure time
2. Compact size
3. A labeling system (if none is available on the system being photographed)
4. A method of preventing double exposure
5. Convenient brightness and contrast controls (not buried inside the camera)
6. A "flat-face" screen (which means that a measurement at the periphery of the image will be reliable)

70- to 100-Millimeter Camera

Cameras using 70- to 100-mm film are cheaper than multiformat cameras but less convenient. The advantages of these systems are that the film is very inexpensive and more than six exposures can be made without changing the film or cassette. However, the system needs a processor. It is inconvenient to photograph a single patient because the roll of film takes many more pictures, and storage is difficult.

DAY-TO-DAY CARE OF CAMERA

Multiformat cameras are not very sturdy and can easily malfunction if mistreated. An important part of practical maintenance is keeping the air filters clean (check daily for dust accumulation). Do not put the multiformat camera in too confined a space because it will tend to overheat. The internal monitor must be adjusted periodically to maintain optimum photographic capability.

Maintenance of Polaroid cameras requires cleaning the rollers with an alcohol swab on a more or less daily basis. The rollers are easily detachable from most Polaroid cameras. Do not unwrap Polaroid film before it is to be used because humidity and heat decrease the sensitivity of the film. Develop the film within a few minutes. If the film is left undeveloped for longer than this, it adheres to the film back. Pull the Polaroid tab straight through the rollers or streaks will occur on the image and paper segments will break off in the rollers.

FILM FOR MULTIFORMAT CAMERAS

There is a choice of film that can be used with multiformat cameras. All manufacturers make both a film with a clear base and one with a blue-green base. We prefer the clear base because we think there is a chance that low-level echoes will be overlooked against a blue-green background, but many feel that the blue-green format is more attractive.

Silver-Coated Paper

Some systems use standard multiformat cameras but use silver-coated paper instead of film. Because paper cannot be viewed through a viewbox, this system is cumbersome for teaching large groups. However, this method is acceptable if showing the image to an audience is not part of your practice because paper is inexpensive and is easily stored.

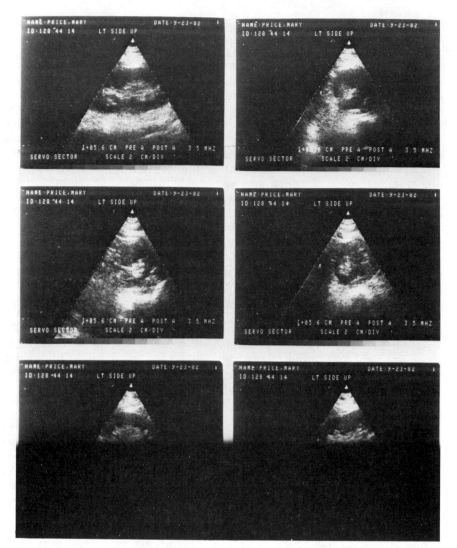

FIGURE 44-2. This film has been partially exposed to light. Check the cassette for cracks and light leaks.

PHOTOGRAPHIC PROBLEMS

1. *Fogging* along the edge of the film may occur (Fig. 44-2). Either the cassette has not been pushed completely into the multiformat camera or there is a light leak along one edge of the cassette. Cassettes are fragile and develop light leaks with rough usage.

2. There may be *white marks* on the film (when using white on black mode), which appear in the same place on sequential films (Fig. 44-3). Dust is present on the camera lens or on the CRT face. Clean the camera.

3. The *film won't expose,* although it seems to be in a good position. Push the cassette properly into its housing.

4. The film may be *unexpectedly dark or light* (Figs. 44-4A,B). The possibilities are (a) that the multiformat camera or ultrasound system has not warmed up, (b) the wrong type of film is in the cassette, (c) the processor has not been warmed up, (d) the developing mixture is wrong, or (e) someone has altered the camera settings.

5. If the processed image is crisscrossed with *diagonal lines* (Fig. 44-5), the horizontal hold of the CRT is out of adjustment. You won't be aware of this unless you look at the camera monitor.

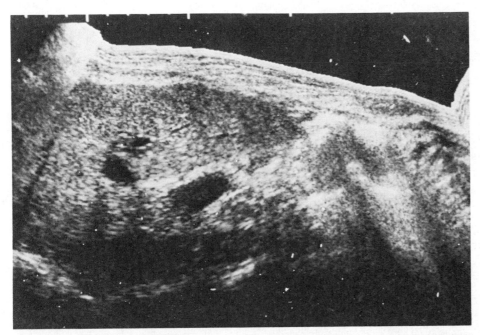

FIGURE 44-3. White marks due to dust on the lens will appear on sequential films in the same area.

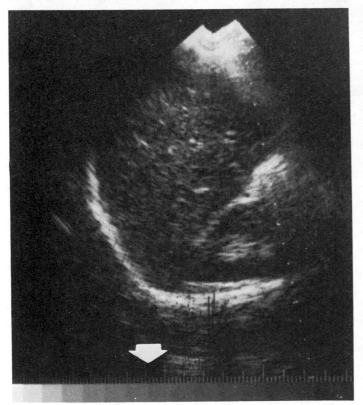

A

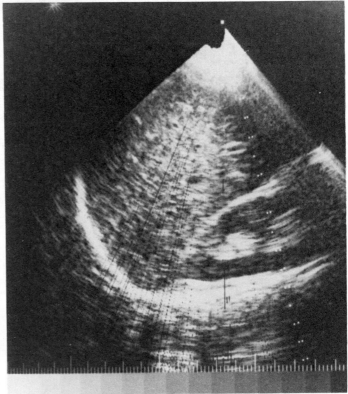

B

FIGURE 44-4. Background problems. A. If the camera is not warmed up, the background will be too dark. Note the suboptimal gray scale. B. The camera is now warmed up. Compare this gray scale with that in A.

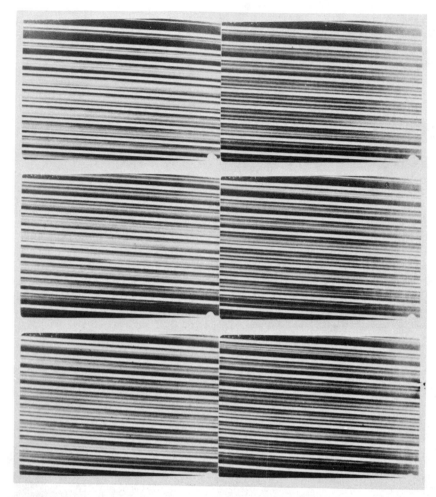

FIGURE 44-5. Diagonal linear artifact usually due to defective horizontal hold on the CRT.

45. ARTIFACTS

ROGER C. SANDERS
MIMI MAGGIO

SONOGRAM ABBREVIATIONS

Bl   Bladder

D   Diaphragm

E   Echoes

GBl   Gallbladder

K   Kidney

L   Liver

P   Pleural effusion

RK   Right kidney

T   Tornado effect

Ut   Uterus

KEY WORDS

Azimuth. Depth axis.

Comet Tail. Artifact due to strong interface in which there is a thin line of echoes within an essentially echo-free area.

Grating Artifacts. Curvilinear artifact seen either in front or behind a strong interface with linear arrays.

Lateral Beam Spread. Widening of the transducer focus as the beam passes through tissue depth.

Main Bang. High-level echo at the skin's surface due partly to the skin and partly to the transducer surface.

Noise. Spurious echoes throughout the image including areas such as the bladder that are known to be echo-free.

Reverberation. Artifactual linear echoes parallel to a strong interface. Sound is returned to the transducer and then into the tissues again.

Ring Down. A particular type of reverberation artifact in which numerous parallel echoes are seen for a considerable distance.

Side Lobes. Secondary off-axis concentrations of energy not parallel to the beam axis; degrades lateral resolution.

Tornado Effect. Artifact due to gas in which there is an absence of echoes with an irregular anterior border due to shadowing.

X-Y Axis. Horizontal axis (transverse axis).

THE PROBLEM

Artifacts in ultrasound can be classified into three categories:

1. *Artifacts related to instrument problems,* which occur when the equipment is not functioning satisfactorily.
2. *Technique-dependent artifacts,* in which the appearance is produced by unsatisfactory operator technique.
3. *Artifacts* that cannot be avoided because of the way in which *sound interacts with tissues.*

Each of these spurious sonographic appearances must be recognized so that the deceptive finding can be disregarded, eliminated, or used as a diagnostic aid.

ARTIFACTS CAUSED BY MALFUNCTION OF EQUIPMENT
Artifactual Noise

Artifactual noise is caused by electrical interference from nearby equipment (e.g., in an intensive care unit; Fig. 45-1).

RECOGNITION. Such "noise" has a repetitive pattern unlike the overall increase in echogenicity seen with too much gain. This type of noise produces a "pattern" over the normal ultrasound image.

CORRECTION TECHNIQUE. Equipment modification can prevent such interference if it occurs in the ultrasound laboratory. You may be able to disconnect the interfering equipment during the scan.

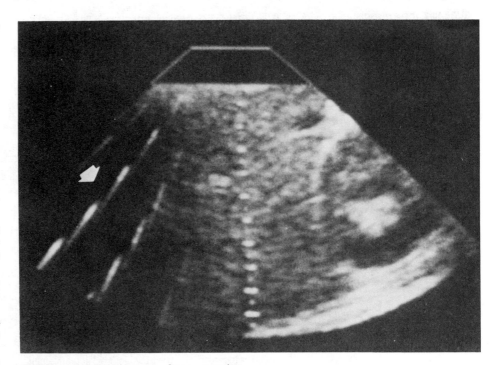

FIGURE 45-1. Interference from nearby equipment causes artifacts on the CRT (arrow).

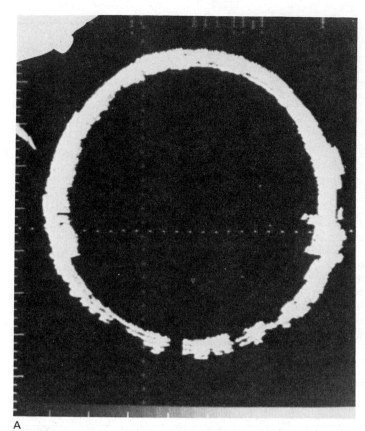

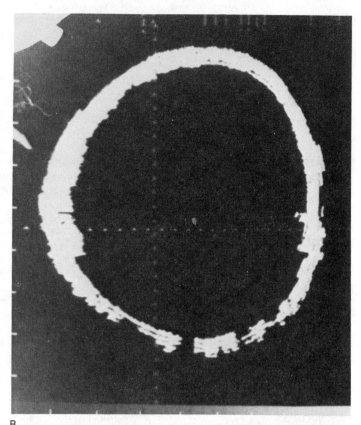

A

B

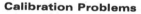

FIGURE 45-2. Incorrect distance markers. A. Normal X-Y dimension image. The spacing of the centimeter marks in both directions is equal. B. X axis is compressed, causing measurements in that direction to be inaccurate. The 1-cm markers in the vertical axis are farther apart than the horizontal 1-cm markers. C. The Y axis is elongated, causing wrong measurements in the vertical axis. The horizontal 1-cm spacing is normal, but the vertical spacing is stretched.

Calibration Problems

INCORRECT DISTANCE MARKERS

Although not apparent on the image, subsequent measurements using another ultrasonic system or phantom may show erroneous caliper measurements.

DIAGNOSTIC CONFUSION. Measurements such as the biparietal diameter may be wrong with tragic clinical consequences (Fig. 45-2A–C).

RECOGNITION. Only by comparison with other systems or by calibration check can such subtle measurement changes be detected.

CORRECTION TECHNIQUE. Calibration checks should be performed frequently (once/month); measurements should be performed in the center of the image where calibration is most correct and not at the edge of the video monitor.

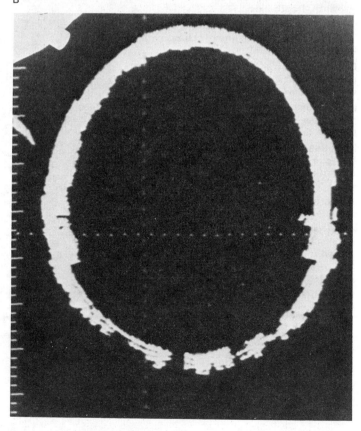

C

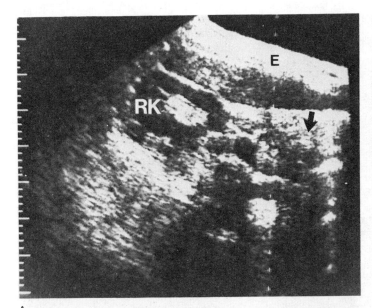

A

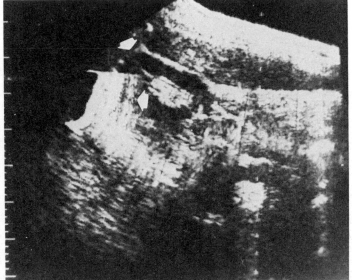

B

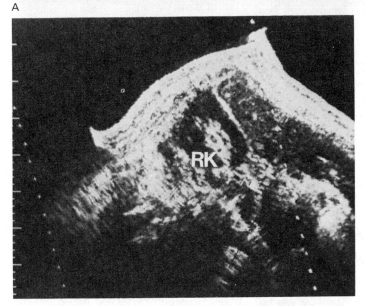

C

**LATERAL PLANE DISTORTION
(X-Y AXIS MISCALIBRATION,
MISREGISTRATION, AND MISALIGNMENT)**

There will be marked distortion of the shape of an organ, causing a round structure to look oval.

DIAGNOSTIC CONFUSION. Organs will assume the wrong shape and look oval rather than round.

RECOGNITION. It will be impossible to scan from either side of the abdomen with a static scanner because two images will not intersect. Quite severe X-Y axis distortion may be present before it is obvious on the scan (Fig. 45-3A–C).

CORRECTION TECHNIQUE. Weekly calibration will show this problem early. A serviceman will be needed to correct it.

FIGURE 45-3. Misregistration. A. Transverse view of the right kidney (RK) scanning in one direction. Note gas-filled bowel to the right of the kidney (arrow) and echoes (E) from main bang artifact at the skin. B. Scanning the right kidney but angling from the other direction. Note the distortion of the kidney borders (arrows) due to misregistration (arrows). C. There is no distortion of the right kidney (RK). Registration is now in alignment. Note irregular shadowing due to gas in bowel adjacent to the kidney.

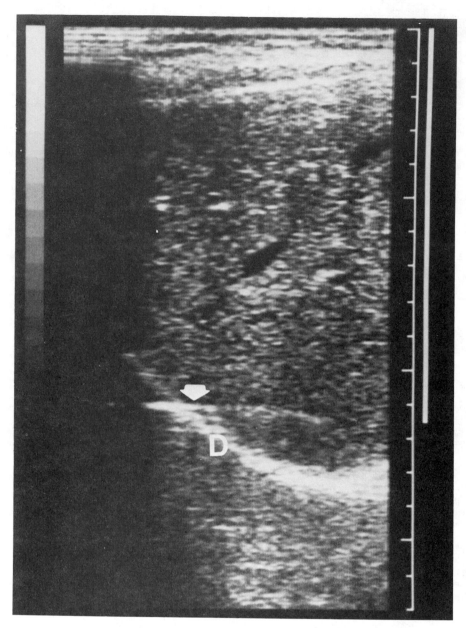

FIGURE 45-4. A grating artifact (arrow) may sometimes occur above or below a strong linear interface (e.g., the diaphragm, D) when using an array system, particularly a linear array.

Focus Problems

With analog systems, poor focusing causes a fuzzy image.

RECOGNITION. Dot markers on the screen are magnified, and the dot boundaries are fuzzy and oval.

CORRECTION TECHNIQUE. Call for service; you may need a new scan converter.

Main Bang Artifact

There are many echoes from the skin-transducer interface in the immediate subcutaneous tissues (Fig. 45-3A). There is such a strong interface between the skin and the transducer that it is almost impossible to avoid this problem completely.

DIAGNOSTIC CONFUSION. Subcutaneous and skin lesions will be hidden within the main bang artifact.

CORRECTION TECHNIQUE. A higher frequency transducer diminishes the problem. Decrease the near field gain. Use of a water bath will avoid a main bang artifact to some extent (see Chapter 33).

Grating Artifact

A line occurs either above or below a strong linear interface with array systems, particularly linear arrays (Fig. 45-4).

DIAGNOSTIC CONFUSION. An apparent septum may be present within an amniotic sac or other cystic process.

RECOGNITION. This septum is usually related to a strong acoustic interface about halfway down the linear array field.

CORRECTION TECHNIQUE. Imaging with a different system such as a B-scanner will show that the supposed echo is artifactual.

ARTIFACTS CAUSED BY TECHNIQUE

Noise

Noise may be created by excess gain (Fig. 45-5). Gain may be turned up to a point where low-level echoes occur in unstructured fluid-filled areas such as the bladder.

DIAGNOSTIC CONFUSION. Excess gain may give the impression that the cystic lesion contains internal material or is solid.

RECOGNITION. All structures will be echogenic at the same depth. Comparison with a known cystic structure such as the urinary bladder will help in deciding whether possible noise is a technical artifact or a real structure.

CORRECTION TECHNIQUE. Decrease gain without losing structural information.

Transducer Selection Problems

TIME GAIN COMPENSATION PROBLEMS

Artifacts created by poor time gain compensation (TGC) technique are common (see Chapter 4). Extra echoes or too few echoes may be introduced owing to wrong use of the TGC curve. Numerous echoes may be created in superficial structures and none in deep structures and vice versa (Fig. 45-5). This appearance may also be caused by the wrong choice of transducer with the result that the focal zone and frequency concentrate on superficial structures.

DIAGNOSTIC CONFUSION. Wrong TGC settings may give rise to apparent anterior placenta previa, creation of a pseudocystic superficial lesion, or masking of a problem by too many echoes.

RECOGNITION. The relative area of increased or decreased echoes extends beyond the natural tissue boundaries.

CORRECTION TECHNIQUE. Observe the principles of TGC usage discussed in Chapter 4.

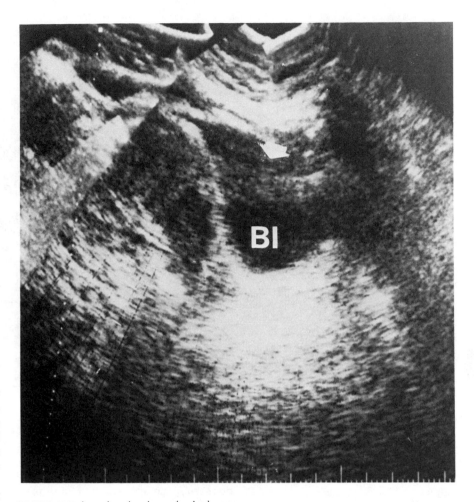

FIGURE 45-5. Low-level echoes (noise) seen in the anterior part (arrow) of the fluid-filled bladder (Bl).

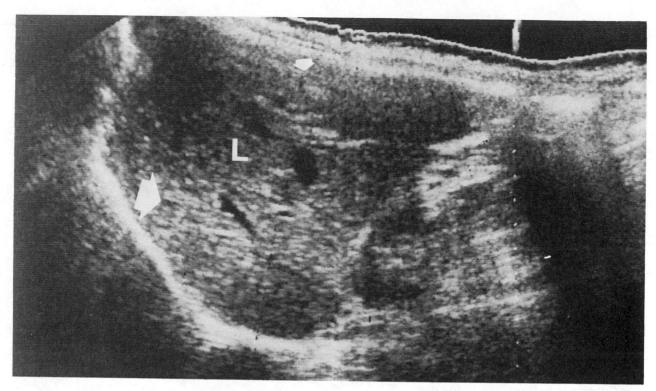

Transducer Artifacts

FRESNEL ZONE ARTIFACT (NEAR FIELD)

The near field of view of a transducer is not imaged ideally because of wave distortion and lack of focusing.

DIAGNOSTIC CONFUSION. An artifactual area exists, for example, in the superficial portion of the liver using standard 3.5-MHz medium focus transducers because the first 1 to 3 cm of the field are distorted by an unequal waveform (Fig. 45-6). Fine echoes in this area usually have no anatomic basis.

CORRECTION TECHNIQUE. The use of a water bath when scanning superficial structures is helpful in correcting this problem and in eliminating the anterior reverberation artifact created from the skin line. Moving the transducer back from the skin surface moves the area of interest into the focal zone. In addition, a short-focus, high-frequency transducer will diminish the extent of the problem.

BEAM DEPTH PROBLEMS

Artifacts will be present beyond the focal zone of the transducer in the far part of the field (Fig. 45-6). The echoes in this region are much coarser, and major lesions may be missed if a long-focus transducer is not used. Because considerable lateral beam spread occurs, small pinpoint structures appear as transverse lines.

DIAGNOSTIC CONFUSION. Subtle small lesions may be missed because of the coarse echogenic structure at depth (e.g., small metastases in the liver).

CORRECTION TECHNIQUE. These artifacts are unavoidable even with the correct TGC settings if the transducer is not changed to one with a more appropriate focal zone.

FIGURE 45-6. The near portion of this liver (L) contains much artifactual information owing to beam distortion (small arrow). A "banding" effect occurs in the midportion of the field because this is the site of maximal focus (large arrow).

BANDING

By using a finely focused transducer or excessively deep anterior time gain compensation suppression, it is easy to create an area of banding across the image (Fig. 45-6). At a standard distance from the transducer face the structures will be more echogenic than structures anterior and posterior to it.

DIAGNOSTIC CONFUSION. The impression of a mass may be created because there are more echoes in the area of banding, for example, a liver metastasis.

CORRECTION TECHNIQUE. Use a transducer with a different frequency and focus and alter the time gain compensation settings.

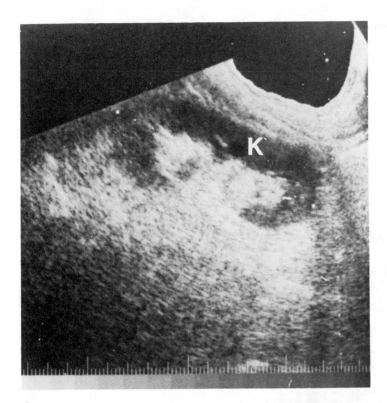

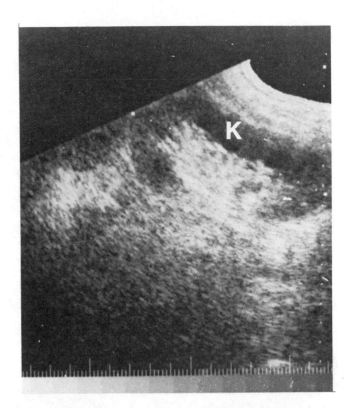

A

B

FIGURE 45-7. Breathing artifacts. A. Allowing the patient to breathe elongates the kidney (K) to 11 cm. B. When the patient holds his breath, the kidney measures 10.4 cm.

Artifacts Caused by Movement

BREATHING

If the patient varies inspiration over the course of a B-scan, the image will be distorted and blurred because part of it will be examined on inspiration and part on expiration.

DIAGNOSTIC CONFUSION. When scanning a kidney, shortening or lengthening may occur if the patient breathes during the scan (Fig. 45-7A,B). The diaphragm and adjacent liver may be interrupted and blurred if the patient takes a breath in the middle of the scan (Fig. 45-8).

CORRECTION TECHNIQUE. Ask the patient to hold his breath.

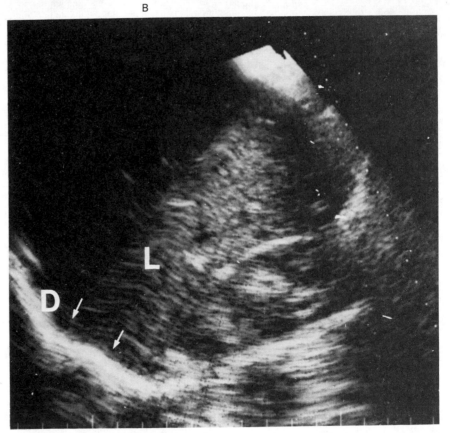

FIGURE 45-8. If the patient is breathing during a scan, the diaphragm (D) may be distorted or blurred (arrows). L = Liver.

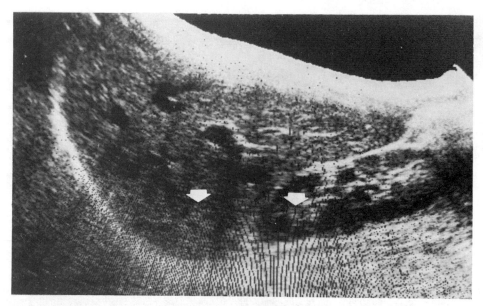

FIGURE 45-9. Drop-out lines (arrows) are created when the scanning speed is too rapid.

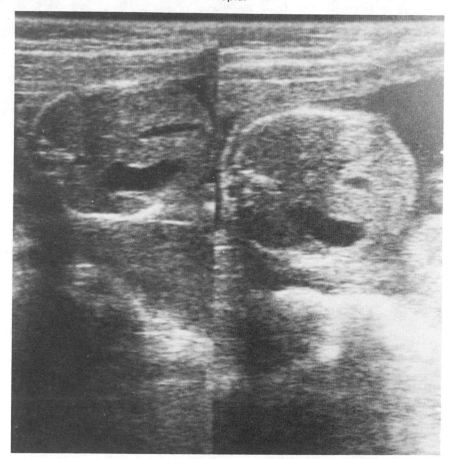

A   B

FIGURE 45-10. Pressure artifacts. A. Too much pressure over the fetal trunk produces a flattened ovoid shape. B. A lighter scanning pressure creates a round trunk and correct measurements.

OPERATOR SCANNING SPEED

If the sonographer scans rapidly, artifacts known as drop-out lines are created (Fig. 45-9). These drop-out lines are seen frequently with analog B-scan units. Most digital units can receive information rapidly enough to avoid this artifact. Some units appear to have gaps between the lines of the image because they have not been "smoothed." Computer processing can eliminate these little gaps between beam lines in a cosmetic but uninformative fashion (i.e., the gaps are filled in with false echoes).

CORRECTION TECHNIQUE. Perform the scan at a lower speed.

OPERATOR PRESSURE

Applying too much or uneven pressure while scanning can distort the image.

DIAGNOSTIC CONFUSION. Scanning the fetal trunk with too much pressure with a linear array may cause a flattened ovoid shape rather than the preferred round trunk (Fig. 45-10).

CORRECTION TECHNIQUE. Use only sufficient pressure to keep the transducer in contact with the skin.

COMPOUNDING

Often the best way to complete a B-scan is to form numerous small sector scans to create one overall image. At the junction of the small sector scans artifact is created because the transducer can be accurately aligned only rarely (see Fig. 45-12).

DIAGNOSTIC CONFUSION. The intersection of two sector scans can be thought to represent a pathologic process.

CORRECTION TECHNIQUES. Repeat the scan using a smoother technique. Recognition of the artifact is possible if one observes where the transducer skin lines join.

Photographic Artifacts

Photographic artifacts are a major problem. If the contrast is set incorrectly, subtle metastatic lesions may be lost in the overall grayness of the image. Undue brightness may also obscure subtle textural alterations (see Chapter 44).

ARTIFACTS CAUSED BY SOUND-TISSUE INTERACTIONS

Artifacts from Strongly Reflective Structures (Shadowing)

Gas, bone, and, to a much lesser extent, muscle do not conduct sound well. When sound strikes a strong interface such as gas or bone, one of two responses may be produced. Either there is no sound conduction through the area (shadowing), or numerous secondary reverberations are produced, causing a series of echogenic lines extending into the tissues (ring down).

DIAGNOSTIC CONFUSION. Large shadowing artifacts may obscure a deep pathologic process (e.g., nodes).

RECOGNITION. The reverberation pattern seen with bone is a series of alternating lines (Fig. 45-11A), whereas that seen with gas is usually a more diffuse, vaguely outlined pattern with considerable noise (Fig. 45-3A, "tornado" effect), although a linear series of bands may also be seen with gas—the "comet" effect (Fig. 45-11B).

CORRECTION TECHNIQUE. The sonographer should attempt to scan around gas or bone, obtaining scans of the areas below these structures from an oblique angle.

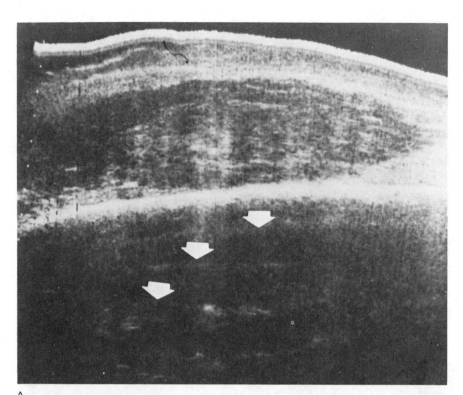

A

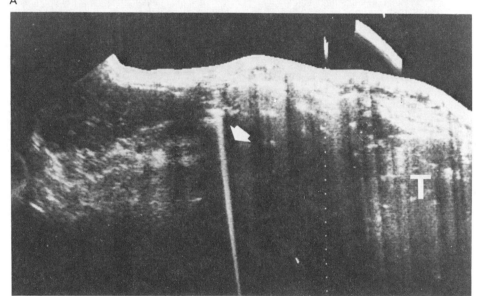

B

FIGURE 45-11. Reverberation artifacts. A. A longitudinal scan of the thigh. Notice the reverberations (alternating lines) extending below the bone interface (arrows). B. Gas may cause the creation of a line of reverberation echoes (arrow), the "comet" effect, or a vague sonolucent area of acoustic shadowing , the tornado effect (T).

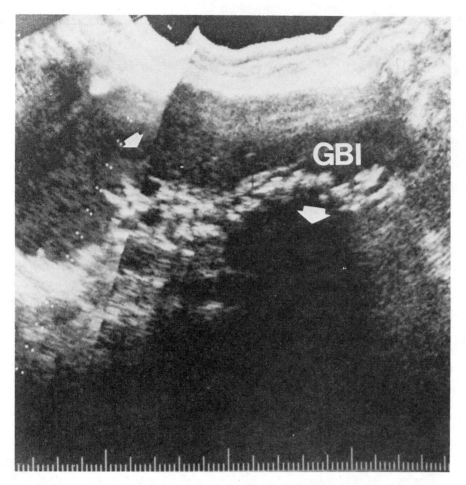

FIGURE 45-12. Large acoustic interfaces due to gallstones are associated with shadowing (large arrow). Note the artifact caused by compound scanning; the image is not aligned (small arrow).

BENEFIT. Shadowing will occur when the sound beam hits a highly reflective surface such as gallstones (Fig. 45-12), renal stones, or surgical clips, allowing a diagnosis of an acoustically dense structure. The shadowing can be made more obvious by increasing the frequency of the transducer.

Reverberation Artifacts

Whenever sound passes out of a structure with an acoustic impedance that is markedly different from its neighbor, a large amount of sound is returned to the transducer. The amount of sound returning may be so great that it is sent from the transducer back into the tissues, causing a duplication of the original structure. The second wave has traveled twice as far as the first one, the third echo three times as far, and so forth. The distance between each successive echo will equal the distance between the original two interfaces (Fig. 45-13). The second echo and each successive echo parallel the original interface.

DIAGNOSTIC CONFUSION. Such reverberation artifacts are most commonly seen adjacent to the bladder anterior wall (Fig. 45-13) but also occur elsewhere in the body in soft tissue as well as fluid; they may mimic a mass.

RECOGNITION. Reverberation artifacts of this type may occur at some distance from the original interface (e.g., behind the posterior wall of the bladder). A second apparent bladder resembling fluid-filled bowel will lie where measurement shows the sacrum should lie (Fig. 45-14).

CORRECTION TECHNIQUE. Distinguishing such artifacts from real structures can be done by (1) using transducers of a different frequency, (2) bouncing the transducer on the abdominal wall and noticing that the second linear structure moves in exactly the same fashion as the strong echo nearest the transducer, and (3) scanning the same area from a different angle.

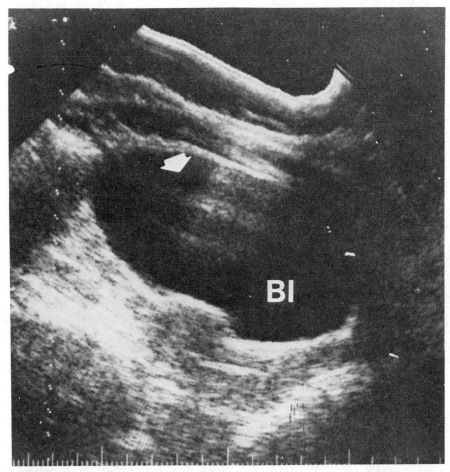

FIGURE 45-13. Eches due to reverberations are parallel to the anterior body wall (arrow) of the bladder (Bl).

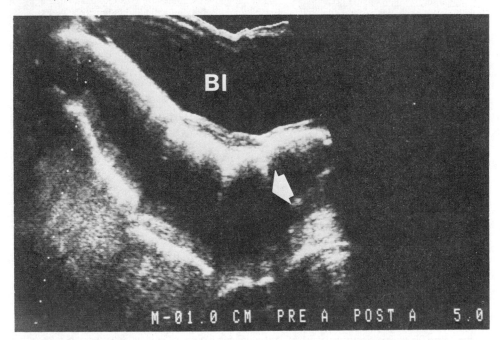

FIGURE 45-14. Reverberation artifact behind the posterior wall of the bladder (Bl) with creation of an apparent cystic lesion posterior to the bladder (arrow).

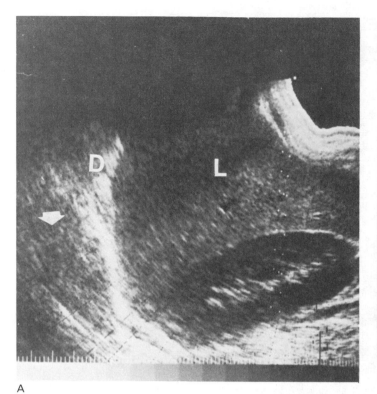

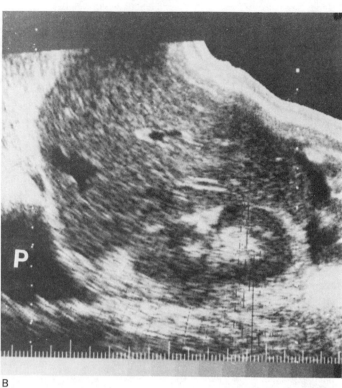

A

B

FIGURE 45-15. Mirror artifacts. A. In the normal patient there is a mirror image of the liver (L) tissue above the diaphragm (D) at the site of the lung (arrow). B. When there is a pleural effusion (P), an echo-free area is seen above the diaphragm.

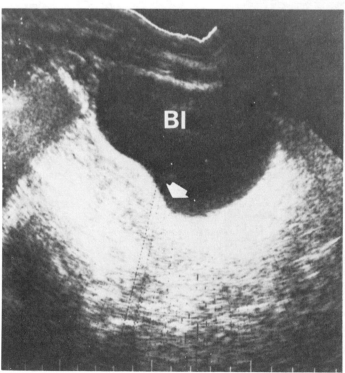

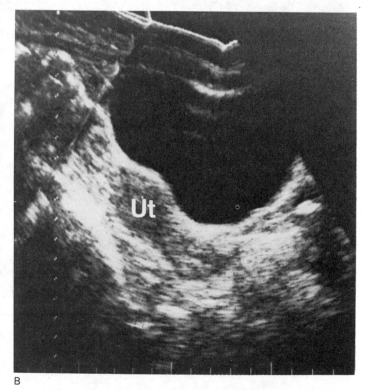

A

B

FIGURE 45-16. Enhancement effect. A. Increased echoes obscure the structures behind the bladder (Bl) owing to enhancement of the sound passing through the bladder (arrow). B. Decreasing the gain allows the uterus (Ut) to be seen clearly.

Mirror Artifacts

If a sonographic structure has a curved appearance, it may focus and reflect the sound like a mirror.

RECOGNITION. This problem occurs most commonly in the diaphragm. Theoretically, there should be no echoes from the lungs because they are full of gas, but in fact, there is a duplication of the structures within the liver above the diaphragm in all normal individuals (Fig. 45-15A). On the left this mirror image can create a false impression of a pleural effusion (see Fig. 38-4) because the diaphragm is also duplicated. This artifact occurs when the patient is scanned in an oblique axis in the coronal position.

BENEFIT. If this mirror image is absent, it can be deduced that a pleural effusion is present (Fig. 45-15B).

CORRECTION TECHNIQUE. Try to scan the same area from another position.

Enhancement Effect

As the sound beam passes through fluid-filled structures or structures containing many cysts, it will not be attenuated and there will be an increase in the amplitude (brightness) of the echoes distal to the fluid (Fig. 45-16A).

DIAGNOSTIC CONFUSION. A true pathologic condition may be obliterated by the increased gain distal to a fluid-filled structure (e.g., the uterus behind the bladder).

BENEFIT. Acoustic enhancement is almost always beneficial and may be useful in differentiating between solid and cystic lesions, in addition to aiding the sonographer in seeing deep structures.

CORRECTION TECHNIQUE. The sonographer should diminish the overall gain, adjust the TGC, and perform a compound scan (Fig. 45-16B). If the area of interest is behind a fluid-filled structure (e.g., a fibroid uterus behind the bladder), many echoes will occur within this area of acoustic enhancement.

Several small sector scans are desirable in such a case. With a single pass only the structures posterior to the bladder are enhanced. Using several small passes, areas not affected by enhancement can be scanned with gain increased, creating an overall cosmetic image.

SELECTED READING

Bartrum, R., and Crow, H. C. (Eds.). *A Manual for Physicians and Technical Personnel: Gray-Scale Ultrasound, Real-time in Ultrasound.* Philadelphia: Saunders, 1983.

Morley, P., Donald, G., and Sanders, R. (Eds.). *Ultrasonic Sectional Anatomy.* Melbourne: Churchill Livingstone, 1983.

APPENDIXES

APPENDIX 1.
Most Commonly Seen Abbreviations on Requisitions
PATRICIA MAY KAPLAN

AAA	Abdominal aortic aneurysm
Ab	Abortion
A's and B's	Apnea and bradycardia
AFM	After fatty meal
AFP	Alpha fetoprotein
ALL	Acute leukocytic leukemia
AML	Acute monocytic leukemia
A-Mode	Amplitude modulation
AODM	Adult onset of diabetes mellitus
AROM	Artificial rupture of membranes
ATB	Antibiotic
ATN	Acute tubular necrosis
BE	Barium enema
B-H	Braxton-Hicks' contraction
BIP (BPD)	Biparietal diameter
B-Mode	Brightness modulation
BMT	Bone marrow transplant
BP	Blood pressure
BPD (BIP)	Biparietal diameter
BPH	Benign prostatic hypertrophy
BSO	Bilateral salpingo-oophorectomy
BTD	Biliary tract disease
BUN	Blood urea nitrogen
Bx	Biopsy
C	Celsius (centigrade)
c̄	With
CBD	Common bile duct
CEC	Central echo complex
CHD	Common hepatic duct
cm	Centimeter
CML	Chronic myeloid leukemia
CNS	Central nervous system
Cr	Creatinine
CRT	Cathode ray tube
C/S	Cesarean section
CST	Contraction stress test
Cx	Cervix
db	Decibel
D & C	Dilatation and curettage
D = E	Dates equal exam
D = E = S	Dates equal exam equal sonogram
D ≠ E	Dates do not equal exam
D < E	Small for dates
D > E	Large for dates
DFHT	Documented fetal heart tone
D.T.'s	Delirium tremens
DTR	Deep tendon reflex
Dx	Diagnosis

EDC	Estimated date of confinement
EFW	Estimated fetal weight
ETOH'er	Ethanol (alcohol) abuser
EUA	Examination under anesthesia
F	Farenheit
FCD	Fibrocystic disease
FDIU	Fetal death in utero
FH	Fundal height, Fetal heart, or Family history
FSH	Follicle-stimulating hormone
FUO	Fever of unknown origin
FTT	Failure to thrive
G	Gravida
GB	Gallbladder
GI	Gastrointestinal
GTD	Gestational trophoblastic disease
GU	Genitourinary
GVHD	Graft versus host disease
Gyn	Gynecology
HBP	High blood pressure
HC	Hepatocellular, or Head circumference
HCG	Human chorionic gonadotropin
HCT	Hematocrit
HSM	Hepatosplenomegaly
Hydro	Hydrocephalus, or Hydronephrosis
IC	Iliac crest
IDDM	Insulin-dependent diabetes mellitus
IUCD (IUD)	Intrauterine contraceptive device
IUGR	Intrauterine growth retardation
IUP	Intrauterine pregnancy
IVC	Inferior vena cava
IVP	Intravenous pyelogram
JODM	Juvenile onset diabetes mellitus
K⁺	Potassium
LE	Lower extremity
LFT	Liver function test (e.g., SGPT, SGOT, alk phos)
LH	Luteinizing hormone
LIF	Long internal focus (transducer)

LK	Left kidney
LLQ	Left lower quadrant
LOLINAD	Little old lady in no apparent distress
LPO	Left posterior oblique
LSO	Left salpingo-oophorectomy
LSU	Left side up
LT	Ligamentum teres
LUQ	Left upper quadrant
MCA	Multiple congenital anomaly
MHz	Megahertz
MIF	Medium internal focus (transducer)
ML	Midline
mm	Millimeter
M-Mode	Time motion modulation
ΔMS	Altered mental status
N	Notch (sternal)
NEFG	Normal external female genitalia
NGT	Nasogastric tube
NPO	Nothing by mouth
NSS	Normal size and shape
NST	Nonstress test
NSVD	Normal spontaneous vaginal delivery
Ob	Obstetrics
OCT	Oxytocin challenge test
OCG	Oral cholecystogram
OR	Operating room
p̄	After
PA	Popliteal artery, or Popliteal aneurysm
Para 1234	(1) Number of full-term pregnancies, (2) number of premature births, (3) number of abortions, (4) number of living children
PE	Pleural effusion, or Pulmonary embolus
PID	Pelvic inflammatory disease
POD#	Post-op day (# __)
PP	Postpartum
PPD	Test for tuberculosis
PROM	Premature rupture of membranes
PSI	Postsaline injection
PT	Pregnancy test
PTA	Prior to admission
PTT	Prothrombin time
PUD	Peptic ulcer disease
PV	Portal vein

RBC Red blood cell
RCM Right costal margin
RK Right kidney
RLL Right lower lobe
RLQ Right lower quadrant
R/O Rule out
ROM Rupture of membranes
RPO Right posterior oblique
RSO Right salpingo-oophorectomy
RT Real-time (dynamic imaging)
RUQ Right upper quadrant
Rx Treatment
$\overline{S}$ Symphysis pubis (SP or P)
$\overline{s}$ Without

SBE Subacute bacterial endocarditis
SIF Short internal focus (transducer)
SMA Superior mesenteric artery
SMV Superior mesenteric vein
SVD Spontaneous vaginal delivery
TAB Therapeutic abortion
TAH Total abdominal hysterectomy
TC Trunk circumference
TCG Time compensation gain
TGC Time gain compensation
TIUV Total intrauterine volume
TOA Tubo-ovarian abscess

TURP Transurethral resection of prostate
TVH Total vaginal hysterectomy
Tx Transplant
U Umbilicus
UE Upper extremity
UGI Upper gastrointestinal series
UPJ Ureteropelvic junction
US Ultrasound
UTI Urinary tract infection
UVJ Ureterovesical junction
VTX vertex presentation
WBC White blood cell
X Xyphoid

APPENDIX 2.

Length of Fetal Long Bones (mm)

Week No.	Humerus Percentile			Ulna Percentile			Radius Percentile			Femur Percentile			Tibia Percentile			Fibula Percentile		
	5	50	95	5	50	95	5	50	95	5	50	95	5	50	95	5	50	95
11	—	6	—	—	5	—	—	5	—	—	6	—	—	4	—	—	2	—
12	3	9	10	—	8	—	—	7	—	—	9	—	—	7	—	—	5	—
13	5	13	20	3	11	18	—	10	—	6	12	19	4	10	17	—	8	—
14	5	16	20	4	13	17	8	13	15	5	15	19	2	13	19	6	11	10
15	11	18	26	10	16	22	12	15	19	11	19	26	5	16	27	10	14	18
16	12	21	25	8	19	24	9	18	21	13	22	24	7	19	25	6	17	22
17	19	24	29	11	21	32	11	20	29	20	25	29	15	22	29	7	19	31
18	18	27	30	13	24	30	14	22	26	19	28	31	14	24	29	10	22	28
19	22	29	36	20	26	32	20	24	29	23	31	38	19	27	35	18	24	30
20	23	32	36	21	29	32	21	27	28	22	33	39	19	29	35	18	27	30
21	28	34	40	25	31	36	25	29	32	27	36	45	24	32	39	24	29	34
22	28	36	40	24	33	37	24	31	34	29	39	44	25	34	39	21	31	37
23	32	38	45	27	35	43	26	32	39	35	41	48	30	36	43	23	33	44
24	31	41	46	29	37	41	27	34	38	34	44	49	28	39	45	26	35	41
25	35	43	51	34	39	44	31	36	40	38	46	54	31	41	50	33	37	42
26	36	45	49	34	41	44	30	37	41	39	49	53	33	43	49	32	39	43
27	42	46	51	37	43	48	33	39	45	45	51	57	39	45	51	35	41	47
28	41	48	52	37	44	48	33	40	45	45	53	57	38	47	52	36	43	47
29	44	50	56	40	46	51	36	42	47	49	56	62	40	49	57	40	45	50
30	44	52	56	38	47	54	34	43	49	49	58	62	41	51	56	38	47	52
31	47	53	59	39	49	59	34	44	53	53	60	67	46	52	58	40	48	57
32	47	55	59	40	50	58	37	45	51	53	62	67	46	54	59	40	50	56
33	50	56	62	43	52	60	41	46	51	56	64	71	49	56	62	43	51	59
34	50	57	62	44	53	59	39	47	53	57	65	70	47	57	64	46	52	56
35	52	58	65	47	54	61	38	48	57	61	67	73	48	59	69	51	54	57
36	53	60	63	47	55	61	41	48	54	61	69	74	49	60	68	51	55	56
37	57	61	64	49	56	62	45	49	53	64	71	77	52	61	71	55	56	58
38	55	61	66	48	57	63	45	49	53	62	72	79	54	62	69	54	57	59
39	56	62	69	49	57	66	46	50	54	64	74	83	58	64	69	55	58	62
40	56	63	69	50	58	65	46	50	54	66	75	81	58	65	69	54	59	62

Source: Jeanty. P. Re: Fetal limb biometry. *Radiology* 147:602, 1983.

APPENDIX 3.

Fetal Crown-Rump Length Against Gestational Age

CRL (mm)	−2 SD	Mean Weeks	+2 SD	CRL (mm)	−2 SD	Mean Weeks	+2 SD
7		6.25	7.15	39	10	10.65	11.35
8		6.45	7.3	40	10.1	10.75	11.45
9		6.7	7.55	41	10.2	10.8	11.55
10	6.25	6.9	7.7	42	10.3	10.9	11.65
11	6.5	7.1	7.9	43	10.4	11.05	11.7
12	6.6	7.25	8.1	44	10.45	11.1	11.8
13	6.85	7.45	8.25	45	10.55	11.2	11.9
14	7.00	7.60	8.45	46	10.66	11.3	12
15	7.15	7.75	8.60	47	10.7	11.35	12.05
16	7.3	7.9	8.70	48	10.8	11.45	12.15
17	7.45	8.1	8.9	49	10.9	11.55	12.25
18	7.60	8.2	9.0	50	10.95	11.6	12.3
19	7.75	8.4	9.15	51	11.1	11.7	12.4
20	7.9	8.5	9.3	52	11.15	11.8	12.5
21	8.05	8.6	9.4	53	11.2	11.85	12.55
22	8.15	8.8	9.55	54	11.3	11.95	12.65
23	8.3	8.9	9.65	55	11.4	12.05	12.75
24	8.4	9.05	9.8	56	11.5	12.1	12.8
25	8.55	9.15	9.9	57	11.55	12.2	12.9
26	8.7	9.3	10	58	11.65	12.3	12.95
27	8.8	9.4	10.1	59	11.7	12.35	13.05
28	8.9	9.5	10.25	60	11.8	12.45	13.15
29	9.05	9.65	10.35	61	11.85	12.5	13.2
30	9.15	9.7	10.45	62	11.9	12.6	13.3
31	9.25	9.85	10.55	63	12	12.65	13.4
32	9.35	9.95	10.65	64	12.05	12.75	13.45
33	9.45	10.05	10.75	65	12.1	12.85	13.55
34	9.55	10.15	10.85	66	12.2	12.9	13.6
35	9.6	10.2	10.95	67	12.3	12.95	13.7
36	9.7	10.35	11.05	68	12.35	13.05	13.75
37	9.8	10.4	11.15	69	12.45	13.1	13.8
38	9.9	10.55	11.25	70	12.5	13.15	13.9

Source: Robinson, H. P., and Fleming, J. E. E.: A critical evaluation of sonar crown-rump length measurements. *Br. J. Obstet. Gynecol., 82*:702, 1975. With permission.

APPENDIX 4.

Fetal Crown-Rump Length Against Gestational Age: Mean ± 2 S.D.

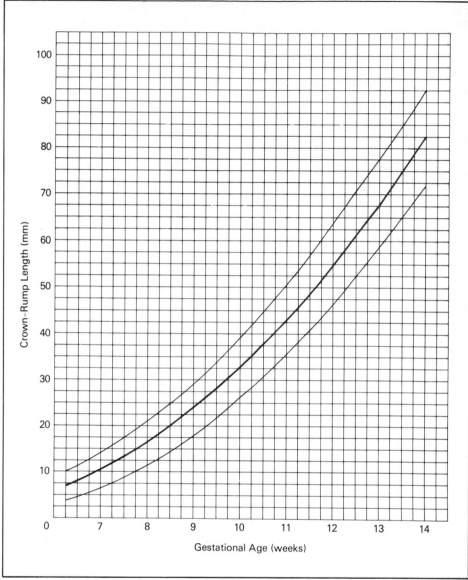

Source: Metreweli, C. Practical Abdominal Ultrasound. London: William Heineman Medical Books Ltd., 1979. (Distributed in the United States by Year Book Medical Publishers, Chicago, IL.)

APPENDIX 5.
Abdominal Circumference: Normal Values

Menstrual Age (weeks)	Lower Limit* (cm)	Predicted Value† (cm)	Upper Limit‡ (cm)	−2 S.D.∥ (cm)	Predicted Value§ (cm)	+ 2 S.D.∥ (cm)
12	5.4	6.3	7.1	3.1	5.6	8.1
13	6.4	7.4	8.3	4.4	6.9	9.4
14	7.4	8.4	9.5	5.6	8.1	10.6
15	8.3	9.5	10.8	6.8	9.3	11.8
16	9.3	10.6	12.0	8.0	10.5	13.0
17	10.2	11.7	13.3	9.2	11.7	14.2
18	11.2	12.8	14.5	10.4	12.9	15.4
19	12.1	13.9	15.7	11.6	14.1	16.6
20	13.1	15.0	17.0	12.7	15.2	17.7
21	14.0	16.1	18.2	13.9	16.4	18.9
22	15.0	17.2	19.5	15.0	17.5	20.0
23	16.0	18.3	20.7	16.1	18.6	21.1
24	16.9	19.4	22.0	17.2	19.7	22.2
25	17.9	20.5	23.2	18.3	20.8	23.3
26	18.8	21.6	24.4	19.4	21.9	24.4
27	19.8	22.7	25.7	20.4	22.9	25.4
28	20.7	23.8	26.9	21.5	24.0	26.5
29	21.7	24.9	28.2	22.5	25.0	27.5
30	22.6	26.0	29.4	23.5	26.0	28.5
31	23.6	27.1	30.6	24.5	27.0	29.5
32	24.6	28.2	31.9	25.5	28.0	30.5
33	25.5	29.3	33.1	26.5	29.0	31.5
34	26.5	30.4	34.4	27.5	30.0	32.5
35	27.4	31.5	35.6	28.4	30.9	33.4
36	28.4	32.6	36.9	29.3	31.8	34.3
37	29.3	33.7	38.1	30.2	32.7	35.2
38	30.3	34.8	39.3	31.1	33.6	36.1
39	31.2	35.9	40.6	32.0	34.5	37.0
40	32.2	37.0	41.8	32.9	35.4	37.9

*Predicted value −.13 (predicted value).
†$AC = -6.9300 + 1.0985 (MA) [R^2 = 95.5\%]$.
‡Predicted value + .13 (predicted value).
§$AC = -10.4997 + 1.4256 (MA) - .00697 (MA)^2 [R^2 = 97.9\%]$.
∥2 S.D. = 2.5 cm.
Source: Adapted from Callen, P. W. *Ultrasonography in Obstetrics and Gynecology.* Boston: Saunders, 1983. With permission.

APPENDIX 6.

Head Circumference: Normal Growth Rates

Menstrual Age Interval (weeks)	−2 S.D. (cm/wk)	Predicted Value (cm/wk)	+2 S.D. (cm/wk)
12–13	1.4	1.6	1.8
13–14	1.3	1.5	1.7
14–15	1.3	1.5	1.7
15–16	1.3	1.5	1.7
16–17	1.3	1.5	1.7
17–18	1.2	1.4	1.6
18–19	1.2	1.4	1.6
19–20	1.2	1.4	1.6
20–21	1.1	1.3	1.5
21–22	1.1	1.3	1.5
22–23	1.2	1.3	1.4
23–24	1.1	1.2	1.3
24–25	1.1	1.2	1.3
25–26	1.1	1.2	1.3
26–27	1.0	1.1	1.2
27–28	1.0	1.1	1.2
28–29	0.9	1.0	1.1
29–30	0.9	1.0	1.1
30–31	0.8	0.9	1.0
31–32	0.8	0.9	1.0
32–33	0.7	0.8	0.9
33–34	0.6	0.8	1.0
34–35	0.5	0.7	0.9
35–36	0.5	0.7	0.9
36–37	0.4	0.6	0.8
37–38	0.4	0.6	0.8
38–39	0.3	0.5	0.7
39–40	0.1	0.4	0.7

Source: Callen, P. W. *Ultrasonography in Obstetrics and Gynecology.* Boston: Saunders, 1983. With permission.

APPENDIX 7.

Head Circumference: Normal Values

Menstrual Age (weeks)	Lower Limit (cm)	Predicted Value (cm)	Upper Limit (cm)	−2 S.D. (cm)	Predicted Value (cm)	+2 S.D. (cm)
12	5.8	7.3	8.8	5.1	7.0	8.9
13	7.2	8.7	10.2	6.5	8.9	10.3
14	8.6	10.1	11.6	7.9	9.8	11.7
15	9.9	11.4	12.9	9.2	11.1	13.0
16	11.3	12.8	14.3	10.5	12.4	14.3
17	12.6	14.1	15.6	11.8	13.7	15.6
18	13.9	15.4	16.9	13.1	15.0	16.9
19	15.2	16.7	18.2	14.4	16.3	18.2
20	16.4	17.9	19.4	15.6	17.5	19.4
21	17.7	19.2	20.7	16.8	18.7	20.6
22	18.9	20.4	21.9	18.0	19.9	21.8
23	20.0	21.5	23.0	19.1	21.0	22.9
24	21.2	22.7	24.2	20.2	22.1	24.0
25	22.3	23.8	25.3	21.3	23.2	25.1
26	23.4	24.9	26.4	22.3	24.2	26.1
27	24.4	25.9	27.4	23.3	25.2	27.1
28	24.4	26.9	29.4	24.3	26.2	28.1
29	25.4	27.9	30.4	25.2	27.1	29.0
30	26.3	28.8	31.3	26.1	28.0	29.9
31	27.2	29.7	32.2	27.0	28.9	30.8
32	28.1	30.6	33.1	27.8	29.7	31.6
33	28.9	31.4	33.9	28.5	30.4	32.3
34	29.7	32.2	34.7	29.3	31.2	33.1
35	30.4	32.9	35.4	29.9	31.8	33.7
36	31.1	33.6	36.1	30.6	32.5	34.4
37	31.7	34.2	36.7	31.1	33.0	34.9
38	32.3	34.8	37.3	31.9	33.6	35.5
39	32.9	35.4	37.9	32.2	34.1	36.0
40	33.4	35.9	38.4	32.6	34.5	36.4

Source: Adapted from Callen, P. W., *Ultrasonography in Obstetrics and Gynecology.* Boston: Saunders, 1983. With permission.

APPENDIX 8.

Correlation of Predicted Menstrual Age Based upon Biparietal Diameters

Menstrual Age (weeks)	Bpd mean values (mm)					
	Composite Sabbagha and Hughey[1]	Composite Kurtz et al.[2]	Kurtz et al.[2] < 1974	Kurtz et al.[2] > 1974	Hadlock et al.[3] 1982	Shepard and Filly[4] 1982
14	28	27	28	26	27	28
15	32	31	31	29	30	31
16	36	34	35	33	33	34
17	39	38	39	36	37	37
18	42	41	42	40	40	40
19	45	45	46	43	43	43
20	48	48	49	46	46	46
21	51	51	52	50	50	49
22	54	54	55	53	53	52
23	58	57	58	56	56	55
24	61	60	61	59	58	57
25	64	63	64	61	61	60
26	67	66	67	64	64	63
27	70	69	69	67	67	65
28	72	71	72	70	70	68
29	75	74	75	72	72	71
30	78	76	77	75	75	73
31	80	79	79	77	77	76
32	82	81	81	79	79	78
33	85	83	83	82	82	80
34	87	85	85	84	84	83
35	88	87	87	86	86	85
36	90	89	89	88	88	88
37	92	91	91	90	90	90
38	93	92	92	92	91	92
39	94	94	94	94	93	95
40	95	95	95	95	95	97

[1]Sabbagha, R. E., and Hughey, M. Standardization of sonar cephalometry and gestational age. *Obstet. Gynecol.* 52:402, 1978.
[2]Kurtz, A. B., Wapner, R. J., Kurtz, R. J., et al. Analysis of biparietal diameter as an accurate indicator of gestational age. *J. Clin. Ultrasound,* 8:319, 1980.
[3]Hadlock, F. P., Deter, R. L., Harrist, R. B., et al. Fetal biparietal diameter: A critical re-evaluation of the relation to menstrual age by means of real-time ultrasound. *J. Ultrasound Med.,* 1:97–104, 1982.
[4]Shepard, M., and Filly, R. A. A standardized plane for biparietal diameter measurement. *J. Ultrasound Med.,* 1:145–150, 1982.
Source: Callen, P. W. *Ultrasonography in Obstetrics and Gynecology.* Boston: Saunders, 1983. With permission.

APPENDIX 9.

Comparison of Predicted Femur Lengths at Points in Gestation

Menstrual Age (weeks)	Femur length (mm)			
	Filly et al.[1] 1981	Jeanty et al.[2] 1981†	Hadlock et al.[3] 1982*	Hadlock et al.[3] 1982†
12		09	14	08
13		12	16	11
14	16	16	19	15
15	19	19	21	18
16	22	23	23	21
17	25	26	26	24
18	28	30	28	27
19	32	33	30	30
20	35	36	33	33
21	38	39	35	36
22	41	42	38	39
23	44	45	40	42
24	47	48	42	44
25	50	51	45	47
26	53	54	47	49
27	55	57	49	52
28	57	59	52	54
29	61	62	54	56
30	63	65	57	58
31		67	59	61
32		70	61	63
33		72	64	65
34		74	66	66
35		77	69	68
36		79	71	70
37		81	73	72
38		83	76	73
39		85	78	75
40		87	80	76

*Linear function
†Linear quadratic function

[1]Filly, R. A., Golbus, M. S., Carey, J. C., et al. Short-limbed dwarfism: Ultrasonographic diagnosis by mensuration of fetal femoral length. *Radiology,* 138:653–656, 1981.
[2]Jeanty, P. Kirkpatrick, C., Dramaix-Wilmet, M., et al. Ultrasonic evaluation of fetal limb growth. *Radiology,* 140:165–168, 1981.
[3]Hadlock, F. P. et al. Fetal femur length as a predictor of menstrual age: Sonographically measured. *Am. J. Roentgenol.,* 138:875–878, 1982.
Source: Callen, P. W. *Ultrasonography in Obstetrics and Gynecology.* Boston: Saunders, 1983. With permission.

APPENDIX 10.

Estimated Fetal Weights*

Biparietal diameter	Abdominal circumference											
	15.5	16.0	16.5	17.0	17.5	18.0	18.5	19.0	19.5	20.0	20.5	21.0
3.1	212	219	227	236	244	253	262	272	282	292	303	314
3.2	218	226	234	243	252	261	270	280	290	301	312	323
3.3	225	233	242	250	260	269	279	289	299	310	321	333
3.4	232	241	249	258	268	277	287	298	308	319	331	343
3.5	239	248	257	266	276	286	296	307	318	329	341	353
3.6	247	256	265	274	284	294	305	316	327	339	351	364
3.7	254	263	273	283	293	303	314	325	337	349	361	374
3.8	262	271	281	291	302	312	324	335	347	359	372	385
3.9	270	280	290	300	311	322	333	345	357	370	383	397
4.0	278	288	299	309	320	331	343	355	368	381	394	408
4.1	287	297	308	318	330	341	353	366	379	392	406	420
4.2	296	306	317	328	340	352	364	377	390	404	418	433
4.3	305	315	326	338	350	362	375	388	401	416	430	445
4.4	314	325	336	348	360	373	386	399	413	428	443	458
4.5	323	334	346	358	371	384	397	411	425	440	455	471
4.6	333	344	356	369	382	395	409	423	438	453	469	485
4.7	343	355	367	380	393	407	421	435	450	466	482	499
4.8	353	365	378	391	404	418	433	448	463	479	496	513
4.9	364	376	389	402	416	431	445	461	477	493	510	527
5.0	374	387	401	414	428	443	458	474	490	507	524	542
5.1	386	399	412	426	441	456	472	488	504	521	539	558
5.2	397	410	424	439	454	469	485	502	519	536	554	573
5.3	409	422	437	452	467	483	499	516	533	551	570	589
5.4	421	435	449	465	480	496	513	531	548	567	586	606
5.5	433	447	463	478	494	511	528	546	564	583	602	622
5.6	446	461	476	492	508	525	543	561	580	599	619	640
5.7	459	474	490	506	523	540	558	577	596	616	636	657
5.8	472	488	504	520	538	555	574	593	612	633	654	675
5.9	486	502	518	535	553	571	590	609	629	650	672	694
6.0	500	516	533	550	568	587	606	626	647	668	690	712
6.1	514	531	548	566	584	604	623	644	665	686	709	732
6.2	529	546	564	582	601	620	641	661	683	705	728	751
6.3	544	561	580	598	618	638	658	679	701	724	747	772
6.4	559	577	596	615	635	655	676	698	721	744	768	792
6.5	575	594	613	632	653	673	695	717	740	764	788	813
6.6	592	610	630	650	671	692	714	737	760	784	809	835
6.7	608	628	648	668	689	711	733	757	780	805	831	857
6.8	626	645	666	686	708	730	753	777	801	827	853	879
6.9	643	663	684	705	727	750	774	798	823	848	875	902
7.0	661	682	703	725	747	771	795	819	845	871	898	926
7.1	680	701	722	745	768	791	816	841	867	894	921	950
7.2	699	720	742	765	789	813	838	863	890	917	945	974
7.3	718	740	763	786	810	835	860	886	913	941	970	999
7.4	738	760	783	807	832	857	883	910	937	966	995	1,025
7.5	758	781	805	829	854	880	906	934	962	991	1,020	1,051
7.6	779	803	827	851	877	903	930	958	987	1,016	1,047	1,078
7.7	801	825	849	874	900	927	955	983	1,012	1,042	1,073	1,105
7.8	823	847	872	898	924	952	980	1,008	1,038	1,069	1,100	1,133
7.9	845	870	895	922	949	977	1,005	1,035	1,065	1,096	1,128	1,161
8.0	868	893	919	946	974	1,002	1,031	1,061	1,092	1,124	1,157	1,190
8.1	892	918	944	971	999	1,028	1,058	1,088	1,120	1,152	1,186	1,220
8.2	916	942	969	997	1,026	1,055	1,085	1,116	1,148	1,181	1,215	1,250
8.3	941	967	995	1,023	1,052	1,082	1,113	1,145	1,177	1,211	1,245	1,281
8.4	966	993	1,021	1,050	1,080	1,110	1,142	1,174	1,207	1,241	1,276	1,312
8.5	992	1,020	1,048	1,078	1,108	1,139	1,171	1,203	1,237	1,272	1,307	1,344
8.6	1,018	1,047	1,076	1,106	1,136	1,168	1,200	1,234	1,268	1,303	1,339	1,377
8.7	1,046	1,074	1,104	1,134	1,166	1,198	1,231	1,265	1,300	1,335	1,372	1,410
8.8	1,073	1,103	1,133	1,164	1,196	1,228	1,262	1,296	1,332	1,368	1,405	1,444
8.9	1,102	1,132	1,162	1,194	1,226	1,259	1,294	1,329	1,365	1,402	1,439	1,478
9.0	1,131	1,161	1,193	1,225	1,257	1,291	1,326	1,361	1,398	1,436	1,474	1,514
9.1	1,161	1,192	1,223	1,256	1,289	1,324	1,359	1,395	1,432	1,470	1,509	1,550
9.2	1,191	1,223	1,255	1,288	1,322	1,357	1,393	1,429	1,467	1,506	1,545	1,586
9.3	1,222	1,254	1,287	1,321	1,355	1,391	1,427	1,464	1,503	1,542	1,582	1,624

*$\text{Log}(BW) = -1.599 + 0.144(BPD) + 0.032(AC) - 0.111(BPD_2 \times AC)/1{,}000$ S. D. = + OR − 106.0 Gm. per kilogram of body weight.

					Abdominal circumference							
21.5	22.0	22.5	23.0	23.5	24.0	24.5	25.0	25.5	26.0	26.5	27.0	27.5
325	337	349	362	375	388	402	417	432	448	464	481	498
335	347	359	372	386	400	414	429	445	461	478	495	513
345	357	370	384	397	412	427	442	458	475	492	509	528
355	368	381	395	409	424	439	455	471	488	506	524	543
366	379	393	407	421	436	452	468	485	503	521	539	559
377	390	404	419	434	449	465	482	499	517	536	555	575
388	402	416	431	446	462	479	496	514	532	551	571	591
399	413	428	443	459	476	493	510	528	547	567	587	608
411	426	441	456	473	489	507	525	543	563	583	603	625
423	438	453	470	486	503	521	540	559	579	599	620	642
435	451	467	483	500	518	536	555	575	595	616	638	660
448	464	480	497	514	533	551	571	591	612	633	656	679
461	477	494	511	529	548	567	587	607	629	651	674	697
474	491	508	526	544	563	583	603	624	646	669	692	716
488	505	522	541	559	579	599	620	642	664	687	711	736
502	519	537	556	575	595	616	637	659	682	706	731	756
516	534	552	572	591	612	633	655	678	701	725	750	776
531	549	568	588	608	629	650	673	696	720	745	771	797
546	564	584	604	625	646	668	691	715	740	765	791	819
561	580	600	621	642	664	687	710	734	760	786	812	840
577	596	617	638	660	682	705	729	754	780	807	834	862
593	613	634	655	678	701	724	749	774	801	828	856	885
609	630	651	673	696	720	744	769	795	822	850	879	908
626	647	669	692	715	739	764	790	816	838	866	895	925	956
643	665	687	710	734	759	784	811	838	866	895	925	956
661	683	706	730	754	779	805	832	860	888	918	949	981
679	702	725	749	774	800	826	854	882	912	942	973	1,006
698	721	745	769	795	821	848	876	905	935	966	998	1,031
717	740	764	790	816	843	870	899	929	959	991	1,023	1,057
736	760	785	811	837	865	893	922	953	984	1,016	1,049	1,084
756	780	806	832	859	887	916	946	977	1,009	1,042	1,076	1,111
776	801	827	854	882	910	940	970	1,002	1,034	1,068	1,103	1,138
797	822	849	876	905	934	964	995	1,027	1,060	1,095	1,130	1,166
818	844	871	899	928	958	989	1,020	1,053	1,087	1,122	1,158	1,195
839	866	894	922	952	982	1,014	1,046	1,079	1,114	1,150	1,186	1,224
861	889	917	946	976	1,007	1,039	1,072	1,106	1,142	1,178	1,215	1,254
884	912	941	970	1,001	1,033	1,065	1,099	1,134	1,170	1,207	1,245	1,284
907	936	965	995	1,027	1,059	1,092	1,126	1,162	1,198	1,236	1,275	1,315
931	960	990	1,021	1,052	1,085	1,119	1,154	1,190	1,227	1,266	1,305	1,346
955	984	1,015	1,046	1,079	1,112	1,147	1,183	1,219	1,257	1,296	1,337	1,378
979	1,009	1,041	1,073	1,106	1,140	1,175	1,212	1,249	1,287	1,327	1,368	1,410
1,004	1,035	1,067	1,100	1,133	1,168	1,204	1,241	1,279	1,318	1,359	1,400	1,443
1,030	1,061	1,094	1,127	1,161	1,197	1,233	1,271	1,310	1,350	1,391	1,433	1,477
1,056	1,088	1,121	1,155	1,190	1,226	1,263	1,302	1,341	1,382	1,424	1,467	1,511
1,083	1,115	1,149	1,184	1,219	1,256	1,294	1,333	1,373	1,414	1,457	1,501	1,546
1,110	1,143	1,177	1,213	1,249	1,286	1,325	1,364	1,405	1,447	1,491	1,535	1,581
1,138	1,172	1,207	1,242	1,279	1,317	1,356	1,397	1,438	1,481	1,525	1,570	1,617
1,166	1,201	1,236	1,273	1,310	1,349	1,389	1,430	1,472	1,515	1,560	1,606	1,653
1,195	1,230	1,266	1,303	1,342	1,381	1,421	1,463	1,506	1,550	1,595	1,642	1,690
1,225	1,260	1,297	1,335	1,374	1,414	1,455	1,497	1,541	1,585	1,632	1,679	1,728
1,255	1,291	1,329	1,367	1,406	1,447	1,489	1,532	1,576	1,621	1,668	1,716	1,766
1,286	1,323	1,361	1,400	1,440	1,481	1,523	1,567	1,612	1,658	1,706	1,755	1,805
1,317	1,355	1,393	1,433	1,473	1,515	1,559	1,603	1,648	1,695	1,744	1,793	1,844
1,349	1,387	1,426	1,467	1,508	1,551	1,594	1,639	1,686	1,733	1,782	1,832	1,884
1,382	1,420	1,460	1,501	1,543	1,586	1,631	1,676	1,723	1,772	1,821	1,872	1,925
1,415	1,454	1,495	1,536	1,579	1,623	1,668	1,714	1,762	1,811	1,861	1,913	1,966
1,449	1,489	1,530	1,572	1,615	1,660	1,705	1,752	1,801	1,850	1,901	1,954	2,007
1,483	1,524	1,565	1,608	1,652	1,697	1,744	1,791	1,840	1,891	1,942	1,995	2,050
1,519	1,560	1,602	1,645	1,690	1,736	1,783	1,831	1,881	1,931	1,984	2,037	2,093
1,554	1,596	1,639	1,683	1,728	1,775	1,822	1,871	1,921	1,973	2,026	2,080	2,136
1,591	1,633	1,677	1,721	1,767	1,814	1,862	1,912	1,963	2,015	2,069	2,124	2,180
1,628	1,671	1,715	1,760	1,807	1,854	1,903	1,953	2,005	2,058	2,112	2,168	2,225
1,666	1,709	1,754	1,800	1,847	1,895	1,945	1,996	2,048	2,101	2,156	2,213	2,270

APPENDIX 10 (continued)

Biparietal diameter	Abdominal circumference											
	15.5	16.0	16.5	17.0	17.5	18.0	18.5	19.0	19.5	20.0	20.5	21.0
9.4	1,254	1,287	1,320	1,354	1,389	1,425	1,462	1,500	1,539	1,579	1,620	1,661
9.5	1,287	1,320	1,354	1,388	1,424	1,461	1,498	1,536	1,576	1,616	1,658	1,700
9.6	1,320	1,354	1,388	1,423	1,460	1,497	1,535	1,574	1,614	1,655	1,697	1,740
9.7	1,354	1,388	1,423	1,459	1,496	1,533	1,572	1,611	1,652	1,694	1,736	1,780
9.8	1,389	1,424	1,459	1,496	1,533	1,571	1,610	1,650	1,691	1,733	1,776	1,821
9.9	1,425	1,460	1,496	1,533	1,571	1,609	1,649	1,690	1,731	1,774	1,817	1,862
10.0	1,461	1,497	1,534	1,571	1,609	1,648	1,689	1,730	1,772	1,815	1,859	1,905

Biparietal diameter	Abdominal circumference											
	28.0	28.5	29.0	29.5	30.0	30.5	31.0	31.5	32.0	32.5	33.0	33.5
3.1	517	535	555	575	596	617	640	663	687	712	738	765
3.2	532	551	571	591	613	635	658	682	707	732	759	786
3.3	547	567	587	608	630	653	677	701	726	753	780	808
3.4	563	583	604	626	648	672	696	721	747	774	802	831
3.5	579	600	621	644	667	691	715	741	768	795	824	853
3.6	595	617	639	662	685	710	735	762	789	817	847	877
3.7	612	634	657	680	705	730	756	783	811	840	870	901
3.8	629	652	675	699	724	750	777	804	833	863	893	925
3.9	647	670	694	719	744	771	798	826	856	886	918	950
4.0	665	689	713	738	765	792	820	849	879	910	942	976
4.1	684	708	733	759	786	813	842	872	903	934	967	1,002
4.2	703	727	753	779	807	835	865	895	927	959	993	1,028
4.3	722	747	773	801	829	858	888	919	951	985	1,019	1,055
4.4	742	767	794	822	851	881	911	943	976	1,011	1,046	1,082
4.5	762	788	816	844	874	904	936	968	1,002	1,037	1,073	1,110
4.6	782	809	838	867	897	928	960	994	1,028	1,064	1,101	1,139
4.7	803	831	860	890	920	952	985	1,019	1,055	1,091	1,129	1,168
4.8	825	853	883	913	945	977	1,011	1,046	1,082	1,119	1,158	1,198
4.9	847	876	906	937	969	1,003	1,037	1,073	1,109	1,148	1,187	1,228
5.0	869	899	930	961	994	1,028	1,064	1,100	1,138	1,177	1,217	1,259
5.1	892	922	954	986	1,020	1,055	1,091	1,128	1,166	1,206	1,247	1,290
5.2	915	946	978	1,012	1,046	1,082	1,118	1,156	1,196	1,236	1,278	1,322
5.3	939	971	1,004	1,038	1,073	1,109	1,146	1,185	1,225	1,267	1,310	1,354
5.4	963	996	1,029	1,064	1,100	1,137	1,175	1,215	1,256	1,298	1,342	1,387
5.5	988	1,021	1,055	1,091	1,127	1,165	1,204	1,245	1,286	1,330	1,374	1,420
5.6	1,013	1,047	1,082	1,118	1,156	1,194	1,234	1,275	1,318	1,362	1,407	1,454
5.7	1,039	1,074	1,109	1,146	1,184	1,224	1,264	1,306	1,350	1,395	1,441	1,489
5.8	1,065	1,100	1,137	1,175	1,213	1,254	1,295	1,338	1,382	1,428	1,475	1,524
5.9	1,092	1,128	1,165	1,203	1,243	1,284	1,326	1,370	1,415	1,462	1,510	1,560
6.0	1,119	1,156	1,194	1,233	1,273	1,315	1,358	1,403	1,449	1,496	1,545	1,596
6.1	1,147	1,184	1,223	1,263	1,304	1,347	1,391	1,436	1,483	1,531	1,581	1,633
6.2	1,175	1,213	1,253	1,293	1,335	1,379	1,424	1,470	1,517	1,567	1,618	1,670
6.3	1,204	1,243	1,283	1,325	1,367	1,411	1,457	1,504	1,553	1,603	1,655	1,708
6.4	1,233	1,273	1,314	1,356	1,400	1,445	1,491	1,539	1,588	1,639	1,692	1,746
6.5	1,263	1,304	1,345	1,388	1,433	1,478	1,526	1,574	1,625	1,677	1,730	1,786
6.6	1,294	1,335	1,377	1,421	1,466	1,513	1,561	1,610	1,662	1,714	1,769	1,825
6.7	1,325	1,367	1,410	1,454	1,500	1,548	1,597	1,647	1,699	1,753	1,808	1,865
6.8	1,356	1,399	1,443	1,488	1,535	1,583	1,633	1,684	1,737	1,792	1,848	1,906
6.9	1,388	1,432	1,476	1,522	1,570	1,619	1,670	1,722	1,776	1,831	1,888	1,947
7.0	1,421	1,465	1,511	1,557	1,606	1,656	1,707	1,760	1,815	1,871	1,929	1,989
7.1	1,454	1,499	1,545	1,593	1,642	1,693	1,745	1,799	1,854	1,912	1,971	2,032
7.2	1,488	1,533	1,580	1,629	1,679	1,730	1,784	1,838	1,895	1,953	2,013	2,075
7.3	1,522	1,568	1,616	1,666	1,716	1,769	1,823	1,878	1,936	1,995	2,055	2,118
7.4	1,557	1,604	1,653	1,703	1,754	1,808	1,862	1,919	1,977	2,037	2,098	2,162
7.5	1,592	1,640	1,690	1,741	1,793	1,847	1,903	1,960	2,019	2,080	2,142	2,207
7.6	1,628	1,677	1,727	1,779	1,832	1,887	1,943	2,001	2,061	2,123	2,186	2,252
7.7	1,665	1,714	1,765	1,818	1,872	1,927	1,985	2,044	2,104	2,167	2,231	2,297
7.8	1,702	1,752	1,804	1,857	1,912	1,968	2,026	2,086	2,148	2,211	2,276	2,344
7.9	1,740	1,791	1,843	1,897	1,953	2,010	2,069	2,130	2,192	2,256	2,322	2,390
8.0	1,778	1,830	1,883	1,938	1,994	2,052	2,112	2,173	2,237	2,302	2,368	2,437
8.1	1,817	1,869	1,923	1,979	2,036	2,095	2,155	2,218	2,282	2,348	2,415	2,485
8.2	1,857	1,910	1,964	2,021	2,079	2,138	2,200	2,263	2,327	2,394	2,463	2,533

Abdominal circumference

21.5	22.0	22.5	23.0	23.5	24.0	24.5	25.0	25.5	26.0	26.5	27.0	27.5
1,705	1,749	1,794	1,840	1,888	1,937	1,987	2,038	2,091	2,145	2,201	2,258	2,316
1,744	1,788	1,834	1,881	1,930	1,979	2,030	2,082	2,135	2,190	2,246	2,304	2,363
1,784	1,829	1,875	1,923	1,972	2,022	2,073	2,126	2,180	2,235	2,292	2,350	2,410
1,824	1,870	1,917	1,966	2,015	2,066	2,117	2,171	2,225	2,281	2,339	2,397	2,458
1,866	1,912	1,960	2,009	2,059	2,110	2,162	2,216	2,271	2,328	2,386	2,445	2,506
1,908	1,955	2,003	2,052	2,103	2,155	2,208	2,262	2,318	2,375	2,433	2,493	2,555
1,951	1,998	2,047	2,097	2,148	2,200	2,254	2,309	2,365	2,423	2,482	2,542	2,604

Abdominal circumference

34.0	34.5	35.0	35.5	36.0	36.5	37.0	37.5	38.0	38.5	39.0	39.5	40.0
792	821	851	882	914	947	981	1,017	1,054	1,092	1,131	1,172	1,215
814	844	875	906	939	973	1,008	1,045	1,082	1,122	1,162	1,204	1,248
837	867	899	931	965	1,000	1,036	1,073	1,112	1,152	1,194	1,237	1,281
860	891	924	957	991	1,027	1,064	1,102	1,142	1,183	1,226	1,270	1,316
884	916	949	983	1,018	1,055	1,093	1,132	1,173	1,215	1,258	1,304	1,350
908	941	975	1,010	1,046	1,083	1,122	1,162	1,204	1,247	1,292	1,338	1,386
933	966	1,001	1,037	1,074	1,112	1,152	1,193	1,236	1,280	1,325	1,373	1,422
958	992	1,028	1,064	1,102	1,142	1,182	1,224	1,268	1,313	1,360	1,408	1,459
984	1,019	1,055	1,093	1,131	1,172	1,213	1,256	1,301	1,347	1,395	1,445	1,496
1,010	1,046	1,083	1,121	1,161	1,202	1,245	1,289	1,335	1,382	1,431	1,481	1,534
1,037	1,074	1,111	1,151	1,191	1,233	1,277	1,322	1,369	1,417	1,467	1,519	1,573
1,064	1,102	1,140	1,181	1,222	1,265	1,310	1,356	1,404	1,453	1,504	1,557	1,612
1,092	1,130	1,170	1,211	1,254	1,298	1,343	1,390	1,439	1,489	1,542	1,596	1,652
1,120	1,160	1,200	1,242	1,285	1,330	1,377	1,425	1,475	1,527	1,580	1,635	1,692
1,149	1,189	1,231	1,274	1,318	1,364	1,411	1,461	1,512	1,564	1,619	1,675	1,734
1,179	1,220	1,262	1,306	1,351	1,398	1,447	1,497	1,549	1,603	1,658	1,716	1,776
1,209	1,250	1,294	1,338	1,385	1,433	1,482	1,534	1,587	1,642	1,698	1,757	1,818
1,239	1,282	1,326	1,372	1,419	1,468	1,519	1,571	1,625	1,681	1,739	1,799	1,861
1,270	1,314	1,359	1,406	1,454	1,504	1,555	1,609	1,664	1,721	1,780	1,842	1,905
1,302	1,346	1,392	1,440	1,489	1,540	1,593	1,647	1,704	1,762	1,822	1,885	1,949
1,334	1,379	1,426	1,475	1,525	1,577	1,631	1,687	1,744	1,804	1,865	1,929	1,994
1,366	1,413	1,461	1,510	1,562	1,615	1,670	1,726	1,785	1,846	1,908	1,973	2,040
1,400	1,447	1,496	1,547	1,599	1,653	1,709	1,767	1,826	1,888	1,952	2,018	2,086
1,433	1,482	1,532	1,583	1,637	1,692	1,749	1,808	1,868	1,931	1,996	2,064	2,133
1,468	1,517	1,568	1,621	1,675	1,731	1,789	1,849	1,911	1,975	2,041	2,110	2,181
1,503	1,553	1,605	1,658	1,714	1,771	1,830	1,891	1,954	2,020	2,087	2,157	2,229
1,538	1,589	1,642	1,697	1,753	1,812	1,872	1,934	1,998	2,065	2,133	2,204	2,277
1,574	1,626	1,680	1,736	1,793	1,853	1,914	1,977	2,043	2,110	2,180	2,252	2,327
1,611	1,664	1,719	1,775	1,834	1,894	1,957	2,021	2,088	2,156	2,227	2,301	2,377
1,648	1,702	1,758	1,816	1,875	1,937	2,000	2,066	2,133	2,203	2,275	2,350	2,427
1,686	1,741	1,798	1,856	1,917	1,979	2,044	2,111	2,179	2,251	2,324	2,400	2,478
1,724	1,780	1,838	1,898	1,959	2,023	2,088	2,156	2,226	2,298	2,373	2,450	2,530
1,763	1,820	1,879	1,939	2,002	2,067	2,133	2,202	2,273	2,347	2,423	2,501	2,582
1,803	1,860	1,920	1,982	2,046	2,111	2,179	2,249	2,321	2,396	2,473	2,552	2,634
1,843	1,901	1,962	2,025	2,090	2,156	2,225	2,296	2,370	2,445	2,524	2,604	2,687
1,883	1,943	2,005	2,068	2,134	2,202	2,272	2,344	2,419	2,495	2,575	2,657	2,741
1,924	1,985	2,048	2,113	2,179	2,248	2,319	2,393	2,468	2,546	2,627	2,710	2,795
1,966	2,028	2,091	2,157	2,225	2,295	2,367	2,441	2,518	2,597	2,679	2,763	2,850
2,008	2,071	2,136	2,202	2,271	2,342	2,415	2,491	2,569	2,649	2,732	2,817	2,905
2,051	2,115	2,180	2,248	2,318	2,390	2,464	2,541	2,620	2,701	2,785	2,871	2,960
2,094	2,159	2,226	2,294	2,365	2,438	2,513	2,591	2,671	2,754	2,839	2,926	3,017
2,138	2,204	2,271	2,341	2,413	2,487	2,563	2,642	2,723	2,807	2,893	2,981	3,073
2,183	2,249	2,318	2,388	2,461	2,536	2,614	2,693	2,776	2,860	2,947	3,037	3,130
2,228	2,295	2,365	2,436	2,510	2,586	2,665	2,745	2,828	2,914	3,002	3,093	3,187
2,273	2,342	2,412	2,485	2,559	2,636	2,716	2,798	2,882	2,969	3,058	3,150	3,245
2,319	2,388	2,460	2,533	2,609	2,687	2,768	2,850	2,936	3,023	3,114	3,207	3,303
2,366	2,436	2,508	2,583	2,659	2,738	2,820	2,904	2,990	3,079	3,170	3,264	3,361
2,413	2,484	2,557	2,633	2,710	2,790	2,872	2,957	3,044	3,134	3,227	3,322	3,420
2,460	2,532	2,606	2,683	2,761	2,842	2,926	3,011	3,099	3,190	3,284	3,380	3,479
2,508	2,581	2,656	2,734	2,813	2,895	2,979	3,066	3,155	3,247	3,341	3,438	3,538
2,557	2,631	2,707	2,785	2,865	2,948	3,033	3,121	3,211	3,303	3,399	3,497	3,598
2,606	2,681	2,757	2,836	2,918	3,001	3,087	3,176	3,267	3,360	3,457	3,556	3,658

APPENDIX 10 (continued)

Biparietal diameter	Abdominal circumference											
	28 0	28.5	29.0	29.5	30.0	30.5	31.0	31.5	32.0	32.5	33.0	33.5
8.3	1,897	1,951	2,006	2,063	2,122	2,182	2,244	2,308	2,374	2,441	2,511	2,582
8.4	1,937	1,992	2,048	2,106	2,165	2,226	2,289	2,354	2,420	2,489	2,559	2,631
8.5	1,978	2,034	2,091	2,149	2,210	2,271	2,335	2,400	2,468	2,537	2,608	2,681
8.6	2,020	2,076	2,134	2,193	2,254	2,317	2,381	2,447	2,515	2,585	2,657	2,731
8.7	2,063	2,120	2,178	2,238	2,300	2,363	2,428	2,495	2,564	2,634	2,707	2,781
8.8	2,106	2,163	2,222	2,283	2,345	2,410	2,475	2,543	2,612	2,684	2,757	2,832
8.9	2,149	2,208	2,267	2,329	2,392	2,457	2,523	2,592	2,662	2,734	2,808	2,884
9.0	2,194	2,252	2,313	2,375	2,439	2,504	2,572	2,641	2,711	2,784	2,859	2,936
9.1	2,238	2,298	2,359	2,422	2,486	2,552	2,620	2,690	2,762	2,835	2,911	2,988
9.2	2,284	2,344	2,406	2,469	2,534	2,601	2,670	2,740	2,812	2,887	2,963	3,041
9.3	2,330	2,391	2,453	2,517	2,583	2,650	2,720	2,791	2,864	2,938	3,015	3,094
9.4	2,376	2,438	2,501	2,566	2,632	2,700	2,770	2,842	2,915	2,991	3,068	3,147
9.5	2,423	2,485	2,549	2,615	2,682	2,750	2,821	2,893	2,967	3,043	3,121	3,201
9.6	2,471	2,534	2,598	2,664	2,732	2,801	2,872	2,945	3,020	3,096	3,175	3,256
9.7	2,519	2,583	2,648	2,714	2,782	2,852	2,924	2,997	3,073	3,150	3,229	3,310
9.8	2,568	2,632	2,698	2,765	2,833	2,904	2,976	3,050	3,126	3,204	3,283	3,365
9.9	2,618	2,682	2,748	2,816	2,885	2,956	3,029	3,103	3,180	3,258	3,338	3,420
10.0	2,668	2,733	2,799	2,867	2,937	3,009	3,082	3,157	3,234	3,313	3,393	3,476

Abdominal circumference

34.0	34.5	35.0	35.5	36.0	36.5	37.0	37.5	38.0	38.5	39.0	39.5	40.0
2,655	2,731	2,809	2,888	2,971	3,055	3,142	3,231	3,323	3,418	3,515	3,615	3,718
2,705	2,782	2,860	2,941	3,024	3,109	3,197	3,287	3,380	3,475	3,573	3,674	3,778
2,756	2,833	2,912	2,994	3,078	3,164	3,252	3,343	3,437	3,533	3,632	3,734	3,838
2,807	2,885	2,965	3,047	3,132	3,219	3,308	3,400	3,494	3,591	3,691	3,794	3,899
2,858	2,937	3,018	3,101	3,186	3,274	3,364	3,457	3,552	3,650	3,750	3,854	3,960
2,910	2,989	3,071	3,155	3,241	3,330	3,420	3,514	3,610	3,708	3,810	3,914	4,021
2,962	3,042	3,125	3,209	3,296	3,385	3,477	3,571	3,668	3,767	3,869	3,974	4,082
3,015	3,096	3,179	3,264	3,352	3,442	3,534	3,629	3,726	3,826	3,929	4,035	4,143
3,068	3,149	3,233	3,319	3,407	3,498	3,591	3,687	3,785	3,886	3,989	4,095	4,204
3,121	3,203	3,288	3,374	3,463	3,555	3,649	3,745	3,844	3,945	4,049	4,156	4,265
3,175	3,258	3,343	3,430	3,520	3,612	3,706	3,803	3,902	4,004	4,109	4,216	4,326
3,229	3,313	3,398	3,486	3,576	3,669	3,764	3,861	3,961	4,064	4,169	4,277	4,388
3,283	3,368	3,454	3,542	3,633	3,726	3,822	3,920	4,020	4,123	4,229	4,338	4,449
3,338	3,423	3,510	3,599	3,690	3,784	3,880	3,979	4,080	4,183	4,289	4,398	4,510
3,393	3,479	3,566	3,656	3,748	3,842	3,938	4,037	4,139	4,243	4,349	4,459	4,571
3,449	3,535	3,623	3,713	3,805	3,900	3,997	4,096	4,198	4,302	4,410	4,519	4,632
3,505	3,591	3,679	3,770	3,863	3,958	4,055	4,155	4,257	4,362	4,470	4,580	4,692
3,561	3,647	3,736	3,827	3,920	4,016	4,114	4,214	4,317	4,422	4,529	4,640	4,753

Source: Warsof, S. T., Gohari, P., Berkowitz, R. L., et al. The estimation of fetal weight by computer assisted analysis. *Am. J. Obstet. Gynecol.,* 128:881, 1977.

APPENDIX 11.

Ratio of Head Circumference to Abdominal Circumference: Normal Values

Menstrual Age (weeks)	−2 S.D.† (cm)	Predicted Value* (cm)	+2 S.D.† (cm)	−2 S.D.§ (cm)	Predicted Value‡ (cm)	−2 S.D.§ (cm)
12	1.16	1.29	1.41	1.12	1.22	1.31
13	1.15	1.28	1.40	1.11	1.21	1.30
14	1.14	1.27	1.39	1.11	1.20	1.30
15	1.13	1.26	1.38	1.10	1.19	1.29
16	1.12	1.25	1.37	1.09	1.18	1.28
17	1.11	1.24	1.36	1.08	1.18	1.27
18	1.10	1.22	1.35	1.07	1.17	1.26
19	1.09	1.21	1.34	1.06	1.16	1.25
20	1.08	1.20	1.33	1.06	1.15	1.24
21	1.07	1.19	1.32	1.05	1.14	1.24
22	1.06	1.18	1.30	1.04	1.13	1.23
23	1.05	1.17	1.29	1.03	1.12	1.22
24	1.04	1.16	1.28	1.02	1.12	1.21
25	1.03	1.15	1.27	1.01	1.11	1.20
26	1.02	1.14	1.26	1.00	1.10	1.19
27	1.01	1.13	1.25	1.00	1.09	1.18
28	1.00	1.12	1.24	.99	1.08	1.18
29	.99	1.11	1.23	.98	1.07	1.17
30	.97	1.10	1.22	.97	1.07	1.16
31	.96	1.09	1.21	.96	1.06	1.15
32	.95	1.08	1.20	.95	1.05	1.14
33	.94	1.07	1.19	.95	1.04	1.13
34	.93	1.05	1.18	.94	1.03	1.13
35	.92	1.04	1.17	.93	1.02	1.12
36	.91	1.03	1.16	.92	1.01	1.11
37	.90	1.02	1.15	.91	1.01	1.10
38	.89	1.01	1.13	.90	1.00	1.09
39	.88	1.00	1.12	.89	.99	1.08
40	.87	.99	1.11	.89	.98	1.08

*HC/AC = 1.42104 − .0106229(MA)[R^2 = 58.9%].
†2 S.D. = 0.12.
‡HC/AC = 1.32293 − .0084471(MA)[R^2 = 67.2%].
§2 S.C. = 0.10

Source: Adapted from Callen, P. W. *Ultrasonography in Obstetrics and Gynecology.* Boston: Saunders, 1983. With permission.

APPENDIX 12.

Mean Values for TIUV as a Quadratic Function of Weeks of Gestation with Upper and Lower 2.5 and 10% Tolerance Limits*

Menstrual Weeks	Lower 2.5%	Lower 10%	Mean	Upper 10%	Upper 2.5%
21	502	789	912	1036	1322
22	507	801	1020	1238	1533
23	536	836	1134	1432	1732
24	589	895	1256	1616	1922
25	667	981	1384	1788	2101
26	771	1091	1520	1949	2269
27	895	1221	1663	2105	2431
28	1033	1364	1813	2262	2593
29	1179	1516	1970	2425	2762
30	1329	1672	2134	2597	2940
31	1483	1832	2306	2780	3129
32	1642	1996	2485	2973	3327
33	1806	2165	2670	3175	3535
34	1980	2345	2863	3381	3746
35	2171	2541	3062	3585	3955
36	2384	2759	3270	3781	4156
37	2623	3004	3484	3965	4346
38	2887	3273	3705	4138	4524
39	3175	3566	3934	4302	4693
40	3484	3880	4170	4459	4855

Source: Filly, R. A. *J. Clin. Ultrasound* 7:24, 1979.

Index

Page numbers in italics refer to figures.